Nursing Student Retention

Understanding the Process and Making a Difference

Nursing Student Retention

Understanding the Process and Making a Difference

Marianne R. Jeffreys, EdD, RN

 Springer Publishing Company

Marianne R. Jeffreys, EdD, RN, is a professor of nursing at The City University of New York College of Staten Island. She received a BS in nursing from the State University of New York College at Plattsburgh, an MA and MEd in nursing education/professorial role from Teachers College, Columbia University, and an EdD in nursing education/nurse executive from Teachers College, Columbia University. Her research interests include nontraditional nursing students, student retention and achievement, self-efficacy, curriculum, psychometrics, and transcultural nursing. Professor Jeffreys may be reached at jeffreys@mail.csi.cuny.edu.

To my son, Daniel W. Edley

Springer Publishing Company, Inc.
536 Broadway
New York, NY 10012-3955

Acquisitions Editor: Ruth Chasek
Production Editor: Betsy Day
Cover design by Joanne Honigman

04 05 06 07 08 / 5 4 3 2 1

Library of Congress Cataloging-in-Publication Data

Jeffreys, Marianne R.
    Nursing student retention : understanding the process and making a difference / Marianne R. Jeffreys
        p. ; cm.
    Includes bibliographical references and index.
    ISBN 0-8261-3445-9
    1. Nursing school dropouts—United States—Prevention. 2. Nursing students—United States—Psychology. 3. Nursing—Study and teaching—United States.
    [DNLM: 1. Student Dropouts. 2. Students, Nursing. 3. Education, Nursing—methods. WY 18 J46n 2004] I. Title.
RT79.J446 2004
610.73'071'173—dc22

2004008870

Printed in the United States of America by Maple-Vail Book Manufacturing Group.

Contents

Preface

This book presents an organizing framework for understanding student retention, identifying at-risk students, developing diagnostic-prescriptive strategies to facilitate success, guiding innovations in teaching and educational research, and evaluating strategy effectiveness. The need for such a book is heightened by the already existing nursing shortage that is predicted to become even more severe. Therefore, nursing student retention is a priority concern for nurse educators, nursing, the health professions, and society. Consequently, government and private agencies have allocated additional funds toward efforts aimed at relieving the nursing shortage and promoting nursing student retention.

The escalating nursing shortage demands a comprehensive approach to understanding retention, with nurse educators actively developing, implementing, and evaluating strategies for facilitating retention and success based on conceptual and empirical support. Graduate students, faculty, and administrators need to learn more about student retention and how to make a positive difference. This book provides essential background information for developing, implementing, and evaluating retention strategies. Its two main purposes are (1) to provide readers with a comprehensive overview of undergraduate nursing student retention, and (2) to offer a guide for retention strategy design, implementation, and evaluation. Accordingly, the book is organized into Part I: "Understanding the Multidimensional Process of Student Retention" and Part II: "Making a Difference: Promoting Retention and Success." Examples, figures, and tables are provided to enhance key points throughout the book. Additionally, the "Educator-in-Action" vignettes following chapter summaries demonstrate practical application strategies and depict the student experience associated with educator actions. Appendices include sample questionnaires, providing additional resources.

Readers are encouraged to pause, reflect, and question throughout the book in order to gain new insights into the multidimensional process of student retention. It is hoped that these new insights, with their holistic and multidimensional approach, will revitalize interest in nursing student retention. The ultimate goal of this book is to motivate others to further explore student retention through continued educational, theoretical, empirical, and practical endeavors. Readers are invited to contribute new insights, creative ideas, innovative strategies, empirical designs, and theoretical inquiries as they embark on the challenging yet rewarding journey toward promoting nursing student retention and success. Let's make a difference!

Acknowledgments

Partial funding for previous research on nursing student retention, and/or the development of an enrichment program and/or nursing student resource center was obtained from The City University of New York (CUNY) College of Staten Island, Division of Science and Technology; the Research Foundation of CUNY, PSC-CUNY Research Award Program; CUNY Faculty Advancement Program; and the New York State Education Department Vocational and Technical Education Act (VATEA).

Understanding the Multidimensional Process of Student Retention

Part I is made up of nine chapters. Chapter 1 begins with an overview of student retention, defines key terms, and presents the Nursing Undergraduate Retention and Success (NURS) conceptual model as an organizing framework. The NURS model proposes that retention decisions will be based on the interaction of student profile characteristics, student affective factors, academic factors, environmental factors, professional integration factors, academic outcomes, psychological outcomes, and outside surrounding factors.

Chapter 2 describes student characteristics prior to beginning a nursing course and includes age, ethnicity and race, gender, language, prior educational experience, family's educational background, prior work experience, and enrollment status. The chapter elaborates upon each of these characteristics, proposing ways that they may influence retention.

Chapter 3 introduces the general concepts underlying cultural values and beliefs, self-efficacy, and motivation that can seriously influence nursing student achievement, persistence, and retention. Several tables and figures illustrate major points significant for practical application in the educational setting. Select cultural values and beliefs especially pertinent to nursing education and student retention are compared and contrasted.

Nurse educators are continually challenged to appraise the influence of academic factors on retention and student success. Chapter 4 discusses personal study skills, study hours, attendance, class schedule, and general academic services (college library, college counseling, and computer laboratory) in relation to undergraduate nursing student retention and aims to assist nurse educators in identifying areas of student strengths and weaknesses. An in-depth exploration of each academic factor reveals several dimensions that can potentially affect students. Special issues unique to nursing education are emphasized.

Chapter 5 presents external environmental factors that may influence students' academic performance, retention, and/or success, and include financial status, family financial support, family emotional support, family responsibilities, child care arrangements, family crisis, employment hours, employment responsibilities, encouragement by outside friends, living arrangements, and transportation. Each environmental factor is analyzed in relation to undergraduate nursing student retention and aims to assist nurse educators in identifying areas of student strengths and weaknesses.

Chapter 6 proposes professional integration factors that enhance students' interaction with the social system of the college environment within the context of professional socialization and career development. These factors include nursing faculty advisement and helpfulness, memberships in professional organizations, professional events, encouragement by friends in class, enrichment programs, and peer mentoring and tutoring. The chapter elaborates upon each of the professional integration factors, proposing ways that they can potentially and directly enhance retention through academic outcomes and psychological outcomes.

The complexity of the nursing educational experience offers unique professional, discipline-specific psychological and developmental opportunities and outcomes beyond course grades or GPA. Both academic and psychological outcomes influence persistence and retention. Chapter 7 addresses pertinent issues surrounding academic and psychological outcomes, presents proposed relationships with other variables in the NURS model, and suggests practical application strategies.

The purpose of Chapter 8 is to enhance awareness of outside surrounding factors (OSF) on student retention, highlight the potential significance of select factors, stimulate further inquiry, and suggest recommendations for nurse educators. Outside surrounding factors exist outside of the academic setting and the individual student's personal environment and can influence retention. They include world, national, and local events; politics and economics; health care system; nursing professional issues; and job certainty.

Chapter 9 introduces select background information and main concepts involved in retention decisions and the decision-making process. Nurse educators are in a strategic position to make a difference by facilitating the process of systematic decision making and enhancing opportunities for retention and success. Steps of the decision-making process specific to nursing student retention are additionally incorporated within an illustration. Implications for nurse educators are proposed.

Chapter 1

Overview of Student Retention*

The nursing profession must be ready to embrace a new age of realism with regard to the changing student population. Currently, the dramatic shift in demographics, the restructured work force, and less academically prepared college applicants have created a more diverse nursing applicant pool (Kelly, 1997; Tayebi, Moore-Jazayeri, & Maynard, 1998). Increasingly, the nontraditional student is replacing the traditional student in nursing. The projected increases in immigration, globalization, and minority population growth have the potential to enrich the diversity of the nursing profession and help meet the needs of an expanding and culturally diverse society (Barbee & Gibson, 2001; Bessent, 1997; DHHS, 2000; Griffiths & Tagliareni, 1999; Tucker-Allen & Long, 1999; Villaruel, Canales, & Torres, 2001; Yoder, 2001). Thus, the untapped potential of the nontraditional student population demands focused attention on promoting nontraditional nursing student success. Unfortunately, the retention rates of nontraditional students are substantially lower than those of traditional students (Barbee & Gibson, 2001; Bessent, 1997; Manifold & Rambur, 2001; Tucker-Allen & Long, 1999; Yurkovich, 2001). Although attrition is financially costly to students, educational institutions, and society, the severest impact can be the adverse psychological costs to the student (Nora, Cabrera, Hagedorn, & Pascarella, 1996; Rowser, 1997; Tinto, 1993).

---

* This chapter was excerpted and adapted from Jeffreys, M. R. (2003). Strategies for promoting nontraditional nursing student retention and success. In M. Oermann & K. Heinrich (Eds.), *Annual Review of Nursing Education, Volume I*. New York, Springer. By permission, Springer.

Enrollment trends, retention rates, professional goals, societal needs, and ethical considerations all declare the need to prioritize the retention of nontraditional students. However, the retention of traditional students must be addressed as well. Nurse educators are in a key position to influence retention positively. As active partners in the complex process of nursing student retention, nurse educators can design theoretically and empirically supported retention strategies targeting specific student populations. Design of a diagnostic-specific strategy first requires an understanding of the dynamic phenomenon of nursing student retention, the complex interaction of influencing variables, and insight into the student's perspective (Harvey & McMurray, 1994; Jeffreys, 2001).

This chapter will provide an overview of undergraduate nursing student retention, define key terms, and present the Nursing Undergraduate Retention and Success (NURS) conceptual model as an organizing framework. The main features will be highlighted in an attempt to succinctly summarize the literature and enhance understanding of the multidimensional phenomenon of undergraduate nursing student retention and success.

UNDERGRADUATE NURSING STUDENT RETENTION AND SUCCESS

Retention has been examined and discussed extensively in both the higher education and nursing literature (Braxton, 2001; Courage & Godbey, 1992; Tinto, 1998). Empirical studies, however, have been more limited and have targeted predominantly traditional students in baccalaureate programs. Many studies have focused on attrition rather than retention through use of autopsy studies, after the student has already withdrawn. Although similar study variables have been examined, inconsistencies between operational definitions have varied extensively, making comparison difficult (Garcia, 1987). Additionally, voluntary attrition, due to personal reasons, and involuntary attrition, due to academic failure, are often undifferentiated (Tucker-Allen, 1989). Diverse sample size, enrollment status, and methodology further compound this interpretive difficulty. Many studies used frameworks originally designed for the traditional student (Eaton & Bean, 1995; Metzner & Bean, 1987). The most persistent trend in student persistence research is that student attrition persists.

An extensive search in the nursing and higher education literature revealed several comprehensive conceptual models to explain undergraduate student attrition (Bean & Metzner, 1985; Metzner & Bean, 1987; Nora, 1987; Pascarella & Chapman, 1983; Spady, 1970; Tinto, 1975).

However, only one model specifically targeted the nontraditional student. No models specifically targeted the nursing student. Subsequently, the Bean and Metzner (1985) model of nontraditional undergraduate student attrition provided the underlying conceptual framework for several studies on nontraditional undergraduate nursing student retention (Jeffreys, 1993, 1998, 2001, 2002). Results from these studies confirmed that nontraditional students often juggled multiple roles such as student, parent, financial provider, and/or employee, and therefore were more influenced by environmental variables than academic variables. Additionally, students perceived family, faculty, friends, tutoring, and an enrichment program as greatly supportive.

Although many of the factors influencing nontraditional students across various disciplines are also relevant to nursing students, there are some distinguishing characteristics of the nontraditional undergraduate nursing student. As a profession, nursing is also different from liberal arts and science disciplines; therefore, applicability of these models to undergraduate nursing students in general is limited. Consequently, the Nontraditional Undergraduate Retention and Success (NURS) model was developed specifically for examining nontraditional undergraduate nursing student retention and success (Jeffreys, 2003). The proposed influencing factors were clustered into variable sets and then incorporated into the original NURS model. With minor modifications, the original NURS model was easily adapted to include the traditional undergraduate nursing student population, resulting in the newly conceptualized model (Figure 1.1). Please note that the acronym NURS was changed from "Nontraditional Undergraduate Retention and Success" to "Nursing Undergraduate Retention and Success" and encompasses components appropriate for both traditional and nontraditional students. Subsequent reference to the NURS model in this book refers to the revised model.

DEFINITIONS

To develop a common knowledge base and avoid discrepancies in definitions, Table 1.1 defines terms important in understanding undergraduate nursing student retention and success.

PURPOSE AND GOAL OF THE NURS MODEL

The purpose of the NURS model is to present an organizing framework for examining the multidimensional factors that affect undergraduate

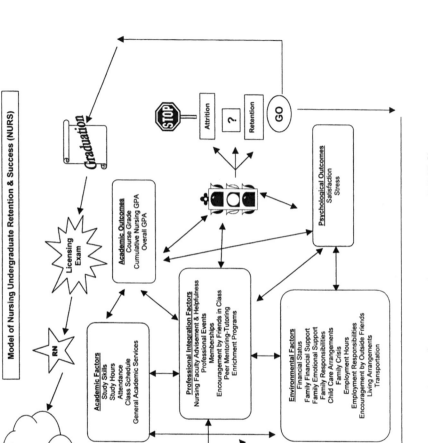

FIGURE 1.1 Model of Nursing Undergraduate Retention & Success (NURS).

TABLE 1.1 Definition of Terms

Nontraditional undergraduate nursing student refers to a nursing student who is enrolled in an entry level undergraduate nursing program (diploma, associate degree, or generic baccalaureate) and who meets one or more of the following criteria: (1) age 25 years or older, (2) commuter, (3) enrolled part-time, (4) male, (5) member of an ethnic and/or racial minority group, (6) speaks English as a second (other) language, (7) has dependent children, (8) has a general equivalency diploma (GED), and (9) required remedial classes.

Traditional undergraduate nursing student refers to a nursing student who is enrolled in an entry level undergraduate nursing program (diploma, associate degree, or generic baccalaureate) and who does not meet the criteria of nontraditional undergraduate nursing student as defined above. Specifically, such a student meets all of the following criteria: (1) age 24 or younger, (2) resides in campus housing or off-campus housing, (3) enrolled full-time, (4) female, (5) white and not a member of an ethnic and/or racial minority group, (6) speaks English as a first language, (7) has no dependent children, (8) has a United States high school diploma, and (9) required no remedial classes.

Course retention is the continuous enrollment in a nursing course without withdrawal.

Course success refers to passing the nursing course.

Continuous program retention is the continuous enrollment in a nursing program (part- or full-time) by taking the required courses sequentially until meeting the program's graduation requirements, possibly including courses repeated for previous withdrawal and/or failure. In **ideal program retention,** the student successfully completes the required courses sequentially, in the specified time period, and without evidence of withdrawal or failure.

Interim program retention is the intermittent enrollment in a nursing program (part- or full-time) by taking the required courses sequentially until meeting the program's graduation requirements, possibly including courses repeated for previous withdrawal and/or failure.

Program success refers to a student's (1) successful completing the program's graduation requirements, (2) passing the RN licensing exam, and (3) obtaining a part- or full-time job as an RN and/or enrolling in a more advanced nursing program. In **ideal program success,** the student successfully completes the program's graduation requirements within the specified time period and without withdrawing or failing, passes the RN licensing exam on the first attempt, and obtains a job as a RN and/or enrolls in a more advanced nursing program.

Withdrawal occurs when students officially withdraw from a college course or courses for personal and/or academic reasons.

(continued)

TABLE 1.1   Definition of Terms *(continued)*

Stopout refers to a break in continuous enrollment for one or more semesters (excluding summer sessions and intercessions).

Attrition refers to students dropping out of the nursing program. **Voluntary attrition** occurs when a student drops out due to personal (nonacademic) reasons, compared to **involuntary attrition** for academic reasons (failure or dismissal).

Student profile characteristics describe student characteristics prior to beginning a nursing course and include age, ethnicity and race, gender, first language, prior educational experience, the family's educational background, prior work experience, and enrollment status.

Student affective factors are students' attitudes, values, and beliefs about learning, including cultural values and beliefs, self-efficacy, and motivation, and their ability to learn and perform the necessary tasks required for course and program success.

Academic factors include personal study skills, study hours, attendance, class schedule (Metzner, 1989), and general academic services (e.g., college library services, college counseling services, and computer laboratory services).

Environmental factors are external to the academic process and may influence students' academic performance and retention (Metzner, 1989) and include financial status, family financial support, family emotional support, family responsibilities, child care arrangements, family crisis, employment hours, employment responsibilities, encouragement by outside friends, living arrangements, and transportation.

Professional integration factors enhance students' interaction with the social system of the college environment within the context of professional socialization and career development. These include nursing faculty advisement and helpfulness, memberships in professional organizations, encouragement by friends in class, professional events, peer mentoring-tutoring, and enrichment programs.

Outside surrounding factors exist outside of the academic setting and the student's personal environment and can influence retention. They include world, national, and local events; politics and economics; the health care system; nursing professional issues; and job certainty.

Academic outcomes are represented by the student's nursing course grade, cumulative GPA for nursing courses, and overall GPA.

Psychological outcomes include satisfaction and stress.

nursing student retention and success in order to identify at-risk students, develop diagnostic-prescriptive strategies to facilitate success, guide innovations in teaching and educational research, and evaluate strategy effectiveness. Although several models have been proposed to examine college student attrition, this model specifically focuses on the aspect of retention (rather than attrition) and targets a specific student population. The main goal of the model is to promote undergraduate nursing student retention and success. The model is tentative and will require modification when new data become available.

ASSUMPTIONS/PREMISES OF THE NURS MODEL

Based on a review of the literature and previous studies of undergraduate nursing student retention, several assumptions underlie the NURS model:

- Undergraduate nursing student retention is a priority concern for nurse educators.
- Student retention is a dynamic and multidimensional phenomenon that is influenced by the interaction of multiple variables (factors).
- For undergraduate nursing students, environmental and professional integration factors greatly influence retention.
- All students, regardless of prior academic performance, can benefit from professional socialization and enrichment throughout preprofessional and professional education.
- Psychological and academic outcomes may interact and influence persistence.

OVERVIEW OF NURS MODEL

The NURS model is presented in Figure 1.1. Briefly, the model indicates that retention decisions will be based on the interaction of student profile characteristics, student affective factors, academic factors, environmental factors, professional integration factors, academic outcomes, psychological outcomes, and outside surrounding factors. Outside surrounding factors have the power to affect student persistence and retention either positively or negatively, despite positive academic and psychological outcomes for nursing. At the beginning of each nursing course, student profile characteristics provide information on the composition of the student group. Individual factors may interact with each other to increase or decrease persistence or risk of attrition.

Similar to the Bean and Metzner (1985) model, it is presumed that environmental factors are more important for nontraditional undergraduate nursing students than are academic factors. Also consistent with the model, academic outcomes interact with psychological outcomes. Good academic performance results in retention only when accompanied by positive psychological outcomes for the nursing program and profession. The voluntary and/or involuntary decision to remain in a course, persist in the nursing program, graduate, take the RN licensing exam, and enter the nursing work force and/or begin a more advanced nursing program occurs during and at the conclusion of each nursing course.

Many models explaining attrition among traditional college students have emphasized the importance of social integration in student adjustment, persistence, and success (Nora, 1987; Pascarella & Chapman, 1983; Spady, 1970; Tinto, 1975). For undergraduate nursing students, a new perspective of social integration is proposed. In the NURS model, professional integration factors are variables that enhance students' interaction with the social system of the college environment within the context of professional socialization and career development. Results from recent studies (Jeffreys, 2001, 2002) have consistently identified professional integration factors, such as nursing faculty advisement and helpfulness, an enrichment program, and peer mentoring-tutoring, as instrumental in assisting with nontraditional nursing student retention. Professional integration factors are at the center of the model because they are at the crossroads of the decision to persist, drop out, or stop out. It is also proposed that professional integration factors are vitally important for both traditional and nontraditional nursing student retention.

Within the NURS model, the proposed factors can be applied to both traditional and nontraditional undergraduate nursing student populations; however, the manner in which they impact upon retention may be different. Such differences will be highlighted throughout Part I of this book. Additionally, the factors interact with each other and with other variable sets in the NURS model. Such interactions will also be addressed throughout Part I.

KEY POINTS SUMMARY

- Current enrollment trends and retention rates, compounded by the escalating nursing shortage and societal health care needs, demand immediate attention toward the development, implementation, and evaluation of retention strategies.

- Nurse educators are in a key position to positively influence retention through the design of theoretically and empirically based retention strategies.
- The Nursing Undergraduate Retention and Success (NURS) model presents an organizing framework for examining the multidimensional factors that affect undergraduate nursing student retention and success in order to identify at-risk students, develop diagnostic-prescriptive strategies to facilitate success, guide innovations in teaching and educational research, and evaluate strategy effectiveness.
- The NURS model proposes that retention decisions will be based on the interaction of student profile characteristics, student affective factors, academic factors, environmental factors, professional integration factors, academic outcomes, psychological outcomes, and outside surrounding factors.
- Academic outcomes interact with psychological outcomes whereby good academic performance results in retention only when accompanied by positive psychological outcomes for the nursing program and profession.
- The voluntary and/or involuntary decision to remain in a course, persist in the nursing program, graduate, take the RN licensing exam, and enter the nursing work force and/or begin a more advanced nursing program occurs during and at the conclusion of each nursing course.
- Professional integration factors are at the center of the model because they are at the crossroads of the decision to persist, drop out, or stopout.
- Detailed appraisal of the various components of the NURS model will enhance overall understanding of nursing undergraduate student retention through a holistic approach.

REFERENCES AND BIBLIOGRAPHY

Barbee, E. L., & Gibson, S. E. (2001). Our dismal progress: The recruitment of non-whites into nursing. *Journal of Nursing Education, 40*(6), 243–245.

Bean, J. P., & Eaton, B. (2001). The psychology underlying successful retention practices. *Journal of College Student Retention: Research, Theory, & Practice, 3*(1), 73–90.

Bean, J. P., & Metzner, B. (1985). A conceptual model of nontraditional undergraduate student attrition. *Review of Educational Research, 55*, 485–540.

Bessent, H. (Ed.). (1997). *Strategies for recruitment, retention, and graduation of minority nurses in colleges of nursing.* Washington, DC: American Nurses Publishing.

Braxton, J. M. (Ed.). (2000). *Reworking the student departure puzzle.* Nashville, TN: Vanderbilt University Press.

Braxton, J. M. (2001). Introduction to special issue: Using theory and research to improve college student retention. *Journal of College Student Retention: Research, Theory, & Practice, 3*(1), 1–2.

Courage, M. M., & Godbey, K. L. (1992). Student retention: Policies and services to enhance persistence to graduation. *Nurse Educator, 17*(2), 29–32.

Department of Health and Human Services. (2000). *Healthy people 2010: Understanding and improving health* (2nd ed.). Washington, DC: U.S. Government Printing Office.

DesJardins, S. L., Ahlburg, D. A., & McCall, B. P. (1999). An event history model of student departure. *Economics of Education Review, 18*(3), 375–390.

Dowell, M. A. (1996). Issues in recruitment and retention of minority nursing students. *Journal of Nursing Education, 35*(7), 293–297.

Eaton, S. B., & Bean, J. P. (1995). An approach/avoidance behavioral model of college student attrition. *Research in Higher Education, 36,* 617–645.

Garcia, M. (1987). *Community college persistence: A field application of the Tinto model.* Unpublished doctoral dissertation, Teachers College, Columbia University, New York.

Griffiths, M. J., & Tagliareni, M. E. (1999). Challenging traditional assumptions about minority students in nursing education. *Nursing & Health Care Perspectives, 20,* 290–295.

Harvey, V., & McMurray, N. (1994). Self-efficacy: A means of identifying problems in nursing education and career progress. *International Journal of Nursing Studies, 31,* 471–485.

Jeffreys, M. R. (1993). *The relationship of self-efficacy and select academic and environmental variables on academic achievement and retention.* Unpublished doctoral dissertation, Teachers College, Columbia University, New York.

Jeffreys, M. R. (1995). Joining together family, faculty, and friends: New ideas for enhancing nontraditional student success. *Nurse Educator, 20*(3), 11.

Jeffreys, M. R. (1998). Predicting nontraditional student retention and academic achievement. *Nurse Educator, 23*(1), 42–48.

Jeffreys, M. R. (2001). Evaluating enrichment program study groups: Academic outcomes, psychological outcomes, and variables influencing retention. *Nurse Educator, 26*(3), 142–149.

Jeffreys, M. R. (2002). Students' perceptions of variables influencing retention: A pretest and post-test approach. *Nurse Educator, 27*(1), 16–19 [Erratum, 2002, 27*(2), 64].

Jeffreys, M. R. (2003). Strategies for promoting nontraditional student retention and success. In M. Oermann & K. Heinrich (Eds.), *Annual review of nursing education: Volume I* (pp. 61–90). New York: Springer.

Kelly, E. (1997). Development of strategies to identify the learning needs of baccalaureate nursing students. *Journal of Nursing Education, 36,* 156–162.

Levin, M. E., & Levin, J. R. (1991). A critical examination of academic retention programs for at-risk minority college students. *Journal of College Student Development, 32,* 322–334.

Manifold, C., & Rambur, B. (2001). Predictors of attrition in American Indian nursing students. *Journal of Nursing Education, 40*(6), 279–281.

Metzner, B. (1989). Perceived quality of academic advising: The effect on freshman attrition. *American Educational Research Journal, 26*, 422–442.

Metzner, B., & Bean, J. P. (1987). The estimation of a conceptual model of nontraditional undergraduate student attrition. *Research in Higher Education, 27*, 15–38.

Nora, A. (1987). Determinants of retention among Chicano college students: A structural model. *Research in Higher Education, 26*, 31–60.

Nora, A., Cabrera, A., Hagedorn, L., & Pascarella, E. (1996). Differential impacts of academic and social experiences on college-related behavioral outcomes across different ethnic and gender groups at four-year institutions. *Research in Higher Education, 37*, 427–451.

Pascarella, E. T., & Chapman, D. W. (1983). Validation of a theoretical model of college withdrawal: Interaction effects in a multi-institutional sample. *Research in Higher Education, 19*, 25–47.

Rowser, J. (1997). Do African American students' perceptions of their needs have implications for retention? *Journal of Black Studies, 27*, 718–726.

Spady, W. (1970). Dropouts from higher education: Toward an empirical model. *Interchange, 2*, 38–62.

Tayebi, K., Moore-Jazayeri, M., & Maynard, T. (1998). From the borders: Reforming the curriculum for the at-risk student. *Journal of Cultural Diversity, 5*, 101–109.

Tinto, V. (1975). Dropout from higher education: A theoretical synthesis of recent research. *Review of Educational Research, 10*, 259–271.

Tinto, V. (1993). *Leaving college: Rethinking the causes and cures of student attrition.* Chicago: University of Chicago Press.

Tinto, V. (1998). College as communities: Taking research on student persistence seriously. *Review of Higher Education, 21*, 167–177.

Tucker-Allen, S. (1989). Losses incurred through minority student nurse attrition. *Nursing & Health Care, 10*, 395–397.

Tucker-Allen, S., & Long, E. (1999). *Recruitment and retention of minority nursing students: Stories of success.* Lisle, IL: Tucker.

Villaruel, A. M., Canales, M., & Torres, S. (2001). Bridges and barriers: Educational mobility of Hispanic nurses. *Journal of Nursing Education, 40*(6), 245–251.

Yoder, M. K. (2001). The bridging approach: Effective strategies for teaching ethnically diverse nursing students. *Journal of Transcultural Nursing, 12*, 319–325.

Yurkovich, E. E. (2001). Working with American Indians toward educational success. *Journal of Nursing Education, 40*(6), 259–269.

Chapter 2

Student Profile Characteristics

The nursing and higher education literature reports numerous background characteristics that influence retention and academic achievement. Often, retention or attrition studies have included one or more background variables to search for predictors of academic success and retention. This approach does not consider the multidimensional phenomenon of student retention. Conceptual models of student attrition in the higher education literature typically include background characteristics as a component in the model (Metzner & Bean, 1987; Nora, 1987; Pascarella & Chapman, 1983; Spady, 1970; Tinto, 1997). Based on the higher education literature, conceptual models, and empirical research, a composite of student profile characteristics relevant for undergraduate nursing student retention is proposed (see Figure 1.1).

Student profile characteristics are described prior to beginning a nursing course and include age, ethnicity and race, gender, language, prior educational experience, family's educational background, prior work experience, and enrollment status. These variables provide information that is integral to determining special student needs and strengths, or identifying at-risk students. Individual variables may interact to increase or decrease risk of attrition. This chapter elaborates upon each of these characteristics, proposing ways that they may influence retention. Such awareness is a necessary first step in understanding the multidimensional process of undergraduate student retention. With a detailed appraisal of student profile characteristics, nurse educators can develop individual and student group composites that will help them design specific retention strategies aimed at maximizing student strengths and addressing student weaknesses. Each section below will explore how the specific characteristic is relevant to undergraduate nursing student retention.

AGE

Greater numbers of older students are entering higher education worldwide, with notable increases reported in Australia, the United Kingdom, and the United States. Almost half of all college students in the United States are over 25 years old (Mancuso, 2001). Consistent with global and multidisciplinary trends, the enrollment of older students in nursing programs has increased over the last decade, with projected increases to persist in the future. Consequently, the variable of age as a predictor in student performance, persistence, and graduation has been explored. Awareness of actual and perceived age-related barriers to retention is necessary if nurse educators are to understand the student retention process.

Several myths about age have served as barriers to retention. A prevalent myth that has been perpetuated by faculty, students, and society alike has been that older students are poorly equipped to meet the challenges of higher education and do not perform as well as traditional-age students. The older student has often been stereotyped and stigmatized in higher education (Richardson, 1994, 1995). On campuses where older students are greatly in the minority, feelings of differential treatment, uncertainty, powerlessness, and low confidence among them have been reported. In contrast, older students' perceptions were more positive on campuses with higher numbers of them (Lynch & Bishop-Clark, 1998). The overall institutional environment, climate, and culture should be examined with respect to age diversity. Age perception in relation to others in the academic environment can influence the academic experience.

Another barrier for older students has been the fact that colleges have typically tailored their academic and support services for the traditional age student. Special services are needed for older students. For example, in adult learner-centered institutions, there is a unique culture that caters to the adult learner through flexible scheduling of classes and support services, active learning experiences, and academic advisement geared to assist them (Mancuso, 2001; Murtaugh, Burns, & Schuster, 1999). Nurse educators should appraise the openness and compatibility of the educational environment for diverse age groups.

For the traditional-age student, social integration and college adjustment within the academic institution are considered to be important predictors in determining retention (Tinto, 1997). Students who adjust well and are socially integrated in activities, clubs, and/or sports are predicted to have higher retention rates than those who feel socially isolated and adjust poorly to the college environment. This is particularly applicable to the traditional-age student who lives away from home at the college. For the older, part-time, commuter student, social integration has been viewed as less critical, especially on commuter campuses (Bean & Metzner, 1985; Metzner & Bean, 1987).

Study findings concerning age as a variable in determining performance, persistence, and retention have been inconsistent in both the nursing and higher education literature. For example, some studies suggested that age is a significant predictor of academic achievement and retention, with older students persisting longer than younger students (DeFelice, 1989; Manifold & Rambur, 2001), whereas other researchers reported contrasting results (Allen, Higgs, & Holloway, 1988; Murtaugh, Burns, & Schuster, 1999). Research contradicting the myth of the older student as disadvantaged and/or at greater risk for attrition has centered on documenting higher academic performance and higher degree attainment. Other reports indicate that older students demonstrate better study habits, more goal commitment, greater motivation, better time management, more self-direction, and preference for adult learning strategies. In contrast, younger students perform better on academic outcomes only when combined with strong indicators of academic aptitude (Hoskins, Newstead, & Dennis, 1997).

Interestingly, Darkenwald and Novak (1997) reported that grades of traditional-age students were higher in classes with greater numbers of older students. This finding contests the myth that older students have a negative impact on classroom environments; in contrast, the older students bring many desirable qualities to class that positively influence the younger students. This finding is important, as younger students have reported and/or demonstrated less effective study and time management strategies (Devlin, 1996), lower self-efficacy, and less self-seeking help behaviors (Gianakos, 1996), variables that can adversely influence performance and retention. Among younger nursing students, lower self-concept was inversely correlated with greater test worry (Waltman, 1997). Clearly, age is a complex variable that needs to be viewed not only in relation to other variables, but also in relation to the interaction of students of diverse ages.

The older student has also been linked to additional role responsibilities that challenge persistence and retention; therefore higher attrition rates have been reported for these students. Overall, the inconsistent findings may be due to one common misperception—that older students are homogeneous and can be viewed as one discrete group. There is great diversity among older students, and so the interaction of other student profile characteristics must be considered. Nurse educators must be cautious in labeling all younger or older students as a homogeneous group. Thorough assessment of the interaction of multiple profile variables will help promote better understanding of the retention process.

ETHNICITY AND RACE

The term *ethnicity* has often been used interchangeably with race (Root, 1992) although ethnicity really should acknowledge the sharing of common cultural values, beliefs, language, literature, food preferences, music, art, norms, and taboos. Race is a way of categorizing people into separate and distinct groups based on physical characteristics, geographical origins of ancestors, and/or social status. Historically, the main purpose of dividing people into groups was to create a hierarchical tier, maintain boundaries between groups, and prevent oppressed (minority) groups from pulling power away from the dominant (non-minority) group (Root, 1992). Within this power imbalance, minority groups have encountered numerous obstacles and struggles for equality in education, privileges, work, housing, lifestyle, status, prestige, and other opportunities. Most minority groups continue to be underrepresented in higher education today (College Board, 2003). However, Ting (2000) indicates that a proportionately higher number of Asian Americans attend college in comparison with the overall Asian-American populations in the United States.

Nursing has not been immune to the struggles within and between minority and non-minority groups, or to the effects of such imbalances. For example, in the United States, the diversity within the nursing profession does not reflect the diversity within society; white nurses of European-American heritage represent approximately 90% of all registered nurses (Barbee & Gibson, 2001; Kimball & O'Neill, 2002). Recent nursing enrollment trends suggest a steady increase among some minority groups. However, no increase has been noted among Hispanic groups (Heller, Oros, & Durney-Crowley, 2000; Villaruel, Canales, & Torres, 2001). Intensive recruitment efforts are imperative.

Even more disturbing are the disparities in minority student persistence. As a group, minority students incur higher attrition rates in college. Unfortunately, this is also true within the nursing discipline (Bessent, 1997; Mills-Wisneski, 2003; Tucker-Allen & Long, 1999). Lack of role models, peer solidarity, and social integration can isolate students, thus presenting another barrier. The underrepresentation of minority groups within the nursing profession can present real and/or perceived added challenges for nursing students, further complicating minority student retention. Inclusion of "ethnicity and race" as a student profile characteristic in the NURS model recognizes that despite the immense diversity between and within ethnic and racial minority and non-minority groups, there are several common barriers that adversely influence nursing student retention, especially among ethnic and racial groups underrepresented in nursing. These barriers include stereotyping, prejudice, discrimination, and racism. "Ethnicity and race" in the NURS model also acknowledges that these factors affect all individuals in some way; anyone may be a potential victim of stereotyping, prejudice, discrimination, and racism.

Prior experiences with stereotyping, prejudice, discrimination, and racism in contemporary society can create fear of repeating such experiences within the academic and professional arena, thus interfering with motivation, achievement, and retention. If nurse educators are to understand the numerous ways in which ethnicity and race impact upon retention, they must openly acknowledge that stereotyping, prejudice, discrimination, and racism exist within nursing education and the nursing profession. The myth that these problems do not exist is a major barrier to understanding. University environments are microcosms of the larger society and may therefore portray and perpetuate ethnically or racially insensitive practices that create feelings of cultural incongruence and isolation among underrepresented groups (Brown & Kurpius, 1997; Constantine, Robinson, Wilton, & Caldwell, 2002; Constantine & Watt, 2002). As a subculture of the university environment, nursing may also overtly or covertly reflect and perpetuate insensitive practices.

It has been well documented that stereotyping, prejudice, discrimination, and racism exist in varying levels in nursing and nursing education (Abrums & Leppa, 2001; Barbee & Gibson, 2001; Farella, 2002; Tucker-Allen & Long, 1999; Yearwood, Brown, & Karlik, 2002). Nurse educators need to move beyond passively tolerating diversity to actively embracing it. Most important, nurse educators need to anticipate student fears and actively dismantle stereotyping, prejudice, discrimination, and racism within academia, nursing, health care, and society. Individual and group self-awareness may reveal that the educational environment has been "unconsciously incompetent" (Purnell, 2003) in cultural sensitivity, cultural competency, and actively anti-racist practices. According to Purnell (2003), the road to cultural competency passes through various stages of being "unconsciously incompetent," "consciously incompetent," "consciously competent," and "unconsciously competent." Cultural values and beliefs will be discussed in greater detail in chapter 3.

Awareness that covert or subtle racism can consciously or unconsciously create feelings of isolation, stress, and cultural pain is extremely important. Nurse educators must also acknowledge that these unwanted feelings can adversely influence retention. One example of subtle racism in nursing and health care is the prevalence of physical examination "norms" that are based on the assessment of a "white" individual (Barbee & Gibson, 2001). Stereotyping subgroups of Asian Americans into one group discounts the diversity within this group; prejudicial views that Asian-American students are the "model minority" and high achiever group not only negate the academic diversity within this group but create additional pressure for these students to reach high levels of achievement with minimal instructor assistance. Such biases can adversely affect retention (Ting, 2000). Assuming that all African-American students are academically underprepared is another common stereotype and prejudice among many nursing faculty (Barbee & Gibson, 2001). Believing that non-minority students are less confident in caring for culturally different clients than minority students are also stereotypical and inaccurate; the danger here is that minority students' special needs concerning care of culturally different clients may never be adequately addressed (Jeffreys & Smodlaka, 1999). Nurse educators' expectations that are more, less, or different, based solely on a student's ethnic or racial background, are discriminatory and racist. Individual student strengths and needs should be objectively appraised.

Ethnicity and race have been used to identify special needs of minority students and have been examined as both sample descriptors and independent variables. The literature abounds with descriptions of minority special needs centered on defining characteristics of the at-risk minority student through the use of precollege and/or at-college predictors. Examples of precollege predictors included measures of academic preparedness (GPA), adaptability, commitment to educational goals, perceptions of progress to goals, willingness to seek academic assistance, self-confidence, reasons for pursuing a degree, and family characteristics (Levin & Levin, 1991). Living environment, classroom experience, advisement, extracurricular activities, financial support, and perceived faculty involvement were described as at-college predictors (Levin & Levin, 1991). This means that ethnicity and race should not be used exclusively to identify at-risk students or to design retention strategies. Ethnicity and race must be examined in relation to the other student profile characteristics and other components of the NURS model. A holistic appraisal will enhance the design of a diagnostic-prescriptive approach to support retention.

GENDER

Bean and Metzner (1985) reported gender as a background and defining variable that influenced nontraditional student attrition. Higher attrition rates were reported for nontraditional male students than for nontraditional female students among multidisciplinary college populations (Bean & Metzner, 1985). Other studies have found no real gender effect (Hoskins, Newstead, & Dennis, 1997). Although the numbers of men in nursing are increasing, they remain an underrepresented minority (6%) within the traditionally female profession (Stevenson, 2003). Due to the disproportionate numbers of men, gender has generally been examined as a sample descriptor in studies of nursing student attrition. One comparison study with approximately equal distribution between men and women reported that male nursing student attrition rate declined from 12% in 1983 to 4% in 1995; attrition rate of women in 1983 was approximately 6% as compared to 4% in 1995 (Kippenbrock, May, & Younes, 1996). One question raised is whether males had higher response rates given the comparatively low numbers of men in nursing. In recent years, because the nursing literature reports the unique experience of the male nursing student, a different examination of gender has been proposed.

Understanding that the experience of the male nursing student is unique is an important step toward enhancing retention (Burtt, 1998). High school counselors' misperceptions and lack of adequate knowledge about the rigors of nursing as a profession have steered many men away from nursing as a viable career option (Kelly, Shoemaker, & Steele, 1996; Sullivan, 2002). Societal misperceptions labeling nursing as a "feminine" profession have been a hindrance in recruiting and retaining men in nursing. In comparison with the recent support for women entering nontraditional work roles, there has been little support for men breaking gender barriers (Baker, 2001; Boughn, 1994). Additionally, the support for women entering the work force has shifted away from encouraging traditional female professions. In fact, Constantine and Watt (2002) reported that gender role perception and feminist identity attitudes may actually create high levels of anger toward women who pursue traditional gender roles.

Gender-related barriers to retention within the nursing profession must be addressed if retention is to be enhanced. Such barriers include overt and covert bias and discrimination. For example, equal opportunities in clinical education and clinical work settings are often lacking for men, sometimes resulting in legal action (Burtt, 1998). Among men, prevalent perceptions of being treated differently from female nurses and/or female students contribute to feelings of loneliness, isolation, and self-doubt (Burtt, 1998; Patterson & Morin, 2002). Fear of being perceived as unmanly and questions by others concerning sexual orientation further isolate men (Boughn, 1994; Burtt, 1998; Kelly, Shoemaker, & Steele, 1996). Social isolation has frequently been reported as adversely influencing retention. Lack of role modeling and professional socialization for male nursing students has been problematic as well.

Boughn (1994) cautions against stereotyping the experiences and needs of male students, noting two distinct groups of men reported in the nursing literature. One group has been described as older, second-career individuals who are often members of a lower socioeconomic class. The second group consists of men in their late teens or early twenties who enter nursing school immediately after high school. Yet, within these two groups, much diversity exists. Like other student profile characteristics, gender must be viewed in context, recognizing the powerful interaction among factors.

LANGUAGE

Global trends and increased immigration around the world have resulted in increased numbers of students whose first language is different from that used in the educational institution (Devlin, 1996). The term *first language* is defined here as the primary, native home language used for listening, speaking, reading, writing, and thinking. Some students who relocate to different countries several times over the course of their primary, secondary, and postsecondary educational process may understand, speak, read, write, and think in several languages on varying levels of fluency and comprehension. Students whose first language is not the same as the one used in school will have special academic and nonacademic needs (Flege & Liu, 2001; Upton & Lee-Thompson, 2001).

For the purposes of this book, the focus will be on English as the language used in the nursing school. Students whose first language is English (EFL) will be differentiated from those whose first language is not English. Although the literal meaning of the term "English as second language" or "ESL" may not truly describe student populations who encounter English as a third, fourth, or fifth language, in this book the term ESL will mean anyone whose first language is other than standard English. Standard English refers to English that is commonly expected on a college level.

Consistent with global and national trends in higher education, nursing programs in the United States have also experienced an increase in ESL populations over the past decade. Canadian schools of nursing have also experienced an ESL student population surge (Jalili-Grenier & Chase, 1997). ESL student populations have been identified as at-risk students, yielding higher rates of attrition and demonstrating unique educational needs. With the emphasis on student retention, the NURS model focuses on identifying the student's first language to help identify subgroups within the ESL group so that appropriate interventions can be designed to enhance retention. Categorizing all ESL students together oversimplifies the complexity of the ESL experience.

It is important to recognize that the ESL focus is not solely on language but involves a multidimensional approach to understanding the ESL student holistically. Students who speak the same first language may be quite diverse in their cultural values and beliefs, ethnic and racial identities, socioeconomic level, and immigration status. Prior educational, lifestyle, and acculturation experiences of an international student are different from those of an immigrant or refugee. Each group may have different first and second language skills that are further complicated by the interaction of diverse factors, all of which put ESL students at greater risk for attrition.

Awareness of the complexities of the ESL experience is a necessary step toward promoting retention. Clearly, although language considerations need to be addressed, nonacademic factors can outweigh language barriers and adversely affect learning, achievement, and retention. Acculturation stress, adaptation, assimilation, cultural values and beliefs about education, experiences with second language, and expectations can impact greatly upon learning, achievement, and retention. These factors will be discussed in greater detail in chapters 3 and 10. Efforts at professional socialization and retention must assess the unique needs of various ESL students on a subgroup and individual basis, integrating language development skills, socialization, and acculturation measures within a culturally congruent framework (Abriam-Yago, Yoder, & Kataoka-Yahiro, 1999; Kataoka-Yahiro & Abriam-Yago, 1997; Upton & Lee-Thompson, 2001).

PRIOR EDUCATIONAL EXPERIENCE

Prior educational experience includes precollege variables (high school performance or GED) and prenursing program variables such as prenursing college course performance and postsecondary education and degrees. For the older student who has never been to college, precollege variables may not be accurate predictors of academic aptitude, achievement, or attrition (Hoskins, Newstead, & Dennis, 1997). They may be more appropriate for traditional students who enter college immediately after high school. Majority students with a high secondary school grade point average (GPA) and excellent attendance records are predicted to have greater academic success in college. High-school performance, however, has been less predictive for minority students (Manifold & Rambur, 2001; Ting, 1997, 2001; Young & Kaplow, 1997), disadvantaged students (Chaney, Muraskin, Cahalan, & Goodwin, 1998), and/or first generation college students (Olenchak & Hebert, 2002).

Use of high school performance or SAT scores as the sole predictor for college success should be avoided (Fleming, 2002). Higher education in general is flooded with academically diverse and less well prepared students worldwide (Ransdell, 2001; Strage et al., 2002). Nursing programs are similarly challenged (Gallagher, Bomba, & Crane, 2001; Heller, Oros, & Durney-Crowley, 2000; Tanner, 1998). Nurse educators will need to develop new measures to assist academically diverse student populations.

Routine assessment of other variables such as the type of secondary school program, gaps in educational experience, place of education, and language used for education will help analyze strengths and weaknesses within today's academically diverse population. Type of secondary school program (college preparatory, honors, advanced placement, vocational, technical, or general) should also be viewed in relation to GPA. Additionally, students from at-risk school districts may have other educational disadvantages that will impact upon college achievement and retention. For example, lack of supplies and materials in impoverished areas may have provided limited educational opportunities, thus creating an educationally disadvantaged environment and increasing risk for poor college performance. Racism, discrimination, lowered teacher expectations, and negative support from peers in at-risk school districts can intensify an educationally disadvantaged environment and limit student success (Olenchak & Hebert, 2002; Rodgers, 1990).

Gaps between the last educational experience and the current enrollment in a nursing program indicate the need for transitional (nonacademic) support as well as refresher knowledge and skills updates or remedial courses. More remedial courses are needed in proportion to older students and with the length of time elapsed between enrollments (Merisotis & Phipps, 2000). Among educators, there is much disagreement about what constitutes remediation. Remedial courses have been defined as reading, writing, and math for college students lacking the necessary skills for performing work at the level stipulated by the educational institution (Merisotis & Phipps, 2000). In nursing and the health sciences, remediation can be extended to include courses in biology, chemistry, and/or physics that would give students the necessary skills and background for performing college-level work in science courses. Test scores usually determine whether a student is able to enter required college-level courses for the nursing major. Unfortunately, scores on an exam may not differentiate among the needs for remedial, refresher, or update courses.

For the purposes of this book, differentiation among terms is important. Remedial coursework is for students who never had an adequate level of skill or knowledge in an area. Refresher courses are for students who previously attained knowledge; however, gaps in education have resulted in "forgetting" information or skills. Update courses are for students who previously attained knowledge and skills in a particular area, have retained the knowledge and skills as presented at their last educational experience, yet are missing essential new knowledge and skills. For example, an older, second-career student with a baccalaureate degree in biology earned twenty years ago may need an update in knowledge rather than a remedial course. In contrast, a recent immigrant who earned a GED after leaving secondary school two years ago may need intensive immersion in remedial work to develop skills and knowledge necessary for beginning college-level biology. Failing grades on a college placement exam may put these two students in the same remedial class, despite the unique needs of each. This type of mismatch can be discouraging to students and interfere with persistence behaviors.

For students educated in other countries, it may be difficult to evaluate learning experiences, grades, standards, degrees, and certifications. The primary language of prior educational experience(s) may also impact upon retention. What can be generalized, however, is that students educated in foreign countries had different educational experiences that may create actual or perceived advantages or disadvantages for them. The learning needs and expectations of foreign-educated students may be very different from what faculty perceive, thus creating another obstacle to learning, achievement, satisfaction, and retention (Jalili-Grenier & Chase, 1997).

Prior educational experience in college includes the learning process, persistence behaviors, and outcomes (grades and degree attainment). Students with prior college degrees are believed to have higher retention rates due to knowledge of what to expect in college, fewer credits needed to complete the degree currently sought, and better financial status (Scott, Burns, & Cooney, 1998). Students with and without college degrees may underestimate the academic rigor and time demands of a nursing program. Prior college transcripts should be reviewed for the number of course withdrawals, repeats, and failures as well as overall GPA, grades achieved in science courses, and transfer history. Some research supports the belief that science course grades serve as strong predictors of success in nursing programs and in passing the NCLEX exam (Brennan, Best, & Small, 1996; Campbell & Dickson, 1996; Griffiths,

Bevil, O'Connor, & Wieland, 1995; Wold & Worth, 1990). Yet other studies over the last 25 years suggest that these variables are not sufficient in explaining student retention and success (Aber & Arathuzik, 1996; Hutcheson, Garland, & Lowe, 1979). Benda (1991) found that the most important predictor of success was whether prerequisite courses were taken at a junior or senior college. Science courses were less predictive if course grades were transferred from another college or if the course was taken more than two years ago (Griffiths et al., 1995). Additionally, transfer history can reveal whether the student had short-term and/or long-term commitments to the previously selected institution(s) and major(s). Strong goal commitment has been identified as a positive predictor of retention (Metzner & Bean, 1987).

Lagtime, or the number of years between a student's last enrollment at another college and the student's entry into college currently, has been explored as a predictor for retention (Malloch & Montgomery, 1996). Among older students, longer lagtime has been correlated with higher GPA; however, among younger students longer lagtime seems to be a disadvantage. Short-term interruptions, or stopouts, appear to be more prevalent among older students, and it is believed that among older students stopouts are viewed as more acceptable than among traditional age students (Malloch & Montgomery). This phenomenon is not surprising, considering that older students often have more responsibilities external to the academic institution. The influence of environmental variables on retention will be discussed in greater detail in chapter 5.

Assessment of prior college experience can identify educationally disadvantaged students at risk for attrition and provide essential information for designing strategies to address weaknesses and to maximize strengths. Academically well prepared students may be put at risk for attrition if emphasis is on the academically weak student. A myopic view of seeing only the academically weak student as at risk for attrition will ignore and isolate the strengths and needs of academically well prepared students. Remembering that even strong students need support is crucial. For example, Olenchak and Hebert (2002) found that gifted first-generation college students often underachieve in college and have high rates of attrition. Capitalizing on student strengths and assessing academically well prepared students for other risk factors for attrition is a necessary step in promoting overall retention.

FAMILY EDUCATIONAL BACKGROUND

With greater numbers of first-generation students entering higher education, exploring the family's educational background deserves attention.

Many studies have indicated that parents' level of formal education is a powerful predictor of traditional student persistence, placing first-generation college students at greater risk than others for attrition (Berger, 2001; Eaton & Bean, 1995; Kuh, 2001). Nursing programs have also seen an increase in first-generation college students, especially among student groups traditionally underrepresented in nursing (Campbell & Davis, 1996; Tayebi, Moore-Jazayeri, & Maynard, 1998; Tucker-Allen & Long, 1999). In the NURS model, family's educational background includes the level of formal education for the student's parents, siblings, spouse, significant other(s), children, and grandchildren.

In two studies of nontraditional nursing student retention, students who selected and actively participated in enrichment program peer mentor-tutor study groups were predominantly the first individuals in their family to attend college (Jeffreys, 2001, 2002). Several explanations may be proposed for this phenomenon of self-selection. These first-generation college students may have perceived themselves at a disadvantage and therefore felt a greater need for peer-mentoring and tutoring than other students. Another explanation may be that they were more motivated, self-directed, and seeking of self-help interventions. Perhaps the opportunity for socialization within college and the nursing profession was quite desirable for first-generation college students. This phenomenon warrants further exploration.

The higher education literature examining traditional age first-generation college student persistence has identified three major areas resulting in disadvantages that increase attrition risk: precollege, transitional, and college experience (Terenzini, Springer, Yaeger, Pascarella, & Nora, 1996). First, differences in planning for college, college selection, and expectations for college put students at an initial disadvantage. Students and families may not have realistic plans, choices, or expectations. Second, the transition between high school or work and college is often a cultural as well as a social and academic one for the first-generation college student. As the first person in a family to enter college, the student experiences losses as well as gains, creating sources of potential conflict and feelings of isolation. Third, first-generation college students have more difficulty than others integrating academically and socially within the college environment, thus increasing the risk for a stressful, unsatisfying, or unhappy college experience (Olenchak & Hebert, 2002; Padilla, Trevino, Gonzalez, & Trevino, 1997; Terenzini et al., 1996). Awareness of the family's educational background, and of the issues surrounding the overall experience of the first-generation college student, can help nurse educators proactively design strategies to assist students during all three phases and enhance retention through positive experiences and realistic expectations.

Several researchers suggest the need to further explore the role parental socialization has in college choice and expectations, especially among Latinos, where college enrollment is lowest (Hernandez, 2000; Hurtado, Inkelas, Briggs, & Rhee, 1997; Villaruel et al., 2001). Family expectations for college, despite the family's educational background, were highest among Asian Americans (Hurtado et al., 1997; Ting, 2000). Although emotional support may be high for the first person in the family to attend college, the student may feel much pressure to succeed, achieve high grades, and fulfill family expectations. As mentioned previously, even gifted first-generation college students often have high rates of attrition (Olenchak & Hebert, 2002). Conversely, in families with multigenerational college degrees, it may also be expected that achieving a college degree is the norm. As a female-dominated profession, nursing may be particularly influenced by the degree attainments of women family members. Family expectations that conflict with student expectations and goals can adversely affect student performance. Nurse educators' sensitivity to student-perceived stress relative to family expectations is important. Additionally, recognizing the potential obstacles faced by first-generation college students is a critical factor.

Among nontraditional populations, women with partners who had earned college degrees perceived less pressure to leave college than did women without such partners (Scott, Burns, & Cooney, 1996). This finding was compounded by the influence of income, as persons with college degrees generally earn higher salaries; people without college degrees usually earn lower salaries and have less realistic expectations and insights about college. It is not surprising that low-income groups apply less frequently to college (Hurtado et al., 1997) and have lower retention rates. Financial status as an environmental factor will be addressed in chapter 5.

PRIOR WORK EXPERIENCE

Examining prior work experience in light of a restructured work force, welfare-to-work initiatives, displaced homemakers, and second career options can be beneficial. Prior work experience suggests that the student had a commitment to a task, needed to meet certain responsibilities within a particular time frame, and is familiar with the workplace environment. Men may enter a nursing program with considerable work experience whereas women may have little or none (Seidl & Sauter, 1990). Displaced homemakers without any prior work experience may feel insecure next to classmates who do have prior work experience.

Housewives and female professionals or paraprofessionals whose work experience was satisfying were more likely to lose interest in college in contrast to women whose prior work experience was dissatisfying, low-paying, low status, and with little chance for career advancement, and thus were more motivated to persist in college and less likely to withdraw (Scott et al., 1996, 1998).

National initiatives aimed at alleviating the nursing shortage emphasize career mobility within the health care field. Although students who work in the health care field as unlicensed personnel, licensed practical nurses (LPNs), or other health care paraprofessionals have prior health care experience, they may have difficulty adjusting to a new role, new world-view, more critical thinking, and decision making within a perspective guided by the professional scope of nursing practice. Linking students with peer mentors who are further along in the career ladder may be beneficial (Hammond, Davis, Marlin, & Montgomery, 1995). Reluctance or inability to change existing views, practices, and work habits may lead to unsafe practices and poor learning outcomes. Overconfidence in self-performance and learning can lead to inadequate preparation, failure, and attrition (see chapter 3).

In nursing programs where high numbers of students have prior health care experience, nurse educators should recognize that those without this experience might perceive themselves at a disadvantage. Low self-efficacy (confidence) may lead to low goal commitment, more stress, and decreased persistence, therefore potentially challenging retention. Focusing on the unique talents and life experiences of all students may help clarify any misperceptions of deficits, particularly in the clinical area. Students with prior experience may feel pressured never to make a mistake; the need to excel may interfere with learning, performance, and retention. Nurse educators must remember that although prior health care experience may provide students with some advantages, the special transitional and socialization needs of these students must be routinely appraised and addressed if all student potentials are to be maximized. Attitudes of faculty toward LPNs and their special needs may also require modification (Hammond et al., 1995).

ENROLLMENT STATUS

Enrollment status refers to whether a student is enrolled full-time (12 or more credits), part-time (fewer than 12 credits), matriculated, nonmatriculated, commuter, or campus resident. Almost half of all college students attend part-time. Consistent with trends in higher education, the number of part-time nursing students has increased (O'Connor & Bevil, 1996; Tanner, 1998). Retention rates are highest among traditional age full-time college students who reside in campus housing (Kuh, 2001; Skahill, 2002). Nonmatriculated and part-time students tend to withdraw more than matriculated and full-time students (Johnson, 1996; St. John, Hu, Simmons, & Musoba, 2001). Purely commuter campuses tend to have the lowest retention rates, with more non-matriculated students attending part-time (Astin, 1997). Part-time commuter students tend to interact less with the academic environment than do traditional, full-time students (Metzner & Bean, 1987; Napoli & Wortman, 1998). Students' enrollment status needs to be viewed in context with the type of institution (commuter versus residential and community college, four-year college, or hospital school of nursing). Matriculated students have a stronger evidence of goal commitment through their already invested time, money, and credits toward the nursing major.

In combination with other environmental variables, enrollment may create role conflicts for part-time but especially full-time students who have other responsibilities. Work-family-student conflict is defined as incompatible pressures arising simultaneously from the work, family, and student roles (Jeffreys, 1993). The influence of environmental variables on retention will be discussed in chapter 5; the influence of stress will be discussed in chapter 7.

INTERACTION WITH OTHER MODEL DIMENSIONS

Student profile characteristics have a direct influence on academic factors, cultural values and beliefs, self-efficacy, motivation, and environmental factors. A bidirectional relationship is proposed between professional integration and professional socialization. This proposition recognizes that individual and combined efforts at professional integration and socialization may positively or negatively influence how student profile characteristics are viewed. For example, a male student who perceives himself to be integrated and positively socialized within the nursing profession may not perceive gender as an obstacle to success. Similarly, an African-American student at a predominantly white university who attends a conference sponsored by the National Black Nurses Association (NBNA) and who is paired with an NBNA mentor may change his or her views about race as an obstacle or as a strength within the nursing profession. Pairing ESL students at varying levels of the educational process can minimize language as a perceived obstacle. Although family educational background at the start of the nursing educational process will remain unchanged, professional socialization and integration efforts can minimize students' concerns about not belonging in college.

KEY POINTS SUMMARY

- Student profile characteristics are described prior to beginning a nursing course and include age, ethnicity and race, gender, language, prior educational experience, family's educational background, prior work experience, and enrollment status.
- Individual variables may interact to increase or decrease risk of attrition.
- Actual and perceived barriers to retention include myths, stereotyping, prejudice, and discrimination based on any of the student profile characteristics.
- Nurse educators' expectations that are more, less, or different, based on a single student profile characteristic are detrimental, since individual student strengths and needs are not objectively appraised.
- Student profile characteristics may strongly identify the need to further explore individual student strengths and weaknesses.
- Student profile characteristics have a direct influence on academic factors, cultural values and beliefs, self-efficacy, motivation, and environmental factors.
- A bidirectional relationship is proposed between professional integration and professional socialization. This proposition recognizes that individual and combined efforts at professional integration and socialization may positively or negatively influence how student profile characteristics are viewed.
- Thorough assessment of the interaction of multiple profile variables will help promote better understanding of the retention process. Each student profile characteristic can have direct and/or indirect impact on retention.

EDUCATOR-IN-ACTION

Without appropriate background knowledge, individual appraisal, and sensitivity, educators' actions may adversely impact upon students' academic and psychological outcomes, persistence, and retention. Consider the possible adverse effects of the following educator actions:

After the preconference prior to the first clinical day, Professor Hurdles individually tells Marsha, a 25-year-old African-American student, that she should go to the college's math and English tutoring center before administering medications and writing nursing progress notes. Marsha earned a baccalaureate degree with honors from a private university and majored in mathematics. For three years, she taught high school algebra, geometry, and AP calculus. After caring for a terminally ill family member, Marsha decided to return to college to become an RN.

Cindy is a 20-year-old white student who lived in many foster homes throughout much of her childhood, resulting in frequent elementary and secondary school transfers. She ran away from her last foster home at age 16 and dropped out of high school; however, she completed her GED one year ago. She feels insecure and has low confidence about her academic ability. She is just about to ask Professor Hurdles where she can get some extra help when Professor Hurdles says, "It's nice to see a young student have all her priorities straight and enter nursing right after high school. I expect you to excel without difficulty."

After several weeks, one male student (Juan) mentions to other students and another clinical instructor, "I wish that I would get the same opportunities as the female students in my clinical group. I haven't been assigned to any female patients. How will I learn to feel comfortable interviewing female patients if I never have the opportunity? Doesn't Professor Hurdles trust me?" Another student, Harry, adds, "I feel the same way. It seems that I always have the assignments with male patients who require heavy lifting and physical care. I thought the nursing profession for men involved more than lifting, moving, and bed baths."

Kim is a foreign student from Korea who has only been in the United States for two years. She currently has a 3.7 GPA in prenursing courses. Her mastery of the English language in such a short time is remarkable, although she speaks with a heavy (but understandable) accent. Professor Hurdles assigns Kim to a Japanese patient (who only speaks Japanese) and says, "I am sure you will have no trouble communicating with your patient now."

In contrast to these examples, educator actions that embrace diverse student profile characteristics, that are knowledgeable, appreciate students as individuals, maximize strengths, and improve weaknesses, have the most potential for promoting positive academic and psychological outcomes, persistence, and retention. For example, during the first clinical preconference, Professor Bridges welcomes all the students, stating, "I look forward to a wonderful semester. We are fortunate to have such a diverse group because each of you undoubtedly has individual strengths, experiences, insights, and talents that can be shared with others, enriching the overall group and ultimately benefiting patient care. On your index card, please write down your personal strengths. We will discuss them in a few minutes."

After 10 minutes, Professor Bridges says, "Everyone may have areas that you may be concerned about or areas that you would like additional help, guidance, or experience with. On the other side of the index card, please write down these areas." During the group discussion, Professor Bridges asks each student to share a perceived strength and an area for professional development, personal growth, or concern. Select student responses follow:

Lucienne: "Many people think I'm African-American, but I came to the United States three years ago after residing in four other countries. Since I speak French and Spanish fluently, I would be happy to help anyone with translations but I don't really know about the cultural customs among the different groups who speak these languages. Multiple choice questions are difficult for me. This is not the type of testing I'm accustomed to, especially on the computer."

Roseanne: "I don't really have anything important to share. I'm 36 and my family questions why I'm going to college to become a nurse. No one in my family ever went to college. I'm just a housewife and mom who attends school part-time. I always wanted to be a nurse. I love talking with people and want to work in pediatrics."

Douglas: "You both could be a big help to me. I worked for ten years in the computer field until the company went bankrupt. I'm really more comfortable with computers than talking with people. Since I lived in a small town my whole life and only moved to this big city recently, I'm not sure how to interact with people of different cultures. Everything seems so fast-paced. I wish I had your lifetime motivation about nursing."

After each presentation, Professor Bridges thanks each student individually for his or her contribution, offers constructive suggestions, and asks for other student input. Individual, paired, and group learning experiences are then developed throughout the semester, with students building on each other's strengths. Although the sharing of student perceptions permits Professor Bridges to gain insight into the individual student experience, she also identifies potential areas of strengths and weaknesses associated with each student profile characteristic (such as acculturation stress and multiple role conflict), appraises students individually, and offers appropriate resources and support accordingly.

REFERENCES AND BIBLIOGRAPHY

Aber, C. S., & Arathuzik, D. (1996). Factors associated with student success in a baccalaureate nursing program within an urban public university. *Journal of Nursing Education, 35*(6), 285–288.

Abriam-Yago, K., Yoder, M., & Kataoka-Yahiro, M. (1999). The Cummins model: a framework for teaching nursing students for whom English is a second language. *Journal of Transcultural Nursing, 10*(2), 143–149.

Abrums, M. E., & Leppa, C. (2001). Beyond cultural competence: Teaching about race, gender, class, and sexual orientation. *Journal of Nursing Education, 40*(6), 270–275.

Adnett, N., & Coates, G. (2000). Mature female entrants to higher education: Closing the gender gap in the UK labour market. *Higher Education Quarterly, 54*(2), 187–201.

Allen, C. B., Higgs, Z. R., & Holloway, J. R. (1988). Identifying students at risk for academic difficulty. *Journal of Professional Nursing, 4*(2), 113–118.

Anderson, L. W. (2001). Predicting academic performance of college students in the United States and in Estonia. *International Journal of Educational Research, 35,* 353–355.

Antonio, A. L. (2001). Diversity and the influence of friendship groups in college. *Review of Higher Education, 25*(1), 63–89.

Astin, A. W. (1997). How "good" is your institution's retention rate? *Research in Higher Education, 38*(6), 647–658.

Baker, C. R. (2001). Role strain in male diploma nursing students: A descriptive quantitative study. *Journal of Nursing Education, 40*(8), 378–380.

Barbee, E. L., & Gibson, S. E. (2001). Our dismal progress: The recruitment of non-whites into nursing. *Journal of Nursing Education, 40*(6), 243–244.

Bean, J. P., & Metzner, B. (1985). A conceptual model of nontraditional undergraduate student attrition. *Review of Educational Research, 55,* 485–540.

Benda, E. J. (1991). The relationship among variables in Tinto's conceptual model and attrition of bachelor's degree nursing students. *Journal of Professional Nursing, 7*(1), 16–24.

Bendixen-Noe, M. K., & Giebelhaus, C. (1998). Nontraditional students in higher education: Meeting their needs as learners. *Mid-Western Educational Researcher, 11*(2), 27–31.

Berger, J. B. (2001). Understanding the organizational nature of student persistence: Empirically based recommendations for practice. *Journal of College Student Retention: Research, Theory, & Practice, 3*(1), 3–22.

Bessent, H. (Ed.). (1997). *Strategies for recruitment, retention, and graduation of minority nurses in colleges of nursing.* Washington, DC: American Nurses Publishing.

Boughn, S. (1994). Why do men choose nursing? *Nursing and Health Care, 15*(8), 406–411.

Boughn, S. (2001). Why women and men choose nursing. *Nursing and Health Care Perspectives, 22*(1), 14–19.

Brennan, A. L., Best, D. G., & Small, S. P. (1996). Tracking student progress in a baccalaureate nursing program: Academic indicators. *Canadian Journal of Nursing Research, 28*(2), 85–97.

Brown, L. L., & Kurpius, S. E. R. (1997). Psychosocial factors influencing academic persistence of American Indian college students. *Journal of College Student Development, 38*(1), 3–12.

Burris, R. F. (2001). Teaching student parents. *Nurse Educator, 26*(2), 64–65, 98.

Burton, D. R. (1997). Alleviating language problems for graduate nursing students from overseas. *Journal of Nursing Education, 36*(7), 330–332.

Burtt, K. (1998). Male nurses still face bias. *American Journal of Nursing, 98*(9), 64–65.

Campbell, A. R., & Davis, S. M. (1996). Faculty commitment: Retaining minority nursing students in majority institutions. *Journal of Nursing Education, 35*(7), 298–303.

Campbell, A. R., & Dickson, C. J. (1996). Predicting student success: A 10-year review using integrative review and meta-analysis. *Journal of Professional Nursing, 12*(1), 47–59.

Campinha-Bacote, J. (1998). *The process of cultural competence in the delivery of healthcare services: A culturally competent model of care* (3rd ed.). Cincinnati, OH: Transcultural C.A.R.E. Associates.

Chaney, B., Muraskin, L. D., Cahalan, M. W., & Goodwin, D. (1998). Helping the progress of disadvantaged students in higher education: The federal student support services program. *Educational Evaluation and Policy Analysis, 20*(3), 197–215.

College Board. (2003). *Challenging times, clear choices: An action agenda for college access and success.* Retrieved February 27, 2003, from http://www.collegeboard.com

Constantine, M. G., Robinson, J. S., Wilton, L., & Caldwell, L. D. (2002). Collective self-esteem and perceived social support as predictors of cultural congruity among black and Latino college students. *Journal of College Student Development, 43*(3), 307–316.

Constantine, M. G., & Watt, S. K. (2002). Cultural congruity, womanist identity attitudes, and life satisfaction among African American college women attending historically black and predominantly white institutions. *Journal of College Student Development, 43*(2), 184–193.

Crawford, L. A., & Olinger, B. H. (1988). Recruitment and retention of nursing students from diverse cultural backgrounds. *Journal of Nursing Education, 27*(8), 379–381.

Darkenwald, G. G., & Novak, R. J. (1997). Classroom age composition and academic achievement in college. *Adult Education Quarterly, 47*(2), 108–116.

Davidhizar, R., & Giger, J. N. (2001). Teaching culture within the nursing curriculum using the Giger-Davidhizar model of transcultural nursing assessment. *Journal of Nursing Education, 40*(6), 282–288.

Davies, P., & Williams, J. (2001). For me or not for me? Fragility and risk in mature students' decision making. *Higher Education Quarterly, 55*(2), 185–204.

DeFelice, C. E. (1989). *The relationship between self-efficacy and academic achievement in associate degree nursing programs.* Unpublished doctoral dissertation, Teachers College, Columbia University, New York.

Devlin, M. (1996). Older and wiser? A comparison of the learning and study strategies of mature age and younger teacher education students. *Higher Education Research and Development, 15*(1), 51–60.

Drevdahl, D. (2001). Teaching about race, racism, and health. *Journal of Nursing Education, 40*(6), 285–288.

Eaton, S. B., & Bean, J. P. (1995). An approach/avoidance behavioral model of college student attrition. *Research in Higher Education, 36*(6), 617–645.

Eppler, M. A., & Harju, B. L. (1997). Achievement motivation goals in relation to academic performance in traditional and nontraditional college students. *Research in Higher Education, 38*(5), 557–573.

Farella, C. (2002). School of hard knocks: Is racism a fixture of nursing academia? *Nursing Spectrum, 14*(12) NY/NJ, 34–35.

Femea, P., Gaines, C., Brathwaite, D., & Abdur-Rahman, V. (1995). Sociodemographic and academic characteristics of linguistically diverse nursing students in a baccalaureate degree nursing program. *Journal of Multicultural Nursing and Health, 1*(3), 24–29.

Flege, J. E., & Liu, S. (2001). The effects of experience on adults' acquisition of a second language. *Studies in Second Language Acquisition, 23*(4), 527–552.

Fleming, J. (2002). Who will succeed in college? When the SAT predicts black students' performance. *Review of Higher Education, 25*(3), 281–296.

Flowers, L. A. (2002). The impact of college racial composition on African American students' academic and social gains: Additional evidence. *Journal of College Student Development, 43*(3), 403–410.

Fries-Britt, S., & Turner, B. (2002). Uneven stories: Successful black collegians at a black and a white campus. *Review of Higher Education, 25*(3), 315–330.

Fuertes, J. N., & Westbrook, F. D. (1996). Using the social, attitudinal, familial, and environmental (S.A.F.E.) acculturation stress scale to assess the adjustment needs of Hispanic college students. *Measurement and Evaluation in Counseling and Development, 29*, 67–76.

Furio, B. J., & Kafka, J. S. (1996). Listening preferences of traditional and nontraditional college students and their relationship to instruction. *The New Jersey Journal of Communication, 4*(1), 99–107.

Galbraith, M. (1991). Attracting men to nursing: What will they find important in their career? *Journal of Nursing Education, 30*(4), 182–186.

Gallagher, P. A., Bomba, C., & Crane, L. R. (2001). Using an admissions exam to predict student success in an ADN program. *Nurse Educator, 26*(3), 132–135.

Gianakos, I. (1996). Career development differences between adult and traditional-aged learners. *Journal of Career Development, 22*(3), 211–223.

Gloria, A. M., & Kurpius, S. E. R. (1996). The validation of the cultural congruity scale and the university environment scale with Chicano/a students. *Hispanic Journal of Behavioral Sciences, 18*(4), 533–549.

Griffiths, M. J., Bevil, C. A., O'Connor, P. C., & Wieland, D. M. (1995). Anatomy and physiology as a predictor of success in baccalaureate nursing students. *Journal of Nursing Education, 34*(2), 61–66.

Hagey, R., & MacKay, R. W. (2000). Qualitative research to identify racist discourse: Towards equity in nursing curricula. *International Journal of Nursing Studies, 37*(1), 45–56.

Hammond, P. V., Davis, B. L., Marlin, B. W., & Montgomery, A. J. (1995). Student upward mobility: Utilization of an educational support model. *Association of Black Nursing Faculty Journal,* March/April, 51–53.

Hansen, G. (1988). Student retention in associate degree nursing education. In *Nursing shortage: Strategies for nursing practice and education.* Washington, DC: Report for the National Invitation Workshop. (ERIC Document Reproduction Service No. ED310257).

Harvey, V. C., & McMurray, N. E. (1997). Students' perceptions of nursing: Their relationship to attrition. *Journal of Nursing Education, 36*(8), 383–389.

Hayes, K., King, E., & Richardson, J. T. E. (1997). Mature students in higher education: III. Approaches to studying in Access students. *Studies in Higher Education, 22*(1), 19–31.

Hayes, S. H., Fiebert, I. M., Carroll, S. R., & Magill, R. N. (1997). Predictors of academic success in a physical therapy program: Is there a difference between traditional and nontraditional students? *Journal of Physical Therapy Education, 11*(1), 10–16.

Heller, B. R., Oros, M. T., & Durney-Crowley, J. (2000). The future of nursing education: 10 trends to watch. *Nursing and Health Care Perspectives, 21*(1), 9–13.

Hernandez, J. C. (2000). Understanding the retention of Latino college students. *Journal of College Student Development, 41*(6), 575–588.

Hinderlie, H. H., & Kenny, M. (2002). Attachment, social support, and college adjustment among black students at predominantly white universities. *Journal of College Student Development, 43*(3), 327–340.

Hoskins, S. L., Newstead, S. E., & Dennis, I. (1997). Degree performance as a function of age, gender, prior qualifications and discipline studied. *Assessment and Evaluation in Higher Education, 22*(3), 317–328.

Hurtado, S., Inkelas, K. K., Briggs, C., & Rhee, B-S. (1997). Differences in college access and choice among racial/ethnic groups: Identifying continuing barriers. *Research in Higher Education, 38*(1), 43–75.

Hutcheson, J. D., Garland, L. M., & Lowe, L. S. (1979). Antecedents of nursing school attrition: Attitudinal dimensions. *Nursing Research, 28*(1), 57–62.

Hyers, A. D., & Joslin, M. N. (1998). The first year seminar as a predictor of academic achievement and persistence. *Journal of the Freshman Year Experience, 10*(1), 7–30.

Ishiyama, J. T., & Hopkins, V. M. (2002). Assessing the impact of a graduate school preparation program on first-generation, low-income college students at a public liberal arts university. *Journal of College Student Retention, Research, Theory, & Practice, 4*(4), 393–405.

Jalili-Grenier, F., & Chase, M. M. (1997). Retention of nursing students with English as a second language. *Journal of Advanced Nursing, 25*, 199–203.

Jeffreys, M. R. (1993). *The relationship of self-efficacy and select academic and environmental variables on academic achievement and retention.* Unpublished doctoral dissertation, Teachers College, Columbia University, New York.

Jeffreys, M. R. (2000). Development and psychometric evaluation of the Transcultural Self-Efficacy Tool: A synthesis of findings. *Journal of Transcultural Nursing, 11*(2), 127–136.

Jeffreys, M. R. (2001). Evaluating enrichment program study groups: Academic outcomes, psychological outcomes, and variables influencing retention. *Nurse Educator, 26*(3), 142–149.

Jeffreys, M. R. (2002). Students' perceptions of variables influencing retention: A pretest and post-test approach. *Nurse Educator, 27*(1), 16–19 [Erratum, 2002, 27(2), 64].

Jeffreys, M. R., & Smodlaka, I. (1998). Exploring the factorial composition of the Transcultural Self-Efficacy Tool. *International Journal of Nursing Studies, 35*, 217–225.

Jeffreys, M. R., & Smodlaka, I. (1999a). Changes in students' transcultural self-efficacy perceptions following an integrated approach to culture care. *Journal of Multicultural Nursing and Health, 5*(2), 6–12. [Erratum, 2000, 6(1), 20].

Jeffreys, M. R., & Smodlaka, I. (1999b). Construct validation of the Transcultural Self-Efficacy Tool. *Journal of Nursing Education, 38*, 222–227.

Johnson, G. M. (1996). Faculty differences in university attrition: A comparison of the characteristics of arts, education and science students who withdrew from undergraduate programs. *Journal of Higher Education Policy and Management, 18*(1), 75–91.

Kasworm, C. E., & Pike, G. R. (1994). Adult undergraduate students: Evaluating the appropriateness of a traditional model of academic performance. *Research in Higher Education, 35*(6), 689–710.

Kataoka-Yahiro, M. R., & Abriam-Yago, K. (1997). Culturally competent teaching strategies for Asian nursing students for whom English is a second language. *Journal of Cultural Diversity, 4*(3), 83–87.

Kelly, N. R., Shoemaker, M., & Steele, T. (1996). The experience of being a male student nurse. *Journal of Nursing Education, 35*(4), 170–174.

Kimball, B., & O'Neil, E. (2002). *Health care's human crisis: The American nursing shortage.* Princeton, NJ: Robert Wood Johnson.

Kippenbrock, T., May, F., & Younes, C. (1996). Nursing students attrition rates decline: A longitudinal study. *Journal of Nursing Science, 1*(5–6), 157–164.

Kuh, G. D. (2001). Organizational culture and student persistence: Prospects and puzzles. *Journal of College Student Retention: Research, Theory, & Practice, 3*(1), 23–40.

Kurz, J. M. (1993). The adult ESL baccalaureate nursing student. *Journal of Nursing Education, 32*(5), 227–229.

Leininger, M. M., & McFarland, M. R. (2002). *Transcultural nursing: Concepts, theories, research, and practice* (3rd ed.). New York: McGraw-Hill.

LeSure-Lester, G. E. (2003). Effects of coping styles on college persistence decisions among Latino students in two-year colleges. *Journal of College Student Retention, Research, Theory, & Practice, 5*(1), 11–22.

Levin, M. E., & Levin, J. R. (1991). A critical examination of academic retention programs for at-risk minority college students. *Journal of College Student Development, 32,* 323–334.

Lynch, J. M., & Bishop-Clark, C. (1998). A comparison of the nontraditional students' experience on traditional versus nontraditional college campuses. *Innovative Higher Education, 22*(3), 217–229.

MacDonald, C., & Stratta, E. (1998). Academic work, gender and subjectivity: Mature non-standard entrants in higher education. *Studies in the Education of Adults, 30*(1), 67–79.

Malloch, D. C., & Montgomery, D. C. (1996). Variation in characteristics among adult students. *Continuing Higher Education Review, 60*(1), 42–53.

Malu, K. F., & Figlear, M. R. (1998). Enhancing the language development of immigrant ESL nursing students. *Nurse Educator, 23*(2), 43–46.

Mancuso, S. (2001). Adult-centered practices: Benchmarking study in higher education. *Innovative Higher Education, 25*(3), 165–181.

Manifold, C., & Rambur, B. (2001). Predictors of attrition in American Indian nursing students. *Journal of Nursing Education, 40*(6), 279–281.

Merisotis, J. P., & Phipps, R. A. (2000). Remedial education in colleges and universities: What's really going on? *Review of Higher Education, 24*(1), 67–85.

Metzner, B., & Bean, J. P. (1987). The estimation of a conceptual model of nontraditional undergraduate student attrition. *Research in Higher Education, 27,* 15–38.

Mills Wisneski, S. M. (2003). African-American baccalaureate nursing students' perceptions of nursing programs and factors that support or restrict academic success. (Doctoral dissertation, Widener University, 2003) *UMI Dissertation Service,* 3083001.

Morales, E. E. (2000). A contextual understanding of the process of educational resilience: High achieving Dominican American students and the "resilience cycle." *Innovative Higher Education, 25*(1), 7–21.

Murtaugh, P. A., Burns, L. D., & Schuster, J. (1999). Predicting the retention of university students. *Research in Higher Education, 40*(3), 355–371.

Napoli, A. R., & Wortman, P. M. (1998). Psychosocial factors related to retention and early departure of two-year community college students. *Research in Higher Education, 39*(4), 419–455.

Nardi, D. A., & Rooda, L. (1992). Student age and measures of success in a nursing education program. *Nurse Educator, 17*(2), 5–6.

Nora, A. (1987). Determinants of retention among Chicano college students: A structural model. *Research in Higher Education, 26,* 31–60.

Nora, A., Cabrera, A., Hagedorn, L. S., & Pascarella, E. (1996). Differential impacts of academic and social experiences on college-related behavioral outcomes across different ethnic and gender groups at four-year institutions. *Research in Higher Education, 37*(4), 427–451.

Nurmi, J-E., & Aunola, K. (2001). How does academic achievement come about? Cross-cultural and methodological notes. *International Journal of Educational Research, 35,* 403–409.

O'Connor, P. C., & Bevil, C. A. (1996). Academic outcomes and stress in full-time day and part-time evening baccalaureate nursing students. *Journal of Nursing Education, 35*(6), 245–251.

Olenchak, F. R., & Hebert, T. P. (2002). Endangered academic talent: Lessons learned from gifted first-generation college males. *Journal of College Student Development, 43*(2), 195–212.

Padilla, R. V., Trevino, J., Gonzalez, K., & Trevino, J. (1997). Developing local models of minority student success in college. *Journal of College Student Development, 38*(2), 125–135.

Pascarella, E. T., & Chapman, D. W. (1983). Validation of a theoretical model of college withdrawal: Interaction effects in a multi-institutional sample. *Research in Higher Education, 19,* 25–47.

Patterson, B. J., & Morin, K. H. (2002). Perceptions of the maternal-child clinical rotation: The male student nurse experience. *Journal of Nursing Education, 41*(6), 266–272.

Phillips, S., & Hartley, J. T. (1990). Teaching students for whom English is a second language. *Nurse Educator, 15*(5), 29–32.

Purnell, L. D. (2003). Purnell's model for cultural competence. In L. D. Purnell & B. J. Paulanka (Eds.), *Transcultural health care: A culturally competent approach* (2nd ed., pp. 8–39). Philadelphia: F.A. Davis.

Ransdell, S. (2001). Predicting college success: The importance of ability and non-cognitive variables. *International Journal of Educational Research, 35,* 357–364.

Ransdell, S., Hawkins, C., & Adams, R. (2001a). Models, modeling, and the design of the study. *International Journal of Educational Research, 35,* 365–372.

Ransdell, S., Hawkins, C., & Adams, R. (2001b). Results of the study. *International Journal of Educational Research, 35,* 373–389.

Richardson, J. T. E. (1994). Mature students in higher education: I. A literature survey on approaches to studying. *Studies in Higher Education, 19,* 309–325.

Richardson, J. T. E. (1995). Mature students in higher education: II. An investigation of approaches to studying and academic performance. *Studies in Higher Education, 20,* 5–17.

Richardson, J. T. E., & King, E. (1998). Adult students in higher education. *Journal of Higher Education, 69*(1), 66–88.

Rodgers, S. G. (1990). Retention of minority nursing students on predominantly white campuses. *Nurse Educator, 15*(5), 36–39.

Root, M. P. P. (1992). Within, between, and beyond race. In M. P. P. Root (Ed.), *Racially mixed people in America* (pp. 3–11). Newbury Park, CA: Sage.

Rosenfeld, P. (1987). Nursing education in crisis—a look at recruitment and retention. *Nursing and Health Care, 5,* 283–286.

Ryan, S., & Porter, S. (1993). Men in nursing: A cautionary comparative critique. *Nursing Outlook, 41,* 262–267.

Scott, C., Burns, A., & Cooney, G. (1996). Reasons for discontinuing study: The case of mature age female students with children. *Higher Education, 31,* 233–253.

Scott, C., Burns, A., & Cooney, G. (1998). Motivation for return to study as a predictor of completion of degree amongst female mature students with children. *Higher Education, 35,* 221–239.

Seidl, A. H., & Sauter, D. (1990). The new non-traditional student in nursing. *Journal of Nursing Education, 29*(1), 13–19.

Shearer, R. A. (1989). Teaching foreign students. *Journal of Nursing Education, 28*(9), 427–428.

Skahill, M. P. (2002). The role of social support network in college persistence among freshman students. *Journal of College Student Retention Research, Theory, & Practice, 4*(1), 39–52.

Smart, J. F., & Smart, D. W. (1995). Acculturative stress: The experience of the Hispanic immigrant. *The Counseling Psychologist, 23,* 25–42.

Sommer, S. (2001). Multicultural nursing education. *Journal of Nursing Education, 40*(6), 276–278.

Spady, W. (1970). Dropouts from higher education: Toward an empirical model. *Interchange, 2,* 38–62.

St. John, E. P., Hu, S., Simmons, A. B., & Musoba, G. D. (2001). Aptitude vs. merit: What matters in persistence. *Review of Higher Education, 24*(2), 131–152.

Stevenson, E. L. (2003). Future trends in nursing employment. *American Journal of Nursing Career Guide 2003,* 19–25.

Strage, A., Baba, Y., Millner, S., Scharberg, M., Walker, E., Williamson, R., & Yoder, M. (2002). What every student affairs professional should know: Student study activities and beliefs associated with academic success. *Journal of College Student Development, 43*(2), 246–266.

Streubert, H. J. (1994). Male nursing students' perceptions of clinical experience. *Nurse Educator, 19*(5), 28–32.

Sullivan, E. (2002). In a woman's world. *Reflections on Nursing Leadership, 28*(3), 10–17.

Tanner, C. A. (1998). The new learner. *Journal of Nursing Education, 37*(6), 239–240.

Tayebi, K., Moore-Jazayeri, M., & Maynard, T. (1998). From the borders: Reforming the curriculum for the at-risk student. *Journal of Cultural Diversity, 5*(3), 101–109.

Terenzini, P. T., Springer, L., Yaeger, P. M., Pascarella, E. T., & Nora, A. (1996). First generation college students: Characteristics, experiences, and cognitive development. *Research in Higher Education, 37*(1), 1–23.

Thompson, C., & Sheckley, B. G. (1997). Differences in classroom teaching preferences between traditional and adult BSN students. *Journal of Nursing Education, 36*(4), 163–170.

Ting, S-M. R. (1997). Estimating academic success in the first year of college for specially admitted white students: A model combining cognitive and psychosocial predictors. *Journal of College Student Development, 38*(4), 401–409.

Ting, S-M. R. (2000). Predicting Asian Americans' academic performance in the first year of college: An approach combining SAT scores and noncognitive variables. *Journal of College Student Development, 41*(4), 442–449.

Tinto, V. (1997). Classrooms as communities. *Journal of Higher Education, 68*(6), 599–623.

Toutkoushian, R. K., & Smart, J. C. (2001). Do institutional characteristics affect student gains from college? *Review of Higher Education, 25*(1), 39–61.

Tucker-Allen, S., & Long, E. (1999). *Recruitment and retention of minority students: Stories of success.* Lisle, IL: Tucker.

Trueman, M., & Hartley, J. (1996). A comparison between the time-management skills and academic performance of mature and traditional-entry university students. *Higher Education, 32,* 199–215.

Upton, T. A., & Lee-Thompson, L-C. (2001). The role of the first language in second language reading. *Studies in Second Language Acquisition, 23*(4), 469–495.

Villaruel, A. M., Canales, M., & Torres, S. (2001). Bridges and barriers: Educational mobility of Hispanic nurses. *Journal of Nursing Education, 40*(6), 245–251.

Waltman, P. A. (1997). Comparison of traditional and non-traditional baccalaureate nursing students on selected components of Meichenbaum and Butler's model of test anxiety. *Journal of Nursing Education, 36*(4), 171–179.

Weaver, H. N. (2001). Indigenous nurses and professional education: Friends or foes? *Journal of Nursing Education, 40*(6), 252–258.

Wolahan, C. G., & Wieczorek, R. R. (1991). Enrichment education: Key to NCLEX success. *Nursing and Health Care, 12*(5), 234–239.

Wold, J. E., & Worth, C. (1990). Baccalaureate student nurse success prediction: A replication. *Journal of Nursing Education, 29*(2), 84–89.

Yearwood, E., Brown, D. L., & Karlik, E. C. (2002). Cultural diversity: Students' perspectives. *Journal of Transcultural Nursing, 13*(3), 237–240.

Young, J. W., & Koplow, S. L. (1997). The validity of two questionnaires for predicting minority students' college grades. *Journal of General Education, 46*(1), 45–55.

Yurkovich, E. E. (2001). Working with American Indians toward educational success. *Journal of Nursing Education, 40*(6), 259–269.

Chapter 3

Cultural Values and Beliefs, Self-Efficacy and Motivation: Important Considerations

Nurse educators must seriously consider the impact of student affective factors on nursing student achievement, persistence, and retention. Student affective factors are attitudes, values, and beliefs about education, nursing, and one's ability to learn and perform the tasks required for course and nursing program success. In the NURS model, these factors include cultural values and beliefs, self-efficacy, and motivation. Student affective factors are different than student profile characteristics in that they deal with variables that may change over time and may be positively or negatively influenced by all other variable sets. This chapter introduces the general concepts underlying cultural values and beliefs, self-efficacy, and motivation that demand sincere consideration in nursing education today.

CULTURAL VALUES AND BELIEFS

Culture refers to patterns of learned values, beliefs, and behaviors that are shared from generation to generation within a group (Leininger, 1978, 1994). All students belong to one or more cultural groups and therefore bring their patterns of learned values, beliefs, and behaviors into the academic and professional setting. Values are standards that have eminent worth, meaning, and importance in one's life; values guide behavior. They are the "powerful directive forces that give order and meaning to people's thinking, decisions, and actions" (Leininger, 1995a). Cultural values influence thinking, decisions, and actions within the student role as well as in other aspects of people's lives.

The inclusion of cultural values and beliefs (CVB) in the NURS model recognizes that students' cultural values and beliefs unconsciously and consciously guide thinking, decisions, and actions that ultimately affect retention. Cultural congruence refers to the degree of fit between students' values and beliefs and the values and beliefs of their surrounding environment (Constantine, Robinson, Wilton, & Caldwell, 2002; Constantine & Watt, 2002; Gloria & Robinson Kurpius, 1996). Here, the surrounding environment refers to the environment of nursing education within the educational institution and the nursing profession. The NURS model proposes that high levels of cultural congruence will serve as a bridge to promoting positive academic and psychological outcomes, thus enhancing persistence behaviors and retention. High levels of cultural incongruence are proposed as inversely related to positive academic and psychological outcomes; thus, cultural incongruence presents a barrier to retention.

Cultural styles are the "recurring elements, expressions, and qualities that characterize a designated cultural group through their [sic] series of action-patterns, beliefs, and values" (Leininger, 1994, p. 155). The dominant values and norms of a cultural group guide the development of cultural styles (Leininger, 1994). Nursing is a unique culture that reflects its own cultural style. Currently (within the United States), the culture of nursing reflects many of the dominant societal values and beliefs held in this country. Similarly, nursing education reflects the Western European value system dominant in American universities. Although increases in culturally diverse students have been noted in higher education and in nursing, the values and beliefs underlying nursing education have been slow to change in accordance with changing student population needs. Furthermore, pedagogical changes in curriculum and teaching–learning strategies have been slow to change from the dominantly used Tylerian model, despite empirical support for active learning strategies (Andrews, 1995; Crow, 1993; Ironside, 2004).

Ethnocentrism and cultural blindness have been major obstacles to the needed changes in nursing education. Ethnocentrism is the idea that the values and beliefs traditionally held within nursing education are supreme. Consequently, traditional teaching–learning practices are upheld. Within the context of nursing education, cultural blindness is the inability to recognize the different CVB that exist among diverse student populations. Because cultural blindness does not acknowledge that differences exist, imposition of dominant nursing education values and beliefs occur. This imposition can cause cultural shock, cultural clashes, and cultural pain among students whose CVB are incongruent with the dominant nursing CVB.

Unfortunately, some nurse educators who acknowledge that differences exist may nevertheless expect students to instantly abandon long-held cultural values and beliefs and to easily adopt new values and beliefs. A nursing student does not simply "take off" old CVB and "put on" new nursing CVB as easily as changing clothes. Lack of cultural fit (cultural incongruence) can result in acculturation stress. Acculturation stress has been well documented among immigrant populations; however, it can occur whenever differences in CVB exist (Constantine, Robinson, et al., 2002; Constantine & Watt, 2002; Fuertes & Westbrook, 1996). Stress resulting from cultural incongruence adversely affects retention directly through negative psychological outcomes and indirectly through poor academic performance (see chapter 7). Poor academic performance can occur as a result of poor psychological outcomes and/or incongruent views concerning education, learning styles, and nursing. Views of nursing and motivation for nursing education can also vary greatly among cultures (Rognstad, 2002).

It is, however, critical to preserve certain values and beliefs within the nursing profession such as the Code of Ethics or standards of practice. Enculturation into nursing is a learning process that must be undertaken by all nursing students. It means that students learn to take on or live by the values, norms, and expectations of the nursing profession (Leininger, 2002). Sufficient assistance can minimize stress and enhance enculturation. Enculturation is more difficult if the student's own CVB are not congruent with those of nursing. For example, a traditional Vietnamese-American student who views the physician as an authority figure may find it difficult to confront one who prescribes a questionable treatment. Over time, it may become easier for that student to become assertive within the professional nursing role while still maintaining traditional CVB in other contexts. Nurse educators are challenged to explore various CVB within nursing, nursing education, and student cultures and to make culturally sensitive and appropriate decisions and actions.

Table 3.1 selectively compares and contrasts CVB of nursing education and four other cultural groups. Based on a review of the literature, traditional views within the identified cultures were included but are in no way meant to stereotype individuals within the cultures. Nurse educators are cautioned about making stereotypes and are reminded to explore cultural values and beliefs of individual students. For the purposes of this chapter, the following categories were selected and deemed most relevant to nursing student retention: individual-group orientation, time perception, verbal communication, nonverbal communication, household responsibilities, health, nurse, education, teacher, work habits, help-seeking behaviors, and persistence. It is beyond the scope of this book to provide in-depth explanations about each category, and yet the importance of an in-depth understanding must be recognized. The selective approach is meant to spark interest, stimulate awareness, and encourage further exploration among nurse educators before attempting the design of culturally relevant and congruent nursing educational strategies. This is critical; the need to understand, respect, maintain, and support the different CVB of culturally diverse students is a precursor to culturally relevant and competent education. Part II of this book will present strategies that incorporate an understanding of how CVB influence retention. Additionally, chapter 10 specifically addresses cultural congruent faculty advisement and helpfulness.

SELF-EFFICACY AND MOTIVATION

Despite the numerous adversities faced by many undergraduate nursing students today, some students persist while others do not. Self-efficacy and motivation can influence persistence and academic performance. Self-efficacy is the student's perceived confidence for learning or performing specific tasks or skills necessary to achieve a particular goal. It is the belief that one can perform or succeed at learning a specific task, despite obstacles and hardships, and that one will expend whatever energy is necessary to accomplish the task (Bandura, 1986). Self-efficacy has been strongly linked to persistence behaviors and motivation. Empirical evidence supports it as a significant variable influencing an individual's actions, performance, and persistence (Bean & Eaton, 2001; Zimmerman, 1995). Motivation has been described as the "power within the student to generate actions that will result in his or her success" (Stage & Hossler, 2000, p. 173).

In nursing, the less frequent study of self-efficacy (confidence) on academic performance and retention of nursing students has demonstrated significant findings (Ford-Gilboe, Laschinger, Laforet-Fliesser, Ward-Griffin, & Foran, 1997; Goldenberg, Iwasiw, & MacMaster, 1997; Harvey & McMurray, 1994; Madorin & Iwasiw, 1999). In the NURS model, self-efficacy is proposed as an important factor influencing retention. Figure 3.1 traces the proposed influences of self-efficacy on student's actions, performance, and persistence for learning tasks. Details will be discussed in the sections that follow.

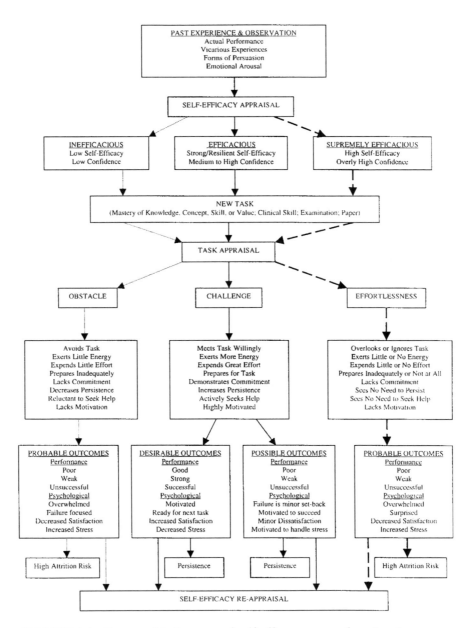

FIGURE 3.1 Proposed influences of self-efficacy on students' actions, performance, and persistence.

Background

A key concept in Bandura's (1986) social cognitive theory is that learning and motivation for learning are directly influenced by self-efficacy perceptions, which are domain-specific and task specific. Individuals with strong self-efficacy perceptions think, feel, and act differently than those who are either inefficacious or overly confident. Strong (resilient) self-efficacy enhances sociocognitive functioning in several ways: (1) new or difficult tasks are viewed as challenges that are accepted willingly, (2) great preparatory efforts are exhibited, (3) strong goal commitment and persistence behaviors are enhanced, (4) failures and setbacks are attributed to insufficient effort, and (5) more energy is expended to overcome failures, hardships, setbacks, and potential stressors in an effort to achieve goals (Bandura, 1986). A strong self-efficacy to withstand failures combined with some uncertainty (task perceived as a challenge rather than self-doubts about capability) will encourage preparatory efforts and thus enhance performance outcomes (Bandura, 1989). Students with this kind of self-efficacy are highly motivated and actively seek help to maximize their abilities.

In contrast, the inefficacious student (one with low confidence levels) is at risk for lowered persistence, poor motivation, and insufficient goal commitment, and may give up when obstacles or hardships are encountered. Such students may easily become discouraged if they do not quickly grasp new concepts, skills, or knowledge. They view academic challenges as overwhelming and insurmountable obstacles, threats, and hardships to be avoided. Consequently, they may decrease their study hours and lower their persistence with study tasks and assignments. Low self-efficacy can affect retention directly, if students give up without even trying and then withdraw from school, or indirectly, through poor academic and/or psychological outcomes. Poor academic outcomes (low grades and/or failure) may be the result of decreased class attendance, inadequate studying, and/or incomplete assignments. Such students become increasingly overwhelmed, focused on failure, dissatisfied, and stressed.

Students with low self-efficacy benefit the most from diagnostic specific interventions designed to enhance self-efficacy and other academic and psychological outcomes (Brown, Lent, & Larkin, 1989; Jeffreys & Smodlaka, 1999a; Zimmerman, 1995). Early identification of inefficacious students, followed by diagnostic-prescriptive interventions, can help students maximize strengths, minimize weaknesses, and facilitate success. For example, students inefficacious about multiple choice test-taking skills will benefit most from intensive test-taking preparation workshops. Because inefficacious students often lose motivation and are reluctant to seek assistance, the nurse educator plays a key role in initiating actions with these students. Although self-efficacy appraisal is task-specific, repeated failures and negative psychological outcomes decrease self-efficacy for learning and performing the necessary tasks for becoming a registered nurse, thereby lowering persistence behaviors overall.

Other at-risk students are those who are supremely efficacious (overly confident). Supremely efficacious students may be totally unaware of their weaknesses, underestimate the task or its importance, overlook the task, and overestimate their abilities and strengths (Bandura, 1989). These students may not see the need for adequate academic preparation, restructuring of priorities, or time management to accommodate academic tasks. Therefore, they may not be adequately prepared. Retention is affected through poor academic and negative psychological outcomes. Poor, weak, or unsuccessful performances can lead to feeling overwhelmed, surprised or shocked, dissatisfied, and stressed.

Supremely efficacious students often lack motivation for the task and see no need to seek assistance; the nurse educator can play a key role in initiating actions with them. Statistically significant findings in one study (Jeffreys, 1993, 1998) indicated that the at-risk students were supremely efficacious; students who perceived academic factors as highly supportive had significantly lower course grades. The results suggested that some students in the study sample did not have accurate perceptions of their academic skills required for professional nursing education. Early identification of supremely efficacious students can help students realistically appraise their strengths and weaknesses and recognize the need for adequate preparation for successful outcomes. Because students, (especially beginning students), may not know what to expect in nursing, they may need guidance in ongoing self-appraisal. Realistic self-efficacy appraisal allows one to seek help to enhance strengths and remedy weaknesses.

Self-Efficacy Appraisal

According to Bandura (1986), past experiences and vicarious experience observing others influence self-efficacy appraisal via four information sources: actual performances, vicarious experiences, forms of persuasion, and emotional arousal (physiological indices). Actual performances are the strongest source of efficacy information. Successful performances can raise efficacy and unsuccessful performances can lower it. Lowered self-efficacy can be psychologically stressful and dissatisfying to students, further impacting negatively on motivation, persistence, and retention. Individuals with low self-efficacy can initially feel devastated by failure or poor performance, and further lowered self-efficacy can cause avoidance behaviors (Bandura, 1986, 1997). Avoidance behaviors in nursing can be dangerous. For example, a student with low self-efficacy for assessing blood pressure reluctantly attempts the assessment, misinterprets findings, and fails to recognize severe hypertension in a client who later strokes. This student may be fearful of attempting other assessments, lack motivation, avoid help-seeking behaviors, and become increasingly dissatisfied and anxious.

Students with strong (realistic) levels of self-efficacy will not be adversely affected by an occasional failure and will view it as a temporary setback or challenge to be overcome with more effort expenditure (Bandura, 1986, 1997). In the above case example, the realistically strong efficacious student would be motivated to seek extra assistance in the skills lab or request additional supervised opportunities in the clinical setting to take blood pressures. Most likely, such a student would initially take the task seriously, view it with some uncertainty, and exert preparatory efforts before attempting to apply blood pressure assessment in the clinical setting. In contrast, the supremely efficacious student (unrealistic and overconfident in self-appraisal) would view the task without uncertainty, prepare inadequately, and potentially jeopardize patient safety. Unsuccessful performances and/or adverse consequences will lower self-efficacy. The supremely efficacious student's new goal should be to view the task seriously and as a challenge that requires adequate preparatory efforts.

Vicarious experience, or modeling, is less influential than actual performance. Models who display effort and perform tasks successfully will be more influential than models who complete the task effortlessly. Self-efficacy perceptions will be further enhanced if models are similar to the individual in background and ability (Bandura, 1986; Schunk, 1987). It would be expected that beginning (novice) students have less astute skills for observing models. With little or no experience in the domain of nursing, such students will be at risk for selective observations that are myopic, slightly skewed, severely distorted, or limited, thereby increasing the risk for unrealistic self-appraisals. Through the use of various structured mentoring strategies, nurse educators can enhance the power of modeling on self-efficacy appraisal and development. (Refer to Part II of this book for strategies.) Furthermore, by assisting students to develop keen observational skills, nurse educators can have a powerful influence on efficacy appraisal.

Forms of persuasion include positive verbal feedback from peers, teachers, and family. Positive persuasion will enhance efficacy only if students' subsequent efforts turn out positively (Schunk, 1987). Therefore, positive verbal feedback should be given judiciously and honestly. In the NURS model, "encouragement" by family, faculty, or friends must be realistic, thus incorporating this important dimension of self-efficacy appraisal.

Physiological indices such as elevated pulse rate and sweating may indicate the emotional arousal of anxiety or fear. Conscious awareness of anxiety symptoms over a particular task may lower efficacy beliefs (Bandura, 1986). For example, if a student repeatedly experiences elevated pulse rate and sweating at the beginning of each clinical day, despite the cognitive and psychomotor ability to perform tasks, the student's efficacy beliefs may be lowered and adversely affect learning, performance, persistence, motivation, and retention. Mild anxiety associated with some uncertainty has some benefits in that students are more attentive to detail, recognize the need for preparatory actions, and actively seek assistance. Lack of any physiological changes would accompany the expected profile of supremely efficacious students and adversely affect task performance.

Self-efficacy changes over time in response to new experiences and observations (Bandura, 1989; Gist & Mitchell, 1992; Saks, 1995). Several studies have supported the fact that culturally diverse nursing students' self-efficacy perceptions were significantly influenced by their educational and health care experiences. For example, in one longitudinal study, self-efficacy perceptions for inefficacious students were raised to medium (strong) levels and self-efficacy perceptions for supremely efficacious students were lowered to medium levels following an educational experience that integrated specific skills (Jeffreys & Smodlaka, 1999a). Students' course level was statistically significant in influencing perceptions in studies examining changes in transcultural self-efficacy perceptions (Jeffreys, 2000a; Jeffreys & Smodlaka, 1996, 1998, 1999a, 1999b). Novice students had overall lower self-efficacy perceptions and more experienced students had overall higher self-efficacy perceptions. Ethnic/racial group identity was statistically insignificant, suggesting that self-efficacy measures can be designed to capture the effect of educational experiences across culturally diverse groups; however further empirical investigation is recommended (Jeffreys, 2000; Jeffreys & Smodlaka, 1998, 1999a, 1999b).

Carefully designed measures (survey tools) can be used to appraise students' initial self-efficacy levels for particular tasks and skills. Situation-specific or task-specific tools must be designed and developed to measure self-efficacy (Bandura, 1989). Consequently, nurse educators should selectively choose a reliable and valid self-efficacy tool specifically designed for their investigation. Often this means that a new tool must be developed. The instrument design process is complex and time-consuming; however, specific steps should be followed to enhance the validity and reliability of findings. Review of survey data to identify inefficacious and supremely efficacious individuals will allow for early intervention and assistance in enhancing realistic self-efficacy appraisal. Empirical support for self-efficacy as a predictor of retention is more difficult to evaluate than conceptually acknowledging that self-efficacy plays an important role in student achievement and retention.

KEY POINTS SUMMARY

- Student affective factors are students' attitudes, values, and beliefs about education, nursing, and one's ability to learn and perform the tasks required for course and nursing program success. In the NURS model, these factors include cultural values and beliefs, self-efficacy, and motivation.
- All students belong to one or more cultural groups and therefore bring their patterns of learned values, beliefs, and behaviors into the academic and professional setting.
- The inclusion of cultural values and beliefs (CVB) in the NURS model recognizes that students' cultural values and beliefs unconsciously and consciously guide thinking, decisions, and actions that ultimately affect retention.
- The NURS model proposes that high levels of cultural congruence will serve as a bridge to promoting positive academic and psychological outcomes, thus enhancing persistence behaviors and retention.
- Stress resulting from cultural incongruence adversely affects retention directly through negative psychological outcomes and indirectly through poor academic performance.
- Despite the numerous adversities faced by many undergraduate nursing students today, some students persist while others do not. Self-efficacy and motivation can influence persistence and academic performance.
- Self-efficacy is the student's perceived confidence for learning or performing specific tasks or skills necessary to achieve a particular goal.
- Students with resilient (strong) self-efficacy beliefs perceive tasks as challenges, exert great effort in overcoming obstacles, are highly motivated, and actively seek help to maximize their abilities.
- Inefficacious students are at risk for lowered persistence, poor motivation, and insufficient goal commitment, and may give up when obstacles or hardships are encountered.

- Supremely efficacious (overly confident) students may be totally unaware of their weaknesses, underestimate the task or its importance, overlook the task, overestimate their abilities and strengths, thereby increasing the risk for inadequate preparation.

EDUCATOR-IN-ACTION

As part of the Writing-Across-the-Curriculum (WAC) initiative, Professor Glass has integrated a low-stakes written "reflection" component in the first introductory nursing fundamentals and medical-surgical nursing course. Students are asked to reflect and then briefly write about a specific topic in class for which they receive class participation credit. During the second week, Professor Glass presents the students with the writing prompt "Nursing is . . ." Responses are diverse, and Professor Glass identifies several students with varying levels of self-efficacy. She sees this as an important opportunity to intervene and promote positive behaviors. Professor Glass returns the assignment the next week, with constructive comments written for each student. Common themes will be addressed generally in class. Select written excerpts and instructor written responses and actions follow:

Morton: ". . . what I should be doing now. I have been a nursing assistant for five years. I really do all the nursing care for the patients in the nursing home except give medications and fill out paperwork. I know what to expect in the nursing program so it will be a lot easier for me."

Analysis: Morton is supremely efficacious, appraises the task of nursing effortlessly, and is at risk for inadequate preparation and undesirable academic and psychological outcomes.

Professor Glass writes, "Thank you for sharing your views. Your work as a nursing assistant has provided you with some valuable experiences with clients and other health care personnel. Some questions to think about may be: What patient assessments must registered professional nurses make before, during, and after medication administration? What background scientific knowledge is pertinent to decision making and planning patient care safely?" Professor Glass then asks to speak with Morton privately after class for further discussion. To help Morton gain a broader perspective, she arranges for Joe, a third-semester student who is also a nursing assistant, to speak with him about the nursing profession, benefits of maximizing opportunities and efforts within the nursing program, and strategies for success. Unfortunately, it is not until

Morton has the actual experience of failing the first exam that he reappraises his situation, seeks to learn vicariously from positive role models, appreciates Professor Glass's constructive feedback and guidance, and exerts greater preparatory efforts.

Natalie: ". . . a very important profession in the health care field. I didn't realize that nurses had so much responsibility and critical decision making. I thought that nurses just carried out the doctor's orders. I realize that nursing is very complex and that I will have to make more time to complete my reading and assignments if I am to be a good nurse."

Analysis: Natalie has strong/resilient self-efficacy.

Professor Glass writes, "You have already gained much insight about the nursing profession. Nursing is complex but can be quite rewarding. Keep up your positive attitude, motivation, and hard work." Intermittently Professor Glass asks Natalie about her perceived clinical progress and continues to encourage her diligent efforts.

Rita: ". . . hard work. It is harder than I expected. The nurses on the unit last week were so knowledgeable and professional. I don't know if I will ever be able to be like them or if I have what it takes to become a nurse. Patients really depend on nurses for their lives. There is so much to know in such a little time."

Analysis: Rita is inefficacious, perceives the task of becoming a nurse as an obstacle, and is at risk for inadequate preparation and undesirable academic and psychological outcomes.

Professor Glass writes, "Thank you for sharing your reflection. I am glad that the nurses last week were such positive role models. Some of those nurses were students here not too long ago and expressed some of the same concerns you have. Nursing is hard work; however, it can be a quite rewarding profession. Please see me for help concerning time management and effective study techniques for maximizing time spent on skill/knowledge mastery and learning." Professor Glass meets with Rita and links her with a culturally diverse study group led by a peer mentor-tutor of similar age and cultural background.

TABLE 3.1 Comparison of Select Cultural Values and Beliefs

	Culture of Nursing Education	Chinese-American	African-American	Mexican-American	Irish-American
Orientation	Individual	Group	Group	Group	Individual
Time perception	Present and future oriented. Punctuality valued.	History of past important. Traditionally lateness for appointments is expected. More recently, lateness is considered rude.	Present oriented. Punctuality less important.	Present oriented. Relaxed punctuality.	Past, present, future. Flexible sense of time.
Verbal communication	Direct, specific, and quick communication preferred. Expects individuals to indicate when something is not understood.	Moderate to low tones preferred. Loud tone associated with anger. Answer "yes" when asked if something is understood. Reluctant to talk about feelings and views.	Loud tones (in comparison to other cultures) are preferred. Views and feelings are shared openly with family and trusted friends.	Personal topics may be taboo. Feelings and views shared only with trusted family and friends. "Small talk" expected to begin communication encounter.	Low contextual language where meaning is explicit rather than implicit. Personal topics are private. Thoughts and feelings shared only with close family and friends.
Nonverbal communication	Most often consistent with dominant societal values, such as direct eye contact, handshaking, and spatial distances.	Avoid direct eye contact, especially with persons of authority and highly respected individuals.	Direct eye contact is sometimes perceived as aggressive.	Avoid direct eye contact, especially with persons of authority and highly respected individuals. Handshaking demonstrates respect.	Direct eye contact is maintained, indicating respect and trust.
Household responsibilities	The "traditional" student did not have household or outside responsibilities. Student role is primary.	Household responsibilities shared; however specific roles expected based on gender. Male is head of family.	Household responsibilities may be divided between men and women and children. Woman is often head of family.	Household responsibilities mainly part of female role. Male dominance with male as head of family. Modesty.	Traditionally household responsibilities part of female role; however in recent years responsibilities shared between men and women.

	Culture of Nursing Education	Chinese-American	African-American	Mexican-American	Irish-American
Health	Professes "holistic" view of health but still strongly based on medical model with focus on symptom alleviation, use of technology, and Western medicine.	Balance between "yin and yang."	"Health is viewed as a harmony with nature."	Balance between "hot and cold."	Determined by external forces.
Nurse	"Professional." Seeking more respect from other health professionals and society.	Respected as authority figures after physicians. Nurses with advanced education are more highly respected than are nurses with less education.	Respected member of the health care team but less important than physicians.	Respected member of the health care team; however often viewed as an outsider.	Nurses are respected as members of a service-oriented field or "occupation."
Education	Within the culture of nursing, disputes surrounding minimal educational requirements still persist.	Highly valued, especially a college education.	Highly valued, especially a college education.	Education is valued; however access to college education has been limited historically. Families often expect females to put family first.	Education is highly valued.
Teacher	Traditional pedagogy viewed teacher as "authority" who "transmits" learning to student. Newer proponents of androgogy view teacher as partner or facilitator of learning who implements learner-centered approaches.	Authority figure. True equality does not exist; therefore concept of "partner" in learning may be difficult to comprehend.	Respected authority figure.	Teacher is viewed as a highly respected superior. Rote learning and memorization predominates education in Mexico, with little emphasis on practical application, analysis, and synthesis.	Respected professional.

(continued)

TABLE 3.1 Comparison of Select Cultural Values and Beliefs (Continued)

	Culture of Nursing Education	Chinese-American	African-American	Mexican-American	Irish-American
Work habits	Speed, accuracy, quality, and cost-effectiveness are valued. Completion of tasks and "keeping busy" are traditionally valued.	Speed in working is not a priority. Hard work is valued.	Hard work is valued.	Work is secondary to family and other life activities. May be uncomfortable with authority persons checking work.	Hard work is highly valued.
Autonomy	Competition with authority. Assertive. Autonomous decision making within the scope of nursing practice expected.	Defers to person in authority, often seeking approval before making decisions. Avoids conflict and values harmony.	Self-reliance and autonomy encouraged within group. Past discrimination experiences may discourage autonomy. Females are often head of household and decision-makers.	Defers to person in authority with males as dominant decision-makers. Input of others is considered in decision-making. Autonomy for females is more difficult than for males. Avoids competition and conflict.	Autonomy and independence outside the family are encouraged while family loyalty is still maintained.
Help-seeking behaviors	Individual is expected to initiate help-seeking behaviors.	Stigma for seeking help for emotional disorders and stress. May be reluctant to approach for help by attempting to "save face."	Varied. May seek help within own social network before seeking outside help.	Varied. May seek help within own social network before seeking outside help.	May delay seeking help. Denial of problems is a way of coping with physical and emotional problems.
Persistence	Nursing is "hard work." Withdrawal from a nursing course is acceptable for academic and/or personal circumstances and should be decided by the individual.	Hard work is highly respected. Withdrawal decisions may be difficult and may include the family.	Withdrawal decisions may be difficult, especially if families have sacrificed greatly to assist student with educational endeavors.	Withdrawal decisions may be difficult, especially if families have sacrificed greatly to assist student with educational endeavors. Decisions may include the family. Withdrawal would be acceptable if interfering with family responsibilities.	Withdrawal decisions may be difficult since academic or personal problem must first be acknowledged.

Some information obtained and adapted from: Andrews & Boyle, 1999; Campinha-Bacote, 1998a; Leininger & McFarland, 2002; Purnell & Paulanka, 2003.

REFERENCES AND BIBLIOGRAPHY

Aber, C. S., & Arathuzik, D. (1996). Factors associated with student success in a baccalaureate nursing program within an urban public university. *Journal of Nursing Education, 35*(6), 285–288.

Abrums, M. E., & Leppa, C. (2001). Beyond cultural competence: Teaching about race, gender, class, and sexual orientation. *Journal of Nursing Education, 40*(6), 270–275.

Albaili, M. A. (1997). Differences among low-, average- and high-achieving college students on learning and study strategies. *Educational Psychology, 17*(1 and 2), 171–177.

Andrew, S. (1998). Self-efficacy as a predictor of academic performance in science. *Journal of Advanced Nursing, 27*, 596–603.

Andrews, M. (1995). Transcultural nursing: Transforming the curriculum. *Journal of Transcultural Nursing, 6*(2), 4–9.

Andrews, M., & Boyle, J. (1999). *Transcultural concepts in nursing.* (3rd ed.). Philadelphia: Lippincott.

Bandura, A. (1986). *Social foundations of thought and action: A social cognitive theory.* Englewood Cliffs, NJ: Prentice-Hall.

Bandura, A. (1989). Regulation of cognitive processes through perceived self-efficacy. *Developmental Psychology, 25*(5), 729–735.

Bandura, A. (1996a). Reflections on human agency. In J. Georgas, M. Manthouli, E. Besevegis, & A. Kokkevi (Eds.), *Contemporary psychology in Europe: Theory, research, and applications (Proceedings of the IVth European Congress of Psychology,* pp. 194–210). Seattle: Hogrefe & Huber.

Bandura, A. (1996b). Regulation of cognitive processes through perceived self-efficacy. In G-H. Jennings (Ed.), *Passages beyond the gate: A Jungian approach to understanding the nature of American psychology at the dawn of the new millennium* (pp. 96–107). Needham Heights, MA: Simon & Schuster Custom Publishing.

Bandura, A. (1997). *Self-efficacy: The exercise of control.* New York: W. H. Freeman.

Bean, J. P., & Eaton, S. B. (2000). A psychological model of student retention. In J. Braxton (Ed.), *Reworking the student departure puzzle* (pp. 48–61). Nashville, TN: Vanderbilt University Press.

Bean, J. P., & Eaton, S. B. (2001). The psychology underlying successful retention practices. *Journal of College Student Retention: Research, Theory, & Practice, 3*(1), 73–90.

Bessent, H. (Ed.). (1997). *Strategies for recruitment, retention, and graduation of minority nurses in colleges of nursing.* Washington, DC: American Nurses Publishing.

Brown, S. D., Lent, R. W., & Larkin, K. C. (1989). Self-efficacy as a moderator of scholastic aptitude: Academic performance relationships. *Journal of Vocational Behavior, 35*(1), 64–75.

Callister, L. C., Khalaf, I., & Keller, D. (2000). Cross-cultural comparison of the concerns of beginning baccalaureate nursing students. *Nurse Educator*, 25(6), 267–271.

Campinha-Bacote, J. (1998a). *The process of cultural competence in the delivery of healthcare services: A culturally competent model of care* (3rd ed.). Cincinnati, OH: Transcultural C.A.R.E. Associates.

Campinha-Bacote, J. (1998b). Cultural diversity in nursing education: Issues and concerns. *Journal of Nursing Education*, 37(1), 3–4.

Chacko, S. B., & Huba, M. E. (1991). Academic achievement among undergraduate nursing students: The development and test of a causal model. *Journal of Nursing Education*, 30(6), 267–273.

Chartrand, J. M. (1990). A causal analysis to predict the personal and academic adjustment of nontraditional students. *Journal of Counseling Psychology*, 37(1), 65–73.

Coffman, D. L., & Gilligan, T. D. (2002). Social support, stress, and self-efficacy: Effects on students' satisfaction. *Journal of College Student Retention: Research, Theory, & Practice*, 4(1), 53–66.

Colbeck, C. L., Cabrera, A. F., & Terenzini, P. T. (2001). Learning professional confidence: Linking teaching practices, students' self-perceptions, and gender. *Review of Higher Education*, 24(1), 173–191.

Constantine, M. G., Robinson, J. S., Wilton, L., & Caldwell, L. D. (2002). Collective self-esteem and perceived social support as predictors of cultural congruity among black and Latino college students. *Journal of College Student Development*, 43(3), 307–316.

Constantine, M. G., & Watt, S. K. (2002). Cultural congruity, womanist identity attitudes, and life satisfaction among African American college women attending historically black and predominantly white institutions. *Journal of College Student Development*, 43(2), 184–193.

Crow, K. (1993). Multiculturalism and pluralistic thought in nursing education: Native American world view and the nursing academic world view. *Journal of Nursing Education*, 32(5), 198–204.

Davidhizar, R., Dowd, S. B., & Giger, J. N. (1998). Educating the culturally diverse healthcare student. *Nurse Educator*, 23(2), 38–42.

Davidhizar, R., & Giger, J. N. (2001). Teaching culture within the nursing curriculum using the Giger–Davidhizar model of transcultural nursing assessment. *Journal of Nursing Education*, 40(6), 282–288.

Ford-Gilboe, M., Laschinger, H. S., Laforet-Fliesser, Y., Ward-Griffin, C., & Foran, S. (1997). The effect of a clinical practicum on undergraduate nursing students' self-efficacy for community-based family nursing practice. *Journal of Nursing Education*, 36(5), 212–219.

Fuertes, J. N., & Westbrook, F. D. (1996). Using the social, attitudinal, familial, and environmental (S.A.F.E.) acculturation stress scale to assess the adjustment needs of Hispanic college students. *Measurement and Evaluation in Counseling and Development*, 29, 67–76.

Gianakos, I. (1996). Career development differences between adult and traditional-aged learners. *Journal of Career Development, 22*(3), 211–223.

Gist, M. E., & Mitchell, T. R. (1992). Self-efficacy: A theoretical analysis of its determinants and malleability. *Academy of Management Review, 17,* 183–211.

Gloria, A. M., & Robinson Kurpius, S. E. (1996). The validation of the cultural congruity scale and the university environment scale with Chicano/a students. *Hispanic Journal of Behavioral Sciences, 18*(4), 533–549.

Greene, B. A., & Miller, R. B. (1996). Influences on achievement: Goals, perceived ability, and cognitive engagement. *Contemporary Educational Psychology, 21,* 181–192.

Goldenberg, D., Iwasiw, C., & MacMaster, E. (1997). Self-efficacy of senior baccalaureate nursing students and preceptors. *Nurse Education Today, 17,* 303–310.

Hackett, G., & Betz, N. (1995). Self-efficacy and career choice and development. In J. E. Maddux (Ed.), *Self-efficacy, adaptation, and adjustment: Theory, research, and application* (pp. 249–280). New York: Plenum.

Hamilton, C. W. (1996). Nature of motivation for educational achievement among African American female college students. *Urban Education, 31*(1), 72–90.

Harrison, A. W., Rainer, R. K., Hochwarter, W. A., & Thompson, K. R. (1997). Testing the self-efficacy–performance linkage of social-cognitive theory. *Journal of Social Psychology, 137*(1), 79–87.

Harvey, V., & McMurray, N. (1994). Self-efficacy: A means of identifying problems in nursing education and career progress. *International Journal of Nursing Studies, 31,* 471–485.

Ironside, P. M. (2004). "Covering content" and teaching thinking: Deconstructing the additive curriculum. *Journal of Nursing Education, 43*(1), 5–12.

Jeffreys, M. R. (1993). *The relationship of self-efficacy and select academic and environmental variables on academic achievement and retention.* Unpublished doctoral dissertation, Teachers College, Columbia University, New York.

Jeffreys, M. R. (1998). Predicting nontraditional student retention and academic achievement. *Nurse Educator, 23*(1), 42–48.

Jeffreys, M. R. (2000). Development and psychometric evaluation of the Transcultural Self-Efficacy Tool: A synthesis of findings. *Journal of Transcultural Nursing, 11*(2), 127–136.

Jeffreys, M. R. (2001). Evaluating enrichment program study groups: Academic outcomes, psychological outcomes, and variables influencing retention. *Nurse Educator, 26*(3), 142–149.

Jeffreys, M. R. (2002). Students' perceptions of variables influencing retention: A pretest and post-test approach. *Nurse Educator, 27*(1), 16–19 [Erratum, 2002, 27(2), 64].

Jeffreys, M. R., & Smodlaka, I. (1996). Steps of the instrument-design process: An illustrative approach for nurse educators. *Nurse Educator, 21*(6), 47–52. [Erratum, 1997, 22(1), 49].

Jeffreys, M. R., & Smodlaka, I. (1998). Exploring the factorial composition of the Transcultural Self-efficacy Tool. *International Journal of Nursing Studies, 35,* 217–225.

Jeffreys, M. R., & Smodlaka, I. (1999a). Changes in students' transcultural self-efficacy perceptions following an integrated approach to culture care. *Journal of Multicultural Nursing and Health, 5*(2), 6–12. [Erratum, 2000, 6(1), 20].

Jeffreys, M. R., & Smodlaka, I. (1999b). Construct validation of the Transcultural Self-efficacy Tool. *Journal of Nursing Education, 38,* 222–227.

Keane, M. (1993). Preferred learning styles and study strategies in a linguistically diverse baccalaureate nursing student population. *Journal of Nursing Education, 32*(5), 214–221.

Labun, E. (2002). The Red River College Model: Enhancing success for native Canadian and other nursing students from disenfranchised groups. *Journal of Transcultural Nursing, 13*(4), 311–317.

Leininger, M. M., & McFarland, M. R. (2002). *Transcultural nursing: Concepts, theories, research, and practice* (3rd ed.). New York: McGraw-Hill.

Leininger, M. M. (1978). *Transcultural nursing: Theories, concepts, and practices.* New York: Wiley.

Leininger, M. M. (1991). *Culture care diversity and universality: A theory of nursing.* New York: National League for Nursing.

Leininger, M. M. (1994). *Transcultural nursing: Concepts, theories, and practices.* Columbus, OH: Greyden.

Leininger, M. M. (1995a). *Transcultural nursing: Concepts, theories, research, and practice.* Blacklick, OH: McGraw-Hill College Custom Services.

Leininger, M. M. (1995b). Teaching transcultural nursing in undergraduate and graduate programs. *Journal of Transcultural Nursing, 6*(2), 10–26.

Leininger, M. M. (2002). Essential transcultural nursing care concepts, principles, examples, and policy statements. In M. M. Leininger & M. R. McFarland (Eds.), *Transcultural nursing: Concepts, theories, research, and practice* (3rd ed., pp. 45–69). New York: McGraw-Hill.

Leininger, M. M., & McFarland, M. R. (2002). *Transcultural nursing: Concepts, theories, research, and practice* (3rd ed.). New York: McGraw-Hill.

Lent, R. W., Brown, S. D., & Gore, P. A. (1997). Discriminant and predictive validity of academic self-concept, academic self-efficacy, and mathematics-specific self-efficacy. *Journal of Counseling Psychology, 44*(3), 307–315.

Lent, R. W., Brown, S. D., & Larkin, K. C. (1987). Comparison of three theoretically derived variables in predicting career and academic behavior: Self-efficacy, interest congruence, and consequence thinking. *Journal of Counseling Psychology, 34*(3), 293–298.

Madorin, S., & Iwasiw, C. (1999). The effects of computer–assisted instruction on the self-efficacy of baccalaureate nursing students. *Journal of Nursing Education, 38*(6), 282–285.

Maddux, J. E. (1995). *Self-efficacy, adaptation, and adjustment: Theory, research, and application.* New York: Plenum.

Manifold, C., & Rambur, B. (2001). Predictors of attrition in American Indian nursing students. *Journal of Nursing Education, 40*(6), 279–281.

Morales, E. E. (2000). A contextual understanding of the process of educational resilience: High achieving Dominican American students and the "resilience cycle." *Innovative Higher Education, 25*(1), 7–21.

Nurmi, J-E., & Aunola, K. (2001). How does academic achievement come about? Cross-cultural and methodological notes. *International Journal of Educational Research, 35*, 403–409.

Parsons, E., & Betz, N. E. (1998). Test-retest reliability and validity studies of the skills confidence inventory. *Journal of Career Assessment, 6*(1), 1–12.

Patterson, C., Crooks, D., & Lunyk-Child, O. (2002). A new perspective on competencies for self-directed learning. *Journal of Nursing Education, 41*(1), 25–31.

Peterson, S. L., & delMas, R. C. (1998). The component structure of career decision-making self-efficacy for underprepared college students. *Journal of Career Development, 24*(3), 209–225.

Pintrich, P. R., & Garcia, T. (1994). Self-regulated learning in college students: Knowledge, strategies, and motivation. In P. R. Pintrich, D. R. Brown, & C. E. Weinstein (Eds.), *Student motivation, cognition, and learning: Essays in honor of Wilbert J. McKeachie* (pp. 113–133). Hillsdale, NJ: Erlbaum.

Purnell, L. D. (2003). Purnell's model for cultural competence. In L. D. Purnell & B. J. Paulanka (Eds.), *Transcultural health care: A culturally competent approach* (2nd ed., pp. 8–39). Philadelphia: F. A. Davis.

Purnell, L. D., & Paulanka, B. J. (2003). *Transcultural health care: A culturally competent approach* (2nd ed). Philadelphia: F. A. Davis.

Ransdell, S. (2001). Predicting college success: The importance of ability and non-cognitive variables. *International Journal of Educational Research, 35*, 357–364.

Ransdell, S., Hawkins, C., & Adams, R. (2001). Results of the study. *International Journal of Educational Research, 35*, 373–389.

Rognstad, M-K. (2002). Recruitment to and motivation for nursing education and the nursing profession. *Journal of Nursing Education, 41*(7), 321–325.

Saks, A. M. (1995). Longitudinal field investigation of the moderating and mediating effects of self-efficacy on the relationship between training and newcomer adjustment. *Journal of Applied Psychology, 80*, 211–225.

Schapiro, S. R., & Livingston, J. A. (2000). Dynamic self-regulation: The driving force behind academic achievement. *Innovative Higher Education, 25*(1), 23–35.

Schunk, D. (1987). *Self-efficacy and cognitive achievement.* Paper presented at the Annual Meeting of the American Psychological Association (New York, August 28–September 1). (ERIC Document Reproduction Service No. ED287880).

Schunk, D. (1995). Self-efficacy and education and instruction. In J. E. Maddux (Ed.), *Self-efficacy, adaptation, and adjustment: Theory, research, and application* (pp. 281–304). New York: Plenum.

Shelton, E. N. (2003). Faculty support and student retention. *Journal of Nursing Education, 42*(2), 68–76.

Solberg, V. S., & Villarreal, P. (1997). Examination of self-efficacy, social support, and stress as predictors of psychological and physical distress among Hispanic college students. *Hispanic Journal of Behavioral Sciences, 19*(2), 182–201.

Solis, E. (1995). Regression and path analysis models of Hispanic community college students' intent to persist. *Community College Review, 23*(3), 3–15.

Sommer, S. (2001). Multicultural nursing education. *Journal of Nursing Education, 40*(6), 276–278.

Stage, F. K., & Hossler, D. (2000). Where is the student? Linking student behaviors, college choice, and college persistence. In J. Braxton (Ed.), *Reworking the student departure puzzle* (pp. 170–195). Nashville, TN: Vanderbilt University Press.

Stark, M. A., Feikema, B., & Wyngarden, K. (2002). Empowering students for NCLEX success: Self-assessment and planning. *Nurse Educator, 27*(3), 103–105.

Stigler, J. W., & Hiebert, J. (1998). Teaching is a cultural activity. *American Educator, (Winter),* 4–11.

Tucker-Allen, S., & Long, E. (1999). *Recruitment and retention of minority students: Stories of success.* Lisle, IL: Tucker.

Villaruel, A. M., Canales, M., & Torres, S. (2001). Bridges and barriers: Educational mobility of Hispanic nurses. *Journal of Nursing Education, 40*(6), 245–251.

Vrugt, A. J., Langereis, M. P., & Hoogstraten, J. (1997). Academic self-efficacy and malleability of relevant capabilities as predictors of exam performance. *Journal of Experimental Education, 66*(1), 61–72.

Weaver, H. N. (2001). Indigenous nurses and professional education: Friends or foes? *Journal of Nursing Education, 40*(6), 252–258.

Williams, R. P., & Calvillo, E. R. (2002). Maximizing learning among students from culturally diverse backgrounds. *Nurse Educator, 27*(5), 222–226.

Winters, C., & Owens, R. (1993). Alternative teaching strategies: Using a health fair to meet tribal college and nursing program needs. *Journal of Nursing Education, 32*(5), 237–238.

Yoder, M. K. (2001). The bridging approach: Effective strategies for teaching ethnically diverse nursing students. *Journal of Transcultural Nursing, 12,* 319–325.

Yoder, M. K., & Saylor, C. (2002). Student and teacher roles: Mismatched expectations. *Nurse Educator, 27*(5), 201–203.

Yurkovich, E. E. (2001). Working with American Indians toward educational success. *Journal of Nursing Education, 40*(6), 259–269.

Zimmerman, B. J. (1995). Self-efficacy and educational development. In A. Bandura (Ed.), *Self-efficacy in changing societies* (pp. 202–231). New York: Cambridge University Press.

Zimmerman, B. J. (1996). Enhancing student academic and health functioning: A self-regulatory perspective. *School Psychology Quarterly, 11*(1), 47–66.

Zimmerman, B. J., & Risemberg, R. (1994). Investigating self-regulatory processes and perceptions of self-efficacy in writing by college students. In P. R. Pintrich, D. R. Brown, & C. E. Weinstein (Eds.), *Student motivation, cognition, and learning: Essays in honor of Wilbert J. McKeachie* (pp. 239–256). IIillsdale, NJ: Erlbaum.

Chapter 4

Academic Factors

Academic factors have been included in conceptual models explaining college student attrition. The conceptual and operational definitions of these academic factors have varied, making comparison of factors between studies and between selected models difficult. Bean and Metzner (1985) describe academic factors as students' primary involvement with the academic process at the college, and purport that among nontraditional students academic factors are less important than environmental factors in influencing retention. Study hours, study skills, academic advising, absenteeism, major and job certainty, and course availability are identified as academic factors (Metzner & Bean, 1987). Academic integration has sometimes been used to describe a cluster of academic factors that can influence retention, and has been defined as "the development of a strong affiliation with the college academic environment both inside and outside of class" (Nora, 1993, p. 235). Use of college services and interaction with college faculty, students, and personnel are included in this definition.

For undergraduate nursing students, the academic factors deemed most important for retention include personal study skills, study hours, attendance, class schedule, and general academic services (college library, college counseling, and computer laboratory). These factors interact with the other variable sets in the NURS model (Figure 1.1). It is essential that nurse educators go beyond a superficial skimming of academic factors to a critical appraisal of how each one can influence retention and student success. An in-depth exploration of each academic factor may reveal several aspects or dimensions that can potentially affect students differently. This chapter discusses each academic factor in relation to undergraduate nursing student retention and aims to assist nurse educators in identifying areas of strengths and weaknesses.

PERSONAL STUDY SKILLS

Personal study skills refer to specific elements (reading skills, writing skills, note-taking, preparing papers, studying for exams, reading notes, listening in class), attitudes about the responsibility for study activities, time management and organization, and effort expended on academic pursuits. However, an alarming one-third of college students surveyed perceived deficits in one or more specific study skills (Strage et al., 2002). Consistent with higher education, the increasingly academically diverse nursing student population presents with varying study skills (Heller, Oros, & Durney-Crowley, 2000; Tanner, 1998). Personal study skills affect nursing student retention through academic performance and psychological outcomes.

Highly developed abilities in reading, writing, note taking, paper preparation, studying for exams, and listening are good personal study skills. However, they are not enough to assure academic success and retention. Attitudes about responsibility for study activities may range from positive, adaptive, and internal locus of control beliefs to negative, maladaptive, and external control beliefs (Nurmi & Aunola, 2001). Adaptive behaviors include self-direction, detailed plans, and task-focused goals relating to study activities and academic pursuits. Maladaptive behaviors include self-handicapping, learned helplessness, task avoidance, and task-irrelevant behaviors for study activities and academic pursuits (Nurmi & Aunola, 2001). Promoting positive, adaptive beliefs in nursing should be a goal for nurse educators.

Excellent time management skills, organizing, and planning are reported as better predictors of academic success than is total number of study hours (Ransdell, 2001a; Strage et al., 2002). Additionally, use of varied study skills has been associated with better academic outcomes (Napoli & Wortman, 1998), which in turn positively influence retention. Effort expended on planning and study activities yields better academic outcomes (Flowers, 2002). Effort expenditure is related to students' self-efficacy perceptions, and not limited to time on task. Conclusively, quality study outweighs study hours, although sufficient study hours are needed to adequately and proficiently achieve desired academic outcomes. Several studies identified a mismatch between students' perceived study skills and study hours whereby study hours were more restrictive to retention in comparison to perceived study skills (Jeffreys, 1993, 2002). Such a mismatch warrants nurse educator intervention.

Student self-appraisal of personal study skills is an advantageous precursor to maximizing strengths, remedying weaknesses, and seeking appropriate assistance. Self-appraisals are usually based upon the student's prior academic experience and performance in terms of successes and failures; however, self-perceptions may be inaccurate and/or may fail to result in appropriate help-seeking behaviors. Researchers have substantiated that many students whose self-perceptions of skills were weak took limited action in seeking help (Alexitch, 2002; Chaney, Muraskin, Cahalan, & Goodwin, 1998). Routinely soliciting student self-appraisals of study skills must be partnered with actively offering appropriate assistance to weaker students. Nurse educators can take an active role in assisting students with specific study skills needed for nursing courses, developing time management and organization, promoting responsible study attitudes and behaviors, and encouraging high quality study effort expenditure.

As mentioned earlier, self-appraisals may not be accurate. In one study, beginning associate degree nursing students overestimated the supportiveness of academic factors. Students with the highest estimates of academic supports had more nursing course failures than did students with more conservative self-appraisals. Personal study skills was only one of the eleven-variable academic cluster used for correlating academic variable strength (AVST) with nursing course grade (Jeffreys, 1993, 1998). Failing students were unable to progress in the nursing program, resulting in attrition.

Guidance with self-appraisal is strongly recommended. Beginning nursing students may need special assistance in evaluating study skills in relation to program requirements. Students moving from preprofessional to professional education need much guidance and often have difficulty with transition into the profession (Schön, 1987). Prior successful study strategies may need to be adapted to meet the special demands of the nursing professional program. Without guidance, students may not recognize the need to adapt, resulting in poor academic, psychological, and retention outcomes.

PERSONAL STUDY HOURS

The importance of personal study hours in relation to academic achievement and retention of college students is well-documented. The nursing literature is filled with reports of student multiple roles that conflict with personal study hours and adversely affect achievement and retention (Bessent, 1997; Griffiths & Tagliareni, 1999; Tucker-Allen & Long, 1999). In the NURS model, personal study hours refer to the number of hours allocated exclusively to positive study activities in which positive study behaviors and attitudes are actively used. Positive behaviors and attitudes are adaptive, self-directed, planned, realistically goal-oriented, and appropriate. Maladaptive behaviors such as procrastination, learned helplessness, unrealistic goal orientation, and defeatist attitudes are not included within personal study hours. Qualifying personal study hours differentiates between desirable and undesirable study activities, behaviors, and attitudes, attempting to measure personal study hours by desirable components rather than by using an accounting mechanism in which all hours are considered equal. All personal study hours are not equal. Students may need guidance in recognizing this difference and in accurately appraising their own personal study hours.

In the NURS model, students with more personal study hours (as operationally defined here) are expected to have more positive academic outcomes and retention than will students with inadequate personal study hours. Adequate study hours are individually based and are defined as the least number of personal study hours needed to achieve the short-term academic outcomes (passing exam, completing accurate care plan, etc.) and long-term academic outcomes (successfully completing nursing course components). Students with inadequate personal study hours are considered to be at risk for academic failure, stress, dissatisfaction, and attrition. Because personal study skills needed for success in nursing may be unknown, undeveloped, underdeveloped, or undervalued, nurse educators are challenged to actively assist students in maximizing personal study hours as defined here.

ATTENDANCE

The Metzner and Bean (1987) model included absenteeism as an academic variable influencing attrition; however, the NURS model focuses on attendance. Attendance was substituted for absenteeism because it is more positive and was considered relevant for retention, as opposed to absenteeism being correlated with attrition. Nevertheless, the literature regarding attendance reveals several interesting phenomena that are relevant for nursing education. First, attendance (or absenteeism) should be monitored to help identify at-risk students. Second, attendance should be monitored in relation to other variables with the purpose of identifying students most at risk for attrition. For example, Bean (1986) notes that among college students with high GPAs, class attendance may not be related to attrition or failure. Among college students with low GPAs, class absence may be a warning sign indicating student dissatisfaction, stress, and/or academic difficulty. Such students are at great risk for attrition and/or failure.

In nursing, attendance is somewhat more complex than it is among the general college population. As an academic factor influencing retention it requires further discussion; thus, specific implications for nursing education will be introduced. First, national and state accreditation guidelines provide a framework for attendance policies; therefore most nursing programs have strict attendance policies. Second, nursing program attendance policies may be stricter than the parent institution's policy. Consequently, students may not comprehend, value, or expect rigid attendance policies in nursing. Additionally, students may not expect that attendance policies will be upheld, especially among beginning students who have had no prior exposure to nursing courses.

Despite strict nursing program attendance policies, students are permitted a maximum number of absences (or a minimum number of attendance hours). Attendance may be further differentiated between various nursing course components such as theoretical (classroom hours), skills laboratory, and/or clinical hours. Clearly, clinical attendance is a valuable dimension to learning and assists the student in connecting theoretical information, nursing skills, and client care. Unlike most college majors, nursing has a humanistic, caring, and life-and-death component. Clinical absences can result in students' being only minimally prepared to care for clients competently. Absences create complicated disadvantages; attendance creates valuable advantages. With limited opportunities to apply learning, students may be at more risk for failure, dissatisfaction, and stress, putting them at greater risk for voluntary or involuntary attrition. By identifying students with minimal attendance and surveying other variables to develop a comprehensive student composite, nurse educators can offer appropriate interventions to enhance academic achievement, satisfaction, stress reduction, and retention.

Early identification suggests the need for an evaluative mechanism for identifying which students are at risk for "minimal" attendance. In one study of nontraditional first semester associate degree students, most students were "highly confident" that they would attend all lecture classes, all skills laboratory classes, and all clinical laboratory classes, although several students were not confident (Jeffreys, 1993). This study did not correlate end-of-semester attendance records with student survey responses; however surveying students' self-expectations for attendance may help identify those students with lower expectations who may be at risk for lower attendance, insufficient academic achievement, and poor retention. Nurse educators could initiate prophylactic interventions to assist at-risk students.

Although attendance is commonly defined as a dichotomous variable, (either one is present or one is not present), upon closer examination, it is more complex. For example, a student may be physically present but mentally absent. Such a student is not benefiting educationally by being present. Another scenario may be the student spectator. Attendance as a spectator limits the potential active learning and critical thinking that occurs with attendance as an active learner. One limitation of mandatory attendance or strict attendance policies is that it may be difficult to differentiate among physical presence, mental presence, spectator attendance, and active attendance. Naturally, active learning will be obvious with group discussions, skills practice, or care of clients in the clinical setting; however it may be more difficult to discern in large classes when lectures, videos, or PowerPoint presentations are the sole means of the passive teaching–learning activity. Attendance needs to be viewed in relation to other variables and to the other dimensions of the NURS model if at-risk students are to be identified early.

Class Schedule

Availability of courses, flexibility of courses, and convenience are factors that can influence retention through academic and psychological outcomes (Bean & Metzner, 1985; Burr, Burr, & Novak, 1999). Consistently, across three study samples, most nursing students have identified "class schedule" as influencing retention. Responses ranged from "severely restrictive" to "greatly supportive" (Jeffreys, 1993, 1998, 2001, 2002). Class schedule is included in the NURS model because students' perceptions of class schedule, with its physical demands and time constraints, can influence retention positively or negatively and in varying degrees. Student perception of class schedule is the most important aspect to assess.

Class schedule interacts with other academic and environmental factors, and professional integration variables in influencing retention. For example, a two-day class schedule compatible with a nursing student's other roles and responsibilities increases the probability for greater class attendance, more study hours, participation in professional events, satisfaction, and academic achievement. In contrast, a four-day class schedule may require a financially challenged single parent to commute three hours to a distant clinical site via public transportation, pay for additional child care services, and change work hours. The incompatible class schedule increases the student's risk for attrition because of multiple role stress, financial strain, and a probability for decreased class attendance, decreased study hours, limited participation in professional events, dissatisfaction, and lowered academic achievement. Some students may have difficulty clearly evaluating the disadvantages and advantages of various class schedules and the effect of class schedule selection on other aspects of their lives. As faculty advisors, nurse educators have a major responsibility to effectively guide students in selecting the class schedule most compatible with balancing other roles and responsibilities, so that students can achieve positive academic outcomes and enhance positive psychological outcomes for nursing.

General Academic Services

General academic services are designed to assist students with their academic goals and are available to all college students, regardless of academic major. They include the library, counseling, and computer laboratories. Although it is important that general academic services have adequate facilities, staffing, and technology to assist college students, it is the students' perception of these services that most strongly influences retention. If students perceive the lack of adequate academic support, attrition will increase. Retention will be enhanced if academic support services follow a student-centered rather than an institutional-centered philosophy, meaning that student academic services must be accessible and convenient, especially to adult learners. General academic services that are convenient, accessible, and helpful will encourage more active use of these support services. Active involvement in the learning process is an important indicator of academic behavior, is essential for academic integration, and enhances student retention (Tinto, 1997).

The assessment of nursing students' perceptions of general academic services is valuable (Lehna, Jackonen, & Wilson, 1996). Consistent findings across three study samples revealed that most undergraduate associate degree nursing students perceived the library, counseling, and computer laboratory to influence retention, stating that these general academic services "moderately support" or "greatly support" retention (Jeffreys, 1993, 1998, 2001, 2002). Students who perceive services to be valuable will expend greater effort in using them. Greater, comprehensive use of services, in conjunction with other academic factors, positively influences retention by enhancing academic and psychological outcomes. For example, maximizing use of various library services appropriate to course objectives can assist with improved study skills and academic integration, thus enhancing retention. Counseling services have been shown to be beneficial to nursing student academic and psychological outcomes (Lehna et al., 1996). Higher education literature reports that counseled students have higher retention rates than non-counseled students (Turner & Berry, 2000; Wilson, Mason, & Ewing, 1997). Kraemer (1997) stated that commuter students who frequently use computer laboratory facilities on campus are more involved in cognitive development than are other students; enhanced cognitive development enhances retention.

To fully comprehend the influence of general academic services on nursing student retention, nurse educators need to assess three dimensions of general academic services. First, they should assess whether students perceive the individual service to be valuable and important to academic achievement, positive psychological outcomes, and retention. Second, they should evaluate whether the services are convenient and accessible from both the student and educator perspective. Third, they should survey the frequency and duration of services used. Even if students do not use general academic services as frequently as nurse educators would recommend, students' perception that the services are available and important is a necessary precursor for strategy design. Strategies should integrate use of these general academic services to enhance nursing outcomes. Mismatches among any of the three dimensions may indicate a need for an intervention strategy aimed at the student, educator, and/or educational institution.

KEY POINTS SUMMARY

- Academic factors include personal study skills, study hours, attendance, class schedule, and general academic services (college library, college counseling, and computer laboratory).
- Personal study skills refer to specific elements (reading skills, writing skills, note taking, preparing papers, studying for exams, reading notes, listening in class), attitudes about the responsibility for study activities, time management and organization, and effort expended on academic pursuits.
- Personal study hours refer to the number of hours allocated exclusively to positive study activities in which positive study behaviors and attitudes are actively used. Positive behaviors and attitudes are adaptive, self-directed, planned, realistically goal-oriented, and appropriate.
- Attendance is presented as a multidimensional variable that differentiates between active learning and the "mentally absent" or "spectators."
- Class schedule interacts with other academic and environmental factors, and professional integration variables in influencing retention.

- General academic services (library, counseling, computer laboratory) are designed to assist with academic goals and are available to all college students, regardless of academic major. Positive academic and psychological outcomes are enhanced through frequent, comprehensive use of general academic services.
- Academic factors interact with each other and with other variable sets in the NURS model.
- Students' perception of academic factors and their influence on retention is a valuable precursor for maximizing academic success and promoting retention.
- Nurse educators should assist students with realistic self-appraisal of academic strengths and weaknesses. Strategies for maximizing success and eliminating deficits can be specifically developed based on individual and group appraisal.

EDUCATOR-IN-ACTION

Several students complain that despite "studying all the time" and completing the required readings, they did not achieve the grade they expected. Sharon states, "For the amount of time I put into nursing, I should have gotten a better grade. All my free time is spent studying and reading nursing. I just don't understand it." Several other students echo the same disconcerting, unhappy sentiments. To guide students with their own personal self-appraisal, Professor Booke asks each student privately to describe details about his/her personal study hours and study skills. Questioning is directed at uncovering adaptive and maladaptive study behaviors and attitudes. Consider Professor Booke's initial questions and the diverse student responses that follow:

Questions

- What were you thinking about before you got ready to read the prerequisite reading (Chapter 12) for the last class? What were you feeling?
- How did you prepare (get ready to read)?
- What were you doing while you were reading Chapter 12?
- How much time was actually spent on reading Chapter 12? How much of this time was uninterrupted?
- How did you read the chapter? Did you engage in active reading or passive reading strategies?

- What did you do after reading the chapter?
- What were you thinking about after you read the chapter? What were you feeling?

Student Responses

Sharon: "I read the chapter from beginning to end while I was riding my exercise bike for 45 minutes. I prepared by selecting the "beginner level" on the exercise bike and positioned my book on the handles. I was thinking that I could exercise my mind and body at the same time. I guess I didn't really engage in active reading since I just read the chapter like a novel. Afterwards I took a shower. I felt as though I got one more thing off my homework list."

Andrew: "I started the chapter while at the bus stop. The bus was crowded so I didn't get a seat for about 15 minutes. Then I finished the main parts of the chapter on the bus. The summary, nursing case study, and practice questions I did the next morning on the bus to class. I guess I had many interruptions, especially since the bus was noisy. Without interruptions, it probably would have taken 45 minutes or longer if I actually stopped to think about what I read as I went along. I felt as though no matter how much I read, I will never understand what the instructor wants me to know."

Barbara: "I read during the warm-up and half-time of my son's football game. I was thinking that I could skim over the chapter during warm-up and then go back to read the important parts during half-time. The chapter has so many details so I highlight the main points and then I go back to skim it again after everyone is asleep. That day I was too tired so I went to bed at 11 p.m. and set my alarm clock for 3 a.m. to get up and finish. I was just thinking about how tired I was and how it took me almost 12 hours to finish Chapter 12."

Jane: "I went to the library and didn't leave until I had written all my notes from the chapter. I don't like to use a highlighter. I spent four hours at the library but most of the time was probably spent writing notes. I stop to think about whether something might be important or not and if it may be something that could be on the next test. I don't really trust myself so I just write down everything."

Tamara: "Honestly, I was still trying to read from the last two classes. I thought that I would get started on my reading during the first week but I kept putting it off so I fell behind. My roommate was really homesick so I tried to spend extra time with her. I start to read in our room but then she wants to talk. I go back and reread the part I just read before I was interrupted to make sure I remember everything. Sometimes I reread the same part ten times and never finish a chapter."

Professor Booke's subsequent questions are directed at identifying individual student strengths and weaknesses:

- What thoughts and actions promote or support positive learning?
- What thoughts and actions interfere with or restrict learning?
- What will you do in the future?

Following a guided, realistic self-appraisal, students in the above scenarios discovered that all personal study hours are not equal. Individual appraisal permitted a mutually developed, diagnostic-prescriptive study plan for the future. To further facilitate ongoing positive study behaviors and attitudes, Professor Booke paired students with peer mentors, encouraged them to join an enrichment program reading and study group, and met with individual students bimonthly.

REFERENCES AND BIBLIOGRAPHY

Alexitch, L. R. (2002). The role of help-seeking attitudes and tendencies in students' preferences for academic advising. *Journal of College Student Development, 43*(1), 5–19.

Baker, R. W., & Siryk, B. (1989). *SACQ Student adaptation to college questionnaire manual.* Los Angeles, CA: Western Psychological Services.

Bean, J. P. (1985). Interaction effects based on class level in an explanatory model of college student dropout syndrome. *American Educational Research Journal, 22*(1), 35–64.

Bean, J. P. (1986). Assessing and reducing attrition. In D. Hossler (Ed.), *Managing college enrollments* (pp. 47–61). New Directions for Higher Education, 53. San Francisco: Jossey-Bass.

Bean, J. P., & Metzner, B. (1985). A conceptual model of nontraditional undergraduate student attrition. *Review of Educational Research, 55,* 485–540.

Berger, J. B. (2001). Understanding the organizational nature of student persistence: Empirically based recommendations for practice. *Journal of College Student Retention: Research, Theory, & Practice, 3*(1), 3–22.

Bessent, H. (Ed.) (1997). *Strategies for recruitment, retention, and graduation of minority nurses in colleges of nursing.* Washington, DC: American Nurses Publishing.

Burr, P. L., Burr, R. M., & Novak, L. F. (1999). Student retention is more complicated than merely keeping the students you have today: Toward a "seamless retention theory." *Journal of College Student Retention, 1*(3), 239–253.

Chaney, B., Muraskin, L. D., Cahalan, M. W., & Goodwin, D. (1998). Helping the progress of disadvantaged students in higher education: The federal student support services program. *Educational Evaluation and Policy Analysis, 20*(3), 197–215.

Dickenson, D. J., & O'Connell, D. J. (1990). Effect of quality and quantity of study on student grades. *Journal of Educational Research, 83,* 227–231.

Flowers, L. A. (2002). The impact of college racial composition on African American students' academic and social gains: Additional evidence. *Journal of College Student Development, 43*(3), 403–410.

Griffiths, M. J., & Tagliareni, M. E. (1999). Challenging traditional assumptions about minority students in nursing education. *Nursing and Health Care Perspectives, 20,* 290–295.

Heller, B. R., Oros, M. T., & Durney-Crowley, J. (2000). The future of nursing education: 10 trends to watch. *Nursing and Health Care Perspectives, 21*(1), 9–13.

Jeffreys, M. R. (1993). *The relationship of self-efficacy and select academic and environmental variables on academic achievement and retention.* Unpublished doctoral dissertation, Teachers College, Columbia University, New York.

Jeffreys, M. R. (1998). Predicting nontraditional student retention and academic achievement. *Nurse Educator, 23*(1), 42–48.

Jeffreys, M. R. (2001). Evaluating enrichment program study groups: Academic outcomes, psychological outcomes, and variables influencing retention. *Nurse Educator, 26*(3), 142–149.

Jeffreys, M. R. (2002). Students' perceptions of variables influencing retention: A pretest and post-test approach. *Nurse Educator, 27*(1), 16–19 [Erratum, 2002, *27*(2), 64].

Karabenick, S. A., & Knapp, J. R. (1991). Relationship of academic help seeking to the use of learning strategies and other instrumental achievement behavior in college students. *Journal of Educational Psychology, 83*(2), 221–230.

Kraemer, B. A. (1997). The academic and social integration of Hispanic students into college. *Review of Higher Education, 20*(2), 163–179.

Lehna, C., Jackonen, S., & Wilson, L. (1996). Navigating a nursing curriculum: Bridges and barriers. *Association for Black Nursing Faculty Journal, 7*(July/August), 98–103.

Mancuso, S. (2001). Adult-centered practices: Benchmarking study in higher education. *Innovative Higher Education, 25*(3), 165–181.

Metzner, B., & Bean, J. P. (1987). The estimation of a conceptual model of nontraditional undergraduate student attrition. *Research in Higher Education, 27,* 15–38.

Napoli, A. R., & Wortman, P. M. (1998). Psychosocial factors related to retention and early departure of two-year community college students. *Research in Higher Education, 39*(4), 419–455.

Nora, A. (1987). Determinants of retention among Chicano college students: A structural model. *Research in Higher Education, 26,* 31–60.

Nora, A. (1993). Two-year colleges and minority students' educational aspirations: Help or hindrance? *Higher Education: Handbook of Theory and Research, 9*, 212–247.

Nora, A. (2001). The depiction of significant others in Tinto's "Rites of Passage": A reconceptualization of the influence of family and community in the persistence process. *Journal of College Student Retention: Research, Theory, & Practice, 3*(1), 41–56.

Nora, A., & Rendon, L. I. (1990). Determinants of predisposition to transfer among community college students: A structural model. *Research in Higher Education, 31*(3), 235–255.

Nurmi, J-E., & Aunola, K. (2001). How does academic achievement come about? Cross-cultural and methodological notes. *International Journal of Educational Research, 35*, 403–409.

Pascarella, E. T., & Chapman, D. W. (1983). Validation of a theoretical model of college withdrawal: Interaction effects in a multi-institutional sample. *Research in Higher Education, 19*, 25–47.

Pitts, J. M., White, W. G., & Harrison, A. B. (1999). Student academic underpreparedness: Effects on faculty. *The Review of Higher Education, 22*(4), 343–365.

Ransdell, S. (2001a). Predicting college success: The importance of ability and non-cognitive variables. *International Journal of Educational Research, 35*, 357–364.

Ransdell, S. (2001b). Discussion and implications. *International Journal of Educational Research, 35*, 391–395.

Ransdell, S., Hawkins, C., & Adams, R. (2001a). Models, modeling, and the design of the study. *International Journal of Educational Research, 35*, 365–372.

Ransdell, S., Hawkins, C., & Adams, R. (2001b). Results of the study. *International Journal of Educational Research, 35*, 373–389.

Ryan, M. P., & Glenn, P. A. (2002). Increasing one-year retention rates by focusing on academic competence: An empirical odyssey. *Journal of College Student Retention: Research, Theory, & Practice, 4*(3), 297–324.

Schön, D. (1987). *Educating the reflective practitioner.* San Francisco: Jossey-Bass.

Strage, A., Baba, Y., Millner, S., Scharberg, M., Walker, E., Williamson, R., & Yoder, M. (2002). What every student affairs professional should know: Student study activities and beliefs associated with academic success. *Journal of College Student Development, 43*(2), 246–266.

Tanner, C. A. (1998). The new learner. *Journal of Nursing Education, 37*(6), 239–240.

Tinto, V. (1997). Classrooms as communities. *Journal of Higher Education, 68*(6), 599–623.

Toutkoushian, R. K., & Smart, J. C. (2001). Do institutional characteristics affect student gains from college? *Review of Higher Education, 25*(1), 39–61.

Tucker-Allen, S., & Long, E. (1999). *Recruitment and retention of minority students: Stories of success.* Lisle, IL: Tucker.

Turner, A. L., & Berry, T. R. (2000). Counseling center contributions to student retention and graduation: A longitudinal assessment. *Journal of College Student Development, 41*(6), 627–636.

Wilson, S. B., Mason, T. W., & Ewing, M. J. M. (1997). Evaluating the impact of receiving university-based counseling services on student retention. *Journal of Counseling Psychology, 44*(3), 316–320.

Chapter 5

Environmental Factors

E nvironmental factors may be defined broadly as factors external to the academic process that may influence students' academic performance and retention (Bean & Metzner, 1985). Traditionally, environmental factors have received little attention in college student attrition or retention studies. Therefore it is not surprising that they have been absent or minimally addressed in college student retention or attrition models. The Bean and Metzner (1985) model of nontraditional undergraduate student attrition proposed that environmental factors, which included finances, hours of employment, outside encouragement, family responsibilities, and opportunity to transfer, were more influential in college attrition than other variable sets. Two compensatory effects or interacting variables are proposed in the model. The first is between environmental variables and academic support. Environmental support is believed to compensate for weak academic support; however, the opposite does not hold true (Metzner & Bean, 1987).

The Bean and Metzner model provided the conceptual framework for several studies on nontraditional undergraduate nursing student retention (Jeffreys, 1993, 1998, 2001, 2002). One aim of the studies was to measure student perceptions of the restrictiveness or supportiveness of select environmental variables and their influence on retention. Several researcher-developed instruments were used to measure student perceptions prospectively (at the beginning of the semester) and/or retrospectively (at the end of the semester). (See Appendices A & B for the instruments used.) Overall, students perceived that environmental variables were more influential than academic variables in their impact on retention.

The environmental factors were then incorporated into the original NURS model (Jeffreys, 2003), which aimed to explain nontraditional undergraduate retention and success. For the traditional student, one major factor influencing retention is college adjustment and social integration into the college residential/life environment. Because "living arrangements" can support or restrict nontraditional student retention and success, it seemed logical to include it in the new NURS model (Figure 1.1). Please note that the acronym NURS was changed from "Nontraditional Undergraduate Retention and Success" to "Nursing Undergraduate Retention and Success" and encompasses components appropriate for both traditional and nontraditional students. In the NURS model, environmental factors are those external to the academic process and include financial status, family financial support, family emotional support, family responsibilities, child care arrangements, family crisis, employment hours, employment responsibilities, encouragement by outside friends, living arrangements, and transportation.

Environmental factors may be applicable to both traditional and non-traditional undergraduate nursing student populations; however, the manner in which they impact upon retention may differ. Differences will be highlighted in this chapter. Additionally, environmental factors interact with each other and with other variable sets in the NURS model. Like the appraisal of academic factors, it is essential that nurse educators critically evaluate how each environmental factor can influence student retention and success. A detailed and holistic appraisal of student profile characteristics and student affective factors is necessary to determine how environmental factors are perceived by individual students and specific student subgroups. This chapter discusses each environmental factor in relation to undergraduate nursing student retention and aims to assist nurse educators in identifying areas of actual and/or perceived student strengths and weaknesses.

FINANCIAL STATUS

Financial status refers to the student's standing in meeting all expenses including tuition, college fees, books and other learning materials, living expenses, financial obligations, and commitments. Nontraditional students, especially older students, generally have greater financial obligations and commitments than do younger students, although all students can potentially be affected by financial status. Financial obligations are expenses that are clearly defined by an external source, such as car payments and car insurance. Financial commitments are expenses that are intrinsically defined and sometimes vague, such as supporting elderly family members who reside in a foreign country. Financial status, if perceived as a barrier, may adversely affect retention directly or indirect-ly. For example, a student who is unable to pay tuition may choose to drop out or to work while attending school. The first option has a direct effect on retention through immediate attrition. The second option may have an indirect effect on retention through academic performance (failure) because of decreased study hours and/or decreased class attendance. Stress and dissatisfaction may also occur and adversely influence retention.

Financial status as a barrier to student academic success and retention has been well documented (College Board, 2003). Various terms have been used to describe this phenomenon: financial burden, financial con-cerns, financial difficulties, financial pressure, financial strain, and finan-cial stress. Numerous empirical approaches have examined financial status as a variable influencing student success. One approach identified particular student profile characteristics that increase the likelihood for financial barriers. Several studies reported that financial status as a barrier is particularly prevalent among nontraditional students, especially minor-ity students (College Board, 2003), older students (Hurtado, Inkelas, Briggs, & Rhee, 1997), women with dependent children (Scott, Burns, & Cooney, 1996, 1998; Williams, 1997), and economically disadvantaged students (Chaney, Muraskin, Cahalan, & Goodwin, 1998).

Nurse educators should avoid stereotyping students as at risk for attri-tion due to financial barriers solely on meeting one of the above demo-graphic categories. A holistic appraisal is needed. For example, assuming that a minority student is economically disadvantaged and confronted with severe financial strain based on the student's ethnic background may not only be inaccurate, but is biased and unethical. Economically disadvantaged students come from many different ethnic, racial, and religious groups.

Economically disadvantaged students perceive financial constraints as a barrier, are less likely to enroll in college, and are even less likely to earn a college degree. However, current financial aid policies and limit-ed scholarships present financial challenges or "resource barriers" for middle-class students (Padilla, Trevino, Gonzalez, & Trevino, 1997) and for students who demonstrate small amounts of financial need (Braxton & McClendon, 2001). Resource barriers are real or perceived obstacles that interfere with the ability to secure adequate finances for anticipated expenses. The uncertainty of receiving financial aid or scholarships, and/or concern about anticipated expenses is another burden that adversely affects retention, either directly or indirectly.

Among diverse samples, student perceptions of the influence of the supportiveness or restrictiveness of financial aid and scholarships on retention have been varied. Although financial problems are often cited as a reason for withdrawal, this is usually done after the student weighs the benefits, costs, and overall academic experience. Student satisfaction or dissatisfaction may tip the scale in favor of retention or attrition (Tinto, 1993). Satisfaction with the academic experience is a desirable outcome that can influence retention; however, being able to meet financial expenses also affects persistence behavior (St. John, Cabrera, Nora, & Asker, 2000).

Student perception of financial status is the most critical element for nurse educators to evaluate in this area. If the student perceives financial status to be a barrier, retention is adversely affected. Student appraisal of financial status and satisfaction in relation to all the other possible interacting variables is complicated. It is an individualized process that is influenced by age, gender, and culture. Perceptions are often influenced externally by political agendas concerning "underprivileged" groups and financial assistance priorities (Nurmi & Aunola, 2001). One study indicated that white middle-class college students perceived greater difficulty in getting loans, grants, and scholarships than did minority middle-class college students. Additionally, white middle-class students who faced the loss of financial aid had greater concerns than other students about dropping out (Nora, Cabrera, Hagedorn, & Pascarella, 1996).

It is not surprising that student perceptions of the influence of financial status on retention are quite varied among diverse ethnic, racial, and socioeconomic groups. Perceived responsibility for paying for college may influence student perceptions and guide decisions on persistence. Cultural values, beliefs, and intergenerational differences within cultures may be influential. For example, whether the student as an individual assumes total financial responsibility for college expenses or whether the family is expected to support the student can influence perceptions.

FAMILY FINANCIAL SUPPORT

Family financial support and assurance of funds should be considered in attrition studies (Eaton & Bean, 1995). Among minority nursing students, family financial support was a perceived asset and often a necessity for academic persistence (Lehna, Jackonen, & Wilson, 1996; Vecchione, 1995). Among students enrolled in professional studies programs, family financial support was also viewed as a significant factor (Hendricks, Smith, Caplow, & Donaldson, 1996). Family financial support for school is more complex than it may initially seem. Several major points will be explored below. Nurse educators are encouraged to consider each point carefully when appraising financial factors influencing retention.

First, family financial support for school should be closely viewed in relation to beliefs about responsibility for paying college expenses. As perceived by the student, does the family have the financial resources to assist with college expenses? Does the family intend to assist the student financially to the best of its ability? Does the family *actually* provide financial assistance to the student to the best of its ability? Finally, does the student perceive the family as financially supportive, adequate, or restrictive? Students may need guidance in evaluating financial status and planning at the beginning of the semester.

Beliefs about gratitude and responsibilities of the student toward family members providing financial support can also affect student perceptions and retention. For example, a student whose family is sacrificing greatly to assist with college expenses may feel extreme pressure to excel academically and persist in school. In contrast, a student whose family has available resources yet is unwilling to assist the student may feel overburdened with financial concerns and frustrated with limited financial aid resources; such perceived barriers can adversely affect persistence behaviors and increase attrition risk.

FAMILY EMOTIONAL SUPPORT

Family emotional support is the active emotional involvement of family members in the student's academic endeavors and career goals. It is manifested by encouraging educational and career goals, promoting feelings of self-worth, believing in the student's ability to succeed, listening to problems and concerns, showing interest in academic progress, expressing optimism, offering assistance, and presence. Presence means caring about the student as a whole person and being available for emotional support. A support person does not actually need to be present bodily, but needs to be perceived as caring and encouraging. Although this is the definition used in the NURS model, surveyed students may define family emotional support differently. Nurse educators may expect a positive correlation between family emotional support for school and academic achievement and retention, but this is not always true. The sections that follow will explore the impact of family emotional support on retention. New perspectives about family emotional support aim to guide nurse educators in closely evaluating it in a variety of contexts. Being open to various worldviews or perspectives will broaden nurse educators' ability to understand the multidimensional process of student retention and assist students appropriately.

Students' perceptions of their family's emotional support are essential to evaluate. They may be realistic, clouded, or unrealistic, and yet they are what will influence decisions to persist or withdraw. They are influenced by previous educational success, struggles, and failures and may change over time and throughout the educational process. The impact of family emotional support on the educational experience will also change. For example, in one study, student perceptions were more optimistic at the beginning of the semester than at the end. When asked prospectively to rate the supportiveness or restrictiveness of family emotional support on their ability to remain in the nursing course that semester, students were optimistic. Initially, none perceived family emotional support as "severely restrictive," yet at the end of the semester 11% of the sample perceived that family emotional support severely restricted their ability to remain in the nursing course. Another 18% perceived that family emotional support would "neither restrict nor support" retention prospectively; however at the end of the semester only 7% of the students responded this way (Jeffreys, 2002). The study was limited to persisters and may have had quite different results if non-persisters had been surveyed. Despite the small sample size, this study offers new information for nurse educators and can provide a basis for further study. Awareness that students may be more optimistic at first or undervalue the impact of family emotional support on retention suggests that students need guidance initially in evaluating their individual situations.

The importance of environmental variables, especially family emotional support, has been thought to be most important for older, commuter students (Metzner & Bean, 1987). However recent literature provides new insights into the impact of family support for different student populations, which needs to be viewed in context with student profile characteristics, cultural values and beliefs, and self-efficacy. Family conflict can adversely affect retention. In contrast, Maville and Huerta (1997) indicated that perceived social support was inversely related to academic progress. Here, a strong family cohesiveness influenced the student to prioritize family first; the allegiance to family was predominant, despite support for school.

Among traditional age minority students residing on college campuses (especially in predominantly white institutions), strong family emotional support was significant for college adjustment and retention (Hinderlie & Kenny, 2002; Tucker-Allen & Long, 1999). Family emotional support was consistently present, despite the absence of family members within students' living environment. Other studies have suggested that strong emotional support may be perceived as an added pressure for students to succeed, especially among traditional age students (Hernandez, 2000; Olenchak & Hebert, 2002; Ting, 2000; Wilkie & Redondo, 1996). Within some cultures, group decision making among immediate and extended family members is the expected norm. Therefore, the decision to go to college, persist, withdraw, or drop out would be influenced by more than just the student's decision.

Lack of family emotional support is not always perceived as a barrier to academic success. Cultural norms, values, and beliefs related to the family role, emotional support, and decision making must be considered. Defining who the family is, from the student's perspective, is an essential step. For example, among African-American traditional age college students who did not choose to identify a paternal figure, lack of a father's support was not perceived as important. Among students who did identify a paternal figure, lack of a father's support was viewed as important (Hinderlie & Kenny, 2002). Nurse educators should be aware that cultural values and beliefs about familial ties, expectations, and emotional support vary; individual variations within cultures frequently occur, as do variations in interfamily dynamics.

Family dynamics may influence the incidence of role conflicts and perceived emotional support. Characteristics of well-functioning families include a strong, stable marital alliance, clear interpersonal boundaries, and the absence of inappropriate coalitions (Lopez, Campbell, & Watkins, 1989). A coalition refers to an "intrafamily alignment wherein two individuals ally against a third person" (Lopez, Campbell, & Watkins, 1989, p. 46). It is well documented that a dysfunctional family environment adversely affects retention and/or college adjustment among traditional age college students; a dysfunctional family environment can also affect nontraditional students adversely.

Family emotional support is a multidimensional environmental factor that interacts with other factors and variable sets within the NURS model and should be viewed in context with the other factors and variable sets. Additionally, family emotional support may have different meanings for different students; therefore generalizations should be avoided. When surveying student perceptions about family emotional support for school, nurse educators should be aware of the potential diversity in responses and varied significance within a cultural context. In some cases, strong family support is not always desirable, and lack of family emotional support is not always a barrier. No support is better than perceived obstacles that are viewed as deliberate and/or insurmountable. What is most desirable is a healthy family support system, especially composed of students' significant other(s) (Nora, 2001).

FAMILY RESPONSIBILITIES

Family responsibilities are the daily tasks, expectations, behaviors, attitudes, and values that are needed to adequately perform the expected role within the family setting/environment. They may or may not be compatible with academic and employment responsibilities. Mutually compatible responsibilities will enhance academic success and minimize stress; incompatible responsibilities will hinder academic success and create multiple role stress. Family responsibilities influence retention indirectly through academic and psychological outcomes and interact with other environmental factors and variable sets in the NURS model. It is presumed that family responsibilities are most applicable for commuter students as residential students do not have daily tasks and responsibilities within the family. Residential students may be influenced adversely if their inability to participate in previously held family responsibilities is perceived negatively.

It is expected that having more family responsibilities interferes with study skills, attendance, academic performance, faculty and peer interaction, satisfaction, academic performance, and retention. Family responsibilities have been identified as a significant obstacle for nontraditional nursing student success (Aber & Arathuzik, 1996; Burris, 2001; Griffiths & Tagliareni, 1999; Hegge, Melcher, & Williams, 1999; Tucker-Allen & Long, 1999). Both time-based pressure and strain-based pressure may result in perceived family–school role conflict. Strain-based pressure refers to strain symptoms (tension) in one role that affect performance in others (Greinhaus & Beutell, 1985). Family responsibilities, combined with school responsibilities, may compete for limited time to complete tasks adequately. Inability to meet family responsibilities adequately may result in decreased ability to concentrate on school responsibilities.

Nursing students may perceive family responsibilities as influencing retention in markedly different ways. For example, in a study of first-semester nontraditional associate degree nursing students, 51% perceived that family responsibilities were moderately restrictive and 6% perceived them as severely restrictive (Jeffreys, 1993, 1998). However, samples composed of associate degree student participants in enrichment program (EP) study groups across varying course levels presented different findings. Most notable was the shift from family responsibilities as moderately restrictive (14%) to severely restrictive (25%) at the end of the semester (Jeffreys, 2002). Beginning students may need additional faculty guidance to manage time, juggle roles, and effectively meet family and academic responsibilities. Approximately 20%–28% of the enrichment program study group participants reported family responsibilities as moderately supportive, yet many family responsibilities may have prevented other students from participating in the EP study groups, thereby skewing the results. It is reasonable to surmise that the general population of associate degree nursing students was faced with multiple family responsibilities that adversely affected retention directly or indirectly. These findings are consistent with the higher education and nursing literature concerning nontraditional students.

Students with dependent children frequently feel overburdened by family and domestic responsibilities. However, perceptions vary with diversity in spousal expectations, cultural expectations, number and ages of children, number and ages of other dependent family members, socioeconomic status, child care arrangements, and other variables (Scott, Burns, & Cooney, 1996; Wycoff, 1996). Students with dependent children have family responsibilities that pertain to child care issues. Combined with other family responsibilities, child care creates further challenges to student success and persistence. Because of its complexity, nurse educators may wish to explore child care arrangements separately in relation to student retention.

CHILD CARE ARRANGEMENTS

Child care arrangements are the needs, concerns, and issues surrounding child care. The increasing number of women who have dependent children and who are enrolled in nursing programs demands attention to child care concerns. Generally, dependent children and child care arrangements have been depicted as a barrier to academic achievement and retention. Often, the presence of dependent children was seen as a predictor for attrition without fully surveying individual differences. Students with dependent children are not a homogenous group, and it behooves the nurse educator to avoid stereotypical assumptions about them.

The number and ages of children, presence of support systems, and student perceptions of child care arrangements are necessary to assess. For example, Scott, Burns, and Cooney (1996, 1998) indicated that younger women with younger children were more likely to leave school due to family responsibilities, financial strain, and child care problems. Quality child care for infants and toddlers is not easily found and is expensive, and thus creates financial strain. Perceived multiple role stress for women who are mothers and students is a complex phenomenon that encompasses emotional role ambiguity, person-role conflict, and inter-role conflict (Gigliotti, 1999, 2001). The issue goes beyond finding a safe, reliable caregiver to the emotional component of nurturance. Child care arrangements in the NURS model take into account the emotional aspect as well as the physical environment and the caregiver.

Insight into student perceptions of child care arrangements as supportive or restrictive for academic achievement and retention is valuable. Consistently, across three study samples, responses were diverse for associate degree nursing students. Among respondents for whom child care was applicable, much disparity between restrictiveness and supportiveness was noted. In one study, almost 60% reported child care as supportive, although approximately 30% reported it as restrictive, both at the beginning of the semester and then again at the end. Others perceived that their child care arrangements did not influence retention in any way. Notably, all of these students remained in nursing courses throughout the semester, successfully passing them (Jeffreys, 2002). Previous studies showed that approximately two-thirds of the students with child care arrangements felt that the arrangements restricted academic achievement and retention.

FAMILY CRISIS

A family crisis is a severe, unexpected family problem that often results in increased family responsibilities, stress, and family–school conflicts. Most literature supports that family crisis adversely affects class attendance, academic performance, and retention. Depending on the type of crisis, effects may be short-term or long-term. For example, a student whose child is rushed to the emergency room for appendicitis may perceive this as a crisis with short-term effects. After the child's successful recovery from the appendectomy, the student can resume usual routines. Long-term effects may be psychological and/or tangible. For example, a student whose husband unexpectedly dies may experience long-term psychological effects (grieving) and tangible effects (lack of husband's income). The student will not be able to resume usual routines (including school) because of emotional distress and financial strain. Repeated crises with short-term effects may take their toll on students' persistence indirectly through stress or directly through failure due to excessive absences.

Surprisingly, some research supports that a family crisis can have a positive effect on persistence behaviors. Napoli and Wortman (1998) found that students with more outside negative life events were more likely to seek support from within the college environment, thereby positively affecting persistence. Strong persistence behaviors are inversely related to voluntary attrition and decrease the risk for involuntary attrition. This rather unexpected finding suggests the reconceptualization of the direction of causality between family crisis and retention. Furthermore, in several studies, it explains the diversity in nursing student responses regarding the effect of family crisis on retention. Upon superficial perusal, the diversity in student responses for this survey item may have raised questions concerning validity. However, upon further scrutiny, the responses make sense. First, most students perceived that a family crisis either would not occur, would neither be restrictive nor supportive, or would be restrictive. Second, post-test data demonstrated a shift from 21% to only 7% perceiving that a family crisis did not influence their ability to remain in the nursing course (Jeffreys, 2002). Finally, four data sets consistently show diversity in responses (Jeffreys, 1993, 1998, 2001, 2002). Unfortunately, further study into the type of family crisis and the psychological and/or tangible impact on student academic performance and retention was not done. In the future, qualitative studies may lend insight into students' perspectives.

EMPLOYMENT HOURS

With the growing number of college students who work at least part-time, employment hours becomes an environmental factor that can influence student performance and retention. In nursing, the number of nontraditional, older students who are employed is also increasing. Work hours, in this context, refer to both the number of hours worked and the compatibility of work hours with school and family responsibilities. Long employment hours and an inflexible work schedule adversely influences academic achievement and retention of nontraditional students.

Several studies correlating the number of work hours with college student outcomes provide interesting findings. One study found that the number of hours worked was only marginally associated with academic success; students who worked 1–5 hours weekly had statistically significant higher GPAs than students who did not work or who worked more hours (Strage et al., 2002). Other researchers reported that the number of work hours adversely affected GPA by decreasing study hours (Ransdell, 2001a, 2001b). The idea of work hours detracting from study hours has also been substantiated by other researchers (Toutkoushian & Smart, 2001). It is logical to acknowledge that the time spent in one role limits the time spent in another.

Although employment hours should be compared closely with work responsibilities and other environmental factors and variable sets, student perception of how work hours influence retention is important. A survey of nursing student perceptions concerning work hours supported the employment trends among college students; approximately two-thirds of the students were employed. (Jeffreys, 1993, 1998, 2001, 2002). Of the employed students, responses were almost equally divided between supportive and restrictive when the students were surveyed at the beginning of the semester. In a study that measured nursing student perceptions at the beginning and at the end of the semester, a shift toward employment hours as restrictive occurred (Jeffreys, 2002). Again, the shift from a more conservative view to a more restrictive view retrospectively is consistent with trends in several other environmental factors. These studies did not differentiate between number of work hours and compatibility of work hours; future researchers may wish to distinguish between the two dimensions.

EMPLOYMENT RESPONSIBILITIES

Employment responsibilities are the tasks, expectations, behaviors, attitudes, and values that are needed to adequately perform the roles within a particular employment setting. Mutually compatible responsibilities will enhance academic success and minimize stress; incompatible responsibilities will hinder academic success and create multiple role stress. Employment responsibilities influence retention indirectly through academic and psychological outcomes and interact with other environmental factors and variable sets in the NURS model. On-campus employment has been linked with positive effects through social integration and values congruent with the academic environment. Off-campus employment has been correlated with decreased persistence (Nora et al., 1996). Similarly, Kraemer (1997) noted that employment responsibilities meant less time on campus and less opportunity for academic and social integration. The nursing literature has not differentiated between types of employment; however, several authors reported employment responsibilities as a hindrance to successful academic outcomes (Aber & Arathuzik, 1996; Maville & Huerta, 1997; Merrill, 1998; Tucker-Allen & Long, 1999; Vecchione, 1995).

Student perceptions about employment responsibilities as restricting or supporting retention are often diverse. The striking change between prospective and retrospective perceptions suggests that students are more optimistic initially. For example, in one study, students initially expected employment responsibilities to be supportive (36%) but later only 14% perceived them as having been supportive (Jeffreys, 2002). Nurse educators can proactively assist students in realistically appraising their employment hours and responsibilities and periodically guide them throughout the semester in effective time management between multiple roles.

ENCOURAGEMENT BY OUTSIDE FRIENDS

Outside friends are those outside of the student's classes and the college environment. They do not include family members. Encouragement by outside friends is their active emotional involvement in relation to the student's academic endeavors and career goals. Positive encouragement is manifested by supporting these goals, promoting feelings of self-worth, believing in the student's ability to succeed, listening to problems and concerns, showing interest in academic progress, expressing optimism, offering assistance, and presence.

The literature presents conflicting evidence about the influence of outside friends on academic performance, persistence, and retention. One study reported that students with more outside friends who attended college were more academically involved than were peers with one-half the number or fewer outside friends who attended college (Strage et al., 2002). Similarly, Hernandez (2000) noted more positive persistence behaviors among Latino students with outside friends who provided them with helpful and substantive information about college and who gave them ongoing encouragement. Other researchers found that outside friends significantly influenced persistence in white college students, whereas minority students were often discouraged because of time spent away from family and friends (Nora, 2001; Nora et al., 1996). What is consistently evident is that "encouragement by those most significant in a student's life is instrumental in affecting the overall college experience and persistence decisions" (Nora, 2001, p. 52). Cultural values and beliefs concerning friendships, views on education, and general worldview need to be considered when evaluating the impact of outside friends on retention.

Pressure by friends to participate in outside (nonacademic) activities, such as social engagements, that conflict with the student's ability to successfully complete academic and career goals is incongruent with positive encouragement behaviors. Difficulty setting limits on friends and social activities negatively influences academic performance and retention (Campbell & Davis, 1996). Among several samples of nontraditional associate degree students, subjects perceived encouragement from outside friends as supportive. Most of the students were older (over 25) and were perhaps more experienced in maintaining friendships with people who provided encouragement (Jeffreys, 1993, 1998, 2001, 2002). Nurse educators may wish to further explore and consider the impact of outside friends in relation to the student's age.

Another dimension to the influence of outside friends is social adjustment and institutional attachment. For example, among European-American students, satisfaction with outside friendships and contacts was negatively correlated with social adjustment and institutional attachment (Kenny & Stryker, 1996). Especially among traditional-age students, strong social adjustment and institutional attachment are expected to enhance academic performance, persistence, and retention. Students who reside at the college, especially those with outside friends who attend other colleges, have more difficulty with college adjustment than do other students, thus creating a potential retention barrier (Turner & Berry, 2000).

LIVING ARRANGEMENTS

Living arrangements include the needs, concerns, and issues concerning students' residential environment while attending college. Generally, living arrangements are quite different for commuter than for non-commuter students. For the campus resident, one major factor influencing retention is college adjustment and social integration into the college residential environment. Living at college is a new experience that requires adjustment. The NURS model takes into account the emotional aspect of living arrangements as well as the physical environment and the other individuals who share it. Consistent with the literature, it is proposed that living arrangements can support or restrict student retention and success.

The literature on college adjustment presents contrasting views. Tinto (1997) proposed that successful adjustment depends on the student's ability to disassociate from past communities of friends and family and to engage in a smooth transition to a new community, developing new friends and creating a new family or community. However, other researchers stated that for minority students, positive family attachments eased transition to the college environment (Cabrera et al., 1999; Hendricks et al., 1996; Nora, 2001). Barriers that impede a smooth transition to a new living environment include far distance from home, friends who attend other colleges, differences in geographic area or size of town, cultural background different from the majority, and difficulty with parental separation. Nurse educators should be aware that the developmental task of parental separation is influenced by culture, gender, family dynamics, and/or interpersonal conflicts. For example, within some families and cultures, parental separation to attend college is valued, encouraged, and expected. In other families and cultures, parental separation for reasons other than marriage is discouraged. Traditional age students from tumultuous living environments may look forward to leaving home; their perceptions may be that their college living arrangements are much improved over their previous ones.

Insight into student perceptions of living arrangements as supportive or restrictive for academic achievement and retention is valuable. Perceived satisfaction with a social support network on campus assists with college adjustment and is particularly crucial for minority students attending predominantly white universities. An environment perceived as uncaring and culturally different has caused feelings of dissatisfaction and difficult college adjustment (Manifold & Rambur, 2001; Villaruel, Canales, & Torres, 2001; Yurkovich, 2001). Positive college adjustment and the perception that living arrangements are conducive to facilitating academic outcomes, satisfaction, and career outcomes will positively influence retention.

Living arrangements can also influence commuter student academic achievement and retention. Lack of a safe, nurturing living environment conducive to studying will affect retention directly or indirectly through academic outcomes. For example, a nursing student living in a homeless shelter will face many adversities in living arrangements that will interfere with academic achievement. A noisy home environment (on or off campus) without adequate study space will also adversely affect retention through academic outcomes and interfere with study hours. Safe, nurturing, and quiet living arrangements that are located far away from the college campus and/or clinical sites present transportation challenges.

TRANSPORTATION

Transportation is more pertinent for commuter students than non-commuter students. However, because nursing programs may require students to travel to sites outside the university setting for clinical experiences, it may also be a concern for residential nursing students. Transportation issues involve dependability, distance, parking, safety, time, energy, and money. In some areas, public transportation is not available and presents challenges to nursing students who need to travel great distances for clinical work and who may not have access to a car. Real or perceived transportation difficulties are a barrier to attendance, punctuality, academic performance, and retention.

Transportation as a barrier may influence retention indirectly through academic and psychological outcomes. Additionally, it interacts with other environmental factors (such as family responsibilities and financial status) and academic factors (attendance and study hours). For example, long travel time will take away from family responsibilities and study hours. Traveling expenses may sometimes prevent students from attending classes in an effort to save money. Financial aid and scholarships usually do not cover transportation expenses, so this can be a serious impediment for economically disadvantaged students. Obviously, transportation issues need to be individually appraised. In several studies conducted at one commuter college, it was not surprising that nursing student perceptions about transportation were quite diverse. The surveyed students commuted various distances, traveled through different neighborhoods, and used one or more modes of transportation (subway, bus, ferry, car, taxi, foot) (Jeffreys, 1993, 1998, 2001, 2002).

KEY POINTS SUMMARY

- In the NURS model, environmental factors are those external to the academic process and include financial status, family financial support, family emotional support, family responsibilities, child care arrangements, family crisis, employment hours, employment responsibilities, encouragement by outside friends, living arrangements, and transportation.
- Financial status refers to the student's standing in meeting all expenses including tuition, college fees, books and other learning materials, living expenses, financial obligations, and commitments.
- Family financial support for school should be closely viewed in relation to beliefs concerning responsibility for paying college expenses.
- Family emotional support is the active emotional involvement of family members in the student's academic endeavors and career goals. It is manifested by encouraging educational and career goals, promoting feelings of self-worth, believing in the student's ability to succeed, listening to problems and concerns, showing interest in academic progress, expressing optimism, offering assistance, and presence.
- Family responsibilities are the daily tasks, expectations, behaviors, attitudes, and values that are needed to adequately perform the expected role within the family setting/environment.
- Child care arrangements are the needs, concerns, and issues surrounding child care, including emotional aspects.
- A family crisis is a severe, unexpected family problem that often results in increased family responsibilities, stress, and family–school conflicts.

- Employment hours refer to the number of hours worked and the compatibility of work hours with school and family responsibilities.
- Employment responsibilities are the tasks, expectations, behaviors, attitudes, and values that are needed to adequately perform the roles within a particular employment setting.
- Encouragement by outside friends is their active emotional involvement in relation to the student's academic endeavors and career goals.
- Living arrangements include the needs, concerns, and issues surrounding students' residential environment while attending college.
- Transportation issues involve dependability, distance, parking, safety, time, energy, and money.
- Each environmental factor is multidimensional, interacting with other variables and variable sets within the NURS model. Environmental factors affect retention directly and indirectly through academic and psychological outcomes.
- A detailed and holistic appraisal of student perceptions concerning the influence of each environmental factor on academic success and retention reveals several dimensions that potentially affect students differently. Whereas some students perceive environmental factors as barriers to retention, other students perceive the same factors as supportive.

EDUCATOR-IN-ACTION

Educators' actions concerning environmental factors can make a considerable difference in student academic and psychological outcomes, persistence, and retention. Without appropriate background knowledge, individual appraisal, and sensitivity, educators' actions may adversely impact upon these areas. Consider the possible adverse effects of the following educator actions:

Pamela's elderly mother-in-law usually cares for Pamela's infant and toddler. However, sudden diarrhea from food poisoning renders her incapable of providing care. Family traditions hold the mother-in-law as the most esteemed family member and head of the family, who must be cared for by the daughter-in-law when ill. Day care is not considered an appropriate option. Pamela has never been late or absent from class, and only two absences are permissible. When she calls Professor Hurdles and tells her that child care and other family responsibilities prevent her from attending class, Professor Hurdles says, "You should have called me yesterday so I wouldn't have made out the patient assignment. That is very unprofessional. If you sent your children to the day care center, you wouldn't have this problem."

Jo-Ann is a 19-year-old student who was abused by her parents until she was adopted at age 10 by her cousin. Her cousin recently died after a lengthy and costly illness. When registering for classes, Jo-Ann says, "If there is an opening, I would like to register for the two-day college class schedule and clinical at Children's Hospital. I live within walking distance from the hospital. Since I'm an independent student, it would save me money." Professor Hurdles replies, "It sounds like you should learn to manage your money better. Why don't you ask your parents?"

In contrast, educator actions that seek to actively acknowledge the importance of environmental factors, appreciate students as individuals, objectively appraise diverse environmental situations, maximize strengths, and improve weaknesses have the most potential for promoting positive academic and psychological outcomes, persistence, and retention. For example, Professor Bridges lists environmental factors on the course orientation agenda, adding credence to their importance. Brief sample student scenarios with various environmental factors are presented in written handouts and then read aloud. Student actions, including the effective use of family, faculty, and friend support networks, are suggested by students and then further discussed.

As the group's interests about the fictitious case scenarios are stimulated, Professor Bridges seizes the opportunity to offer guidance and assist the current students. "If there are any environmental factors that you would like to talk with me about, or would like further guidance with, please write them down on your index card. If there is something you would like me to address in class further, please let me know. There is no need to write down your name. If there is something you would like to speak with me about individually, please include your name. Feel free to see me during office hours, call me, or send an e-mail." Several students write:

Trina: "After our class discussion, I realized that I may need help with balancing my work, family, and school responsibilities. Maybe applying for a student loan would allow me to work fewer hours and have more time for school and my family. Previously, I thought that student loans were only for young students. Is it too late to get a loan for this semester?"

Anna: "At first I felt overwhelmed by my family responsibilities. I thought that I was alone. The discussion and handouts made me realize that I wasn't alone and didn't have to struggle through this by myself. Thanks."

Leon: "My parents didn't want me to apply for financial aid or loans. I've been working full-time to pay for school. I get passing grades, but I want to do better in school. The nurse externship program combines work and a forgivable loan without needing parental permission and financial aid forms. Thanks for telling us about it. Can you help me with the application process?"

Jackie: "I don't have any questions now but it's helpful knowing that instructors think factors other than school are important in our lives. It's nice to know that faculty care."

Professor Bridges follows up with individual student requests and refers students to additional resources as appropriate. In class, she continues to remind students about the importance of ongoing self-appraisal of environmental factors and their effect on academic responsibilities, achievement, stress, satisfaction, and progress in nursing.

REFERENCES & BIBLIOGRAPHY

Aber, C. S., & Arathuzik, D. (1996). Factors associated with student success in a baccalaureate nursing program within an urban public university. *Journal of Nursing Education, 35*(6), 285–288.

Antonio, A. L. (2001). Diversity and the influence of friendship groups in college. *Review of Higher Education, 25*(1), 63–89.

Astin, A. W. (1997). How "good" is your institution's retention rate? *Research in Higher Education, 38*(6), 647–658.

Baum, S. (2003a). *The financial aid partnership: Strengthening the federal government's leadership role.* Retrieved February 27, 2003, from http://www.collegeboard.com

Baum, S. (2003b). *The role of student loans in college access.* Retrieved February 27, 2003, from http://www.collegeboard.com

Bean, J. P. (1985). Interaction effects based on class level in an explanatory model of college student dropout syndrome. *American Educational Research Journal, 22*(1), 35–64.

Bean, J. P., & Metzner, B. (1985). A conceptual model of nontraditional undergraduate student attrition. *Review of Educational Research, 55,* 485–540.

Beck, C. T. (2001). Caring within nursing education: A metasynthesis. *Journal of Nursing Education, 40*(3), 101–109.

Benda, E. J. (1991). The relationship among variables in Tinto's conceptual model and attrition of bachelor's degree nursing students. *Journal of Professional Nursing, 7*(1), 16–24.

Bessent, H. (Ed.) (1997). *Strategies for recruitment, retention, and graduation of minority nurses in colleges of nursing.* Washington, DC: American Nurses Publishing.

Braxton, J. M., & McClendon, S. A. (2001). The fostering of social integration and retention through institutional practice. *Journal of College Student Retention: Research, Theory, & Practice, 3*(1), 57–72.

Braxton, J. M., & Mundy, M. E. (2001). Powerful institutional levers to reduce college student departure. *Journal of College Student Retention: Research, Theory, & Practice, 3*(1), 91–118.

Brown, L. L., & Kurpius, S. E. R. (1997). Psychosocial factors influencing academic persistence of American Indian college students. *Journal of College Student Development, 38*(1), 3–12.

Burris, R. F. (2001). Teaching student parents. *Nurse Educator, 26*(2), 64–65; 98.

Cabrera, A. F., Nora, A., Terenzini, P. T., Pascarella, E. T., & Hagedorn, L. S. (1999). Campus racial climate and the adjustment of students to college: A comparison between white students and African American students. *Journal of Higher Education, 70*(2), 134–160.

Campbell, A. R., & Davis, S. M. (1996). Faculty commitment: Retaining minority nursing students in majority institutions. *Journal of Nursing Education, 35*(7), 298–303.

Campbell, A. R., & Dickson, C. J. (1996). Predicting student success: A 10-year review using integrative review and meta-analysis. *Journal of Professional Nursing, 12*(1), 47–59.

Chaney, B., Muraskin, L. D., Cahalan, M. W., & Goodwin, D. (1998). Helping the progress of disadvantaged students in higher education: The federal student support services program. *Educational Evaluation and Policy Analysis, 20*(3), 197–215.

Cole, D. A., & Jordan, A. E. (1989). Assessment of cohesion and adaptability in component family dyads: A question of convergent and discriminant validity. *Journal of Counseling Psychology, 36*(4), 456–463.

College Board. (2003). *Challenging times, clear choices: An action agenda for college access and success.* Retrieved February 27, 2003, from http://www.collegeboard.com

Constantine, M. G., Robinson, J. S., Wilton, L., & Caldwell, L. D. (2002). Collective self-esteem and perceived social support as predictors of cultural congruity among black and Latino college students. *Journal of College Student Development, 43*(3), 307–316.

Courage, M. M., & Godbey, K. L. (1992). Student retention: Policies and services to enhance persistence to graduation. *Nurse Educator, 17*(2), 29–32.

Crawford, L. A., & Olinger, B. H. (1988). Recruitment and retention of nursing students from diverse cultural backgrounds. *Journal of Nursing Education, 27*(8), 379–381.

Eaton, S. B., & Bean, J. P. (1995). An approach/avoidance behavioral model of college student attrition. *Research in Higher Education, 36*(6), 617–645.

Fleming, J. (2002). Who will succeed in college? When the SAT predicts black students' performance. *Review of Higher Education, 25*(3), 281–296.

Flowers, L. A. (2002). The impact of college racial composition on African American students' academic and social gains: Additional evidence. *Journal of College Student Development, 43*(3), 403–410.

Fuertes, J. N., & Westbrook, F. D. (1996). Using the social, attitudinal, familial, and environmental (S.A.F.E.) acculturation stress scale to assess the adjustment needs of Hispanic college students. *Measurement and Evaluation in Counseling and Development, 29,* 67–76.

Gianakos, I. (1996). Career development differences between adult and traditional-aged learners. *Journal of Career Development, 22*(3), 211–223.

Gigliotti, E. (1999). Women's multiple role stress: Testing Neuman's flexible line of defense. *Nursing Science Quarterly, 12*(1), 36–44.

Gigliotti, E. (2001). Development of the perceived multiple role stress scale (PMRS). *Journal of Nursing Measurement, 9*(2), 163–180.

Griffiths, M. J., & Tagliareni, M. E. (1999). Challenging traditional assumptions about minority students in nursing education. *Nursing & Health Care Perspectives, 20,* 290–295.

Harvey, V. C., & McMurray, N. E. (1997). Students' perceptions of nursing: Their relationship to attrition. *Journal of Nursing Education, 36*(8), 383–389.

Hegge, M., Melcher, P., & Williams, S. (1999). Hardiness, help-seeking behavior, and social support of baccalaureate nursing students. *Journal of Nursing Education, 38*(4), 179–182.

Heller, B. R., Oros, M. T., & Durney-Crowley, J. (2000). The future of nursing education: 10 trends to watch. *Nursing and Health Care Perspectives, 21*(1), 9–13.

Hendricks, A. D., Smith, K., Caplow, J. H., & Donaldson, J. F. (1996). A grounded theory approach to determining the factors related to the persistence of minority students in professional programs. *Innovative Higher Education, 21*(2), 113–126.

Hernandez, J. C. (2000). Understanding the retention of Latino college students. *Journal of College Student Development, 41*(6), 575–588.

Hinderlie, H. H., & Kenny, M. (2002). Attachment, social support, and college adjustment among black students at predominantly white universities. *Journal of College Student Development, 43*(3), 327–340.

Hoffman, J. A., & Weiss, B. (1987). Family dynamics and presenting problems in college students. *Journal of Counseling Psychology, 34*(2), 157–163.

Hurtado, S., Inkelas, K. K., Briggs, C., & Rhee, B-S. (1997). Differences in college access and choice among racial/ethnic groups: Identifying continuing barriers. *Research in Higher Education, 38*(1), 43–75.

Jeffreys, M. R. (1993). *The relationship of self-efficacy and select academic and environmental variables on academic achievement and retention.* Unpublished doctoral dissertation, Teachers College, Columbia University, New York.

Jeffreys, M. R. (1998). Predicting nontraditional student retention and academic achievement. *Nurse Educator, 23*(1), 42–48.

Jeffreys, M. R. (2001). Evaluating enrichment program study groups: Academic outcomes, psychological outcomes, and variables influencing retention. *Nurse Educator, 26*(3), 142–149.

Jeffreys, M. R. (2002). Students' perceptions of variables influencing retention: A pretest and post-test approach. *Nurse Educator, 27*(1), 16–19 [Erratum, 2002, 27(2), 64].

Jeffreys, M. R. (2003). Strategies for promoting nontraditional student retention and success. In M. Oermann & K. Heinrich (Eds.), *Annual Review of Nursing Education: Volume I* (pp. 1–90). New York: Springer.

Johnstone, D. B. (2003). *Fundamental assumptions and aims underlying the principles and policies of federal financial aid to students.* Retrieved February 27, 2003, from http://www.collegeboard.com

Kenny, M. E., & Stryker, S. (1996). Social network characteristics and college adjustment among racially and ethnically diverse first-year students. *Journal of College Student Development, 37*(6), 649–658.

Kirkland, M. L. S. (1998). Stressors and coping strategies among successful female African American baccalaureate nursing students. *Journal of Nursing Education, 37*(1), 5–12.

Kraemer, B. A. (1997). The academic and social integration of Hispanic students into college. *Review of Higher Education, 20*(2), 163–179.

Kuh, G. D. (2001). Organizational culture and student persistence: Prospects and puzzles. *Journal of College Student Retention: Research, Theory, & Practice, 3*(1), 23–40.

Lam, P. C., Doverspike, D., & Mawasha, P. R. (1997). Increasing diversity in engineering academics (IDEAs): Development of a program for improving African American representation. *Journal of Career Development, 24*(1), 55–70.

Langston-Moss, R. (1997). Experiences and perceptions of Black American female nursing students attending predominantly white nursing programs. *Journal of National Black Nurses Association, 9*(2), 21–30.

Lehna, C., Jackonen, S., & Wilson, L. (1996). Navigating a nursing curriculum: Bridges and barriers. *Association of Black Nursing Faculty Journal, 7*(July/August), 98–103.

Levin, M. E., & Levin, J. R. (1991). A critical examination of academic retention programs for at-risk minority college students. *Journal of College Student Development, 32*, 323–334.

Loerch, K. J., Russell, J. E. A., & Rush, M. C. (1989). The relationships among family domain variables and work-family conflict for men and women. *Journal of Vocational Behavior, 35*, 288–308.

Lopez, F. G., Campbell, V. L., & Watkins, C. E. (1988). Family structure, psychological separation, and college adjustment: A canonical analysis and cross-validation. *Journal of Counseling Psychology, 35*(4), 402–409.

Lopez, F. G., Campbell, V. L., & Watkins, C. E. (1989). Effects of marital conflict and family coalition patterns on college student adjustment. *Journal of College Student Development, 30*, 46–52.

Malveaux, J. (2003). *What's at stake: The social and economic benefits of higher education.* Retrieved February 27, 2003, from http://www.collegeboard.com

Manifold, C., & Rambur, B. (2001). Predictors of attrition in American Indian nursing students. *Journal of Nursing Education, 40*(6), 279–281.

Maville, J., & Huerta, C. G. (1997). Stress and social support among Hispanic student nurses: Implications for academic achievement. *Journal of Cultural Diversity, 4*(1), 18–25.

McPherson, M. S., & Schapiro, M. O. (2003). *Getting the most out of federal student aid spending—encouraging colleges and universities to promote the common good.* Retrieved February 27, 2003, from http://www.collegeboard.com

Merrill, E. B. (1998). Culturally diverse students enrolled in nursing: Barriers influencing success. *Journal of Cultural Diversity, 5*(2), 58–67.

Metzner, B. S. (1989). Perceived quality of academic advising: The effect on freshman attrition. *American Educational Research Journal, 26,* 422–442.

Metzner, B., & Bean, J. P. (1987). The estimation of a conceptual model of nontraditional undergraduate student attrition. *Research in Higher Education, 27,* 15–38.

Milem, J. F., & Berger, J. B. (1997). A modified model of college student persistence: Exploring the relationship between Astin's theory of involvement and Tinto's theory of student departure. *Journal of College Student Development, 38*(4), 387–400.

Mohr, J. J., Eiche, K. D., & Sedlacek, W. E. (1998). So close, yet so far: Predictors of attrition in college seniors. *Journal of College Student Development, 39*(4), 343–354.

Napoli, A. R., & Wortman, P. M. (1998). Psychosocial factors related to retention and early departure of two-year community college students. *Research in Higher Education, 39*(4), 419–455.

Nora, A. (1987). Determinants of retention among Chicano college students: A structural model. *Research in Higher Education, 26,* 31–60.

Nora, A. (2001). The depiction of significant others in Tinto's "Rites of Passage": A reconceptualization of the influence of family and community in the persistence process. *Journal of College Student Retention: Research, Theory, & Practice, 3*(1), 41–56.

Nora, A., Cabrera, A., Hagedorn, L. S., & Pascarella, E. (1996). Differential impacts of academic and social experiences on college-related behavioral outcomes across different ethnic and gender groups at four-year institutions. *Research in Higher Education, 37*(4), 427–451.

Nurmi, J-E., & Aunola, K. (2001). How does academic achievement come about? Cross-cultural and methodological notes. *International Journal of Educational Research, 35,* 403–409.

O'Connor, P. C., & Bevil, C. A. (1996). Academic outcomes and stress in full-time day and part-time evening baccalaureate nursing students. *Journal of Nursing Education, 35*(6), 245–251.

Olenchak, F. R., & Hebert, T. P. (2002). Endangered academic talent: Lessons learned from gifted first-generation college males. *Journal of College Student Development, 43*(2), 195–212.

Padilla, R. V., Trevino, J., Gonzalez, K., & Trevino, J. (1997). Developing local models of minority student success in college. *Journal of College Student Development, 38*(2), 125–135.

Ransdell, S. (2001a). Predicting college success: The importance of ability and non-cognitive variables. *International Journal of Educational Research, 35,* 357–364.

Ransdell, S. (2001b). Discussion and implications. *International Journal of Educational Research, 35,* 391–395.

Ransdell, S., Hawkins, C., & Adams, R. (2001a). Models, modeling, and the design of the study. *International Journal of Educational Research, 35,* 365–372.

Ransdell, S., Hawkins, C., & Adams, R. (2001b). Results of the study. *International Journal of Educational Research, 35,* 373–389.

Rodgers, S. G. (1990). Retention of minority nursing students on predominantly white campuses. *Nurse Educator, 15*(5), 36–39.

Rosenfeld, P. (1987). Nursing education in crisis—a look at recruitment and retention. *Nursing and Health Care, 5,* 283–286.

Rowser, J. F. (1997). Do African American students' perceptions of their needs have implications for retention? *Journal of Black Studies, 27*(5), 718–725.

Scott, C., Burns, A., & Cooney, G. (1996). Reasons for discontinuing study: The case of mature age female students with children. *Higher Education, 31,* 233–253.

Scott, C., Burns, A., & Cooney, G. (1998). Motivation for return to study as a predictor of completion of degree amongst female mature students with children. *Higher Education, 35,* 221–239.

St. John, E. P., Cabrera, A. F., Nora, A., & Asker, E. H. (2000). Economic influences on persistence reconsidered: How can finance research inform the reconceptualization of persistence models? In J. Braxton (Ed.), *Reworking the student departure puzzle.* Nashville, TN: Vanderbilt University Press.

St. John, E. P., Hu, S., Simmons, A. B., & Musoba, G. D. (2001). Aptitude vs. merit: What matters in persistence. *Review of Higher Education, 24*(2), 131–152.

Strage, A., Baba, Y., Millner, S., Scharberg, M., Walker, E., Williamson, R., & Yoder, M. (2002). What every student affairs professional should know: Student study activities and beliefs associated with academic success. *Journal of College Student Development, 43*(2), 246–266.

Terenzini, P. T., Springer, L. Yaeger, P. M., Pascarella, E. T., & Nora, A. (1996). First generation college students: Characteristics, experiences, and cognitive development. *Research in Higher Education, 37*(1), 1–23.

Ting, S-M. R. (1997). Estimating academic success in the first year of college for specially admitted white students: A model combining cognitive and psychosocial predictors. *Journal of College Student Development, 38*(4), 401–409.

Ting, S-M. R. (2000). Predicting Asian Americans' academic performance in the first year of college: An approach combining SAT scores and noncognitive variables. *Journal of College Student Development, 41*(4), 442–449.

Tinto, V. (1993). *Leaving college: Rethinking the causes and cures of student attrition.* Chicago: University of Chicago Press.

Tinto, V. (1997). Classrooms as communities. *Journal of Higher Education, 68*(6), 599–623.

Toutkoushian, R. K., & Smart, J. C. (2001). Do institutional characteristics affect student gains from college? *Review of Higher Education, 25*(1), 39–61.

Tucker-Allen, S. (1989). Losses incurred through minority student nurse attrition. *Nursing and Health Care, 10*(7), 395–397.

Tucker-Allen, S., & Long, E. (1999). *Recruitment and retention of minority students: Stories of success.* Lisle, IL: Tucker.

Turner, A. L., & Berry, T. R. (2000). Counseling center contributions to student retention and graduation: A longitudinal assessment. *Journal of College Student Development, 41*(6), 627–636.

Vecchione, E. (1995). Looking at problems that hinder nontraditional students' achievements. *Nursing Leadership Forum, 1*(3), 94–98.

Villaruel, A. M., Canales, M., & Torres, S. (2001). Bridges and barriers: Educational mobility of Hispanic nurses. *Journal of Nursing Education, 40*(6), 245–251.

Wilkie, C., & Redondo, B. (1996). Predictors of academic success and failure of first-year college students. *Journal of the Freshman Year Experience, 8*(2), 17–32.

Williams, E. (1997). How women experience social support as mature adult learners in a vocational setting. *Journal of Vocational Education Research, 22*(1), 39–53.

Williams, R. P. (1993). The concerns of beginning nursing students. *Nursing and Health Care, 14*(4), 178–184.

Wycoff, S. E. M. (1996). Academic performance of Mexican American women: Sources of support that serve as motivating variables. *Journal of Multicultural Counseling and Development, 24*, 146–155.

Yurkovich, E. E. (2001). Working with American Indians toward educational success. *Journal of Nursing Education, 40*(6), 259–269.

Chapter 6

Professional Integration and Socialization

Many models explaining attrition among traditional age college students have emphasized the importance of social integration in college in student adjustment, persistence, and success. Social integration refers to the "degree of congruency between the student and the social system of the college" (Tinto, 1975, p. 107). It is achieved through formal and informal faculty interactions, peer interactions, and extracurricular activities. Students with limited social integration experience greater isolation, thus adversely impacting upon academic performance and retention. Difficulty with integration may result in increased stress and anxiety (negative psychological outcomes), increasing the risk for academic difficulty and attrition (Wilson, Mason, & Ewing, 1997).

In the higher education literature, the importance of social integration and academic integration in college student retention is frequently discussed. Researchers have noted the powerful influence of social integration with specific populations of students such as African-American males (Davis, 1995), minority students (Fleming, 2002; Hinderlie & Kenny, 2002; Nora & Cabrera, 1996), adult students (Mancuso, 2001), first-generation minority students (Olenchak & Hebert, 2002), and Hispanic students (Hernandez, 2000; Kraemer, 1997). Bean and Metzner (1985; Metzner & Bean, 1987) propose that for nontraditional (older, part-time, and/or commuter students), social integration is less influential than environmental factors on retention, although it may have indirect effects through psychological outcomes. Conclusively, social integration is a factor that should be closely considered among all populations; however, the conceptualization and the significance of social integration may vary within and between specific student subgroups.

For undergraduate nursing students, a new perspective of social integration is proposed in the NURS model (Figure 1.1). Professional integration factors are those that enhance students' interaction with the social system of the college environment within the context of professional socialization and career development. These factors include nursing faculty advisement and helpfulness, memberships in professional organizations, professional events, encouragement by friends in class, enrichment programs, and peer mentoring and tutoring. Results from recent studies have identified nursing faculty advisement and helpfulness, enrichment program, and peer-mentor-tutoring as instrumental in assisting with nursing student retention (Jeffreys, 1993, 1998, 2001, 2002). Other reports have documented the significance of enrichment programs that incorporate nonacademic components and recognize the power of faculty, peer, and professional mentoring (Bessent, 1997; Hesser, Pond, Lewis, & Abbott, 1996; Ramsey, Blowers, Merriman, Glenn, & Terry, 2000; Tucker-Allen & Long, 1999). Professional socialization is important for professional growth and development as well as retention. It is particularly powerful in encouraging students underrepresented in the nursing profession, such as men and minority students.

Professional integration factors are at the center of the NURS model because it is believed that they are at the crossroads of the decision to persist, drop out, or stop out. Lack of professional integration increases the risk of attrition, whereas strong professional integration increases commitment, persistence behaviors, and retention. It is also proposed that professional integration factors are vitally important for both traditional and nontraditional nursing student retention; however, students must be actively involved in such activities throughout the educational process. Nurse educators are the key initiators and advocates of professional integration because they have the power to actively promote enrichment programs, professional events, memberships, encouragement by friends in class, and peer mentoring-tutoring. Faculty can make a difference by increasing professional integration and eliminating social isolation.

Nurse educators must first recognize that professional integration is a multidimensional process that incorporates cognitive, affective, and practical dimensions, and that it will be best enhanced through the careful orchestration and planned coordination of activities that creatively combine these dimensions. It is also proposed that it will be exponentially augmented through the ongoing use of various professional integration factors that complement each other. This complementary coordination can be emphasized through faculty interventions that aim to maximize students' experience with these factors. Although each individual factor can have a positive influence on retention, the combined effect greatly outweighs the individual effect. This is consistent with the holistic perspective that views the whole dimension of professional integration as greater than the mere total of each separate and distinct part. Affective growth and development, leading to holistic changes, will occur cumulatively after the combination of various strategies (Terenzini, Pascarella, & Blimling, 1996).

Before designing strategies, nurse educators must understand the potential power of each professional integration factor. This chapter elaborates upon each of these factors, proposing ways that they can potentially and directly enhance retention through academic and psychological outcomes. The individual benefits of each professional integration factor will be highlighted. Potential barriers to successful professional integration will conclude the chapter. Awareness of actual and perceived barriers to professional integration strategies is necessary if nurse educators are to understand the student retention process and to develop ways of preventing obstacles and removing barriers before designing strategies. Strategies for promoting retention and success will be discussed in Part II of this book.

FACULTY ADVISEMENT AND HELPFULNESS

Faculty advisement and helpfulness means the active involvement of nursing faculty in the student's academic endeavors, career goals, and professional socialization. Faculty advisement involves the interaction with students in formal, preset meetings, such as in the classroom or during weekly office hours. Faculty helpfulness goes beyond the formal domain into the informal setting when, for example, a faculty member stops in the hallway to talk with a student about an upcoming professional conference or congratulates a student about an excellent performance with a challenging hospitalized client. Faculty helpfulness is offering to meet with students outside scheduled hours for a study group or for a résumé writing workshop. Faculty advisement and helpfulness are manifested by encouraging educational and career goals, promoting positive feelings of self-worth, believing in the student's ability to succeed, listening to problems and concerns, showing interest in academic progress, presenting a realistic outlook, expressing optimism, offering assistance, and presence. Presence means caring about the student as a whole person and being available as a resource, making appropriate referrals when needed.

Although the faculty member needs to be present at designated (expected) times, such as in class or in the faculty office, the most important factor is that the student perceives the faculty member as caring and encouraging. Student perceptions and expectations about advisement vary and can be influenced by student profile characteristics, and environmental, academic, and affective factors. Similarly, faculty expectations and perceptions of the advisor role may be quite varied. The faculty advisor role may be undervalued and the significance of the quality of faculty interactions may be underestimated among faculty. However, the advisor role is pivotal in promoting socialization and retention. The faculty advisor is often the first person the student encounters within the educational institution and perhaps the nursing profession. The faculty advisor has the potential to help students prevent problems, develop strengths, eliminate weaknesses, and feel integrated within the nursing profession. A negative first experience with a faculty advisor can turn away students who could ultimately make a significant contribution to the nursing profession and health care.

Although the developmental advisement approach is strongly supported in the literature as offering the most benefits to enhance student academic and psychological growth and development, not all nursing faculty may value, support, or practice developmental advisement. In a developmental approach, student–faculty relationships encourage open communication, shared responsibility and power, caring, mentoring, total student development, self-direction, active help-seeking behaviors, and decision making. Developmental advisement is more focused on the *process* of learning, whereas prescriptive advisement is grade-oriented, or focused on the attainment of a prescribed product. Prescriptive advisement views the faculty advisor as the authority person who dispenses information and prescribes the measures needed for students to complete their curriculum requirements (Alexitch, 2002; Herndon, Kaiser, & Creamer, 1996).

The NURS model advocates developmental advisement, which necessitates a commitment on the part of both faculty member and student. The advisor–advisee relationship changes over the educational process. Developmental advisement and helpfulness is proactive, with faculty members often initiating contacts with students and encouraging informal contacts. Lack of preparation in effective advisement strategies appropriate for various students throughout the educational process has led to the design of faculty development workshops. Faculty advisement strategies will be discussed in chapter 10.

Although the developmental approach is advocated in the NURS model, students may view faculty advisement and helpfulness differently. Not all students may value a developmental advisement approach. Often, student perceptions and expectations about the faculty advisement role are different from those of the faculty (Baldwin & Wold, 1993; Lehna, Jackonen, & Wilson, 1996; Trent, 1997; Winters, 1990). Additionally, expectations about helpfulness can be different than those of faculty (Poorman, Webb, & Mastorovich, 2002). A mismatch between student and faculty expectations and perceptions creates another barrier, whereby students become disappointed and dissatisfied and poor psychological outcomes for the nursing program increase the risk for attrition. The value of student perceptions about faculty advisement and helpfulness is critical in determining whether satisfaction or dissatisfaction will result. For example, in several studies, student perceptions of faculty advisement and helpfulness were consistently found to be one of the top three "greatly supportive" factors for student retention (Jeffreys, 1993, 1998, 2001, 2002).

The most important experiences to students are often the informal faculty–student interactions that occur outside the classroom, routine advisement, and scheduled office hours (Diekelmann, 1993). In general, out-of-classroom experiences have a powerful influence on retention (Campbell & Campbell, 1997; Milem & Berger, 1997; Terenzini et al., 1996), but especially among minority students in predominantly white institutions (Nora, 2001; Tucker-Allen & Long, 1999) and among adult students (Mancuso, 2001). The informal socialization process helps nurture professional growth, development, and integration into the nursing culture. The nursing culture refers to "the learned and transmitted lifeways, values, symbols, patterns, and normative practices of members of the nursing profession of a particular society" (Leininger, 1995a, p. 208). Students are invited into the nursing culture and are guided by expert mentors through the open sharing of nursing values, beliefs, norms, and practices.

Nurse educators must recognize students' holistic needs, expand the teaching and advisor role into a mentor role, and create innovative strategies to enhance student success. However, the nurse educator alone cannot best promote professional socialization. Capitalizing on the strengths of other professional integration factors can only help broaden the supportive collaborative network for students.

MEMBERSHIPS

Membership in one's professional association is an essential activity for professional career growth, development, and mobility, as well as one that promotes an added opportunity for professional socialization and integration (Betts & Cherry, 2002; Joel & Kelly, 2002). Within the NURS

model, memberships refer to affiliation or participation in nursing organizations or associations as a member, as prescribed by the respective
bylaws. Nursing organizations/associations include the National Student
Nurses Association (NSNA), the school's student nurse club (SNC), and
specialty nursing organizations that permit student nurse membership.
Memberships promote professional integration through various benefits
and privileges that may include voting rights, newsletters, journals, free
items, listserv announcements of professional issues, discounts at professional events, networking, referrals, mentoring services, job postings,
and legal advice.

The NSNA provides an opportunity for student nurses to be actively involved in professional nursing issues, health care issues, and nursing
student/education issues. Active involvement includes a variety of activities such as voting for NSNA officers, writing a letter to the editor of
the NSNA journal, *Imprint,* representing the nursing program at a
NSNA meeting, or running for a NSNA office. Because the NSNA is
exclusively for undergraduate nursing students throughout the United
States, students may feel a common bond with other nursing students
beyond the limited enclaves of one nursing program. Positive solutions
from student role models and the knowledge that nursing students
throughout the country may be experiencing similar anxieties, concerns,
obstacles, fears, and feelings can enhance professional integration, self-
efficacy, motivation, persistence behaviors, and retention. Additionally,
the NSNA provides unique opportunities for mentoring by nursing
leaders and student leaders (Vance & Olson, 1998).

One benefit of the school's student nurse club (SNC) may be that all
nursing (and sometimes prenursing) students are usually considered
automatic members; new students are often welcomed by more advanced
students at a special event or ceremony. A second benefit is that students
can develop close networks and feelings of solidarity with other students
throughout the stages of the nursing program, thereby enhancing professional integration. Students involved in the SNC are often aware of
special nuances pertinent to that particular nursing program. Another
benefit of the SNC is the opportunity to interact with peers, faculty,
and/or nurses during SNC-sponsored social events. If positive psychological outcomes result, student motivation, persistence, and retention
will be enhanced.

Many specialty nursing organizations, such as the international
Transcultural Nursing Society, permit, solicit, and/or actively encourage
student nurse membership and participation. Other specialty nursing
organizations that permit student membership include the American
Association of Critical Care Nurses, the Association of Child and

Adolescent Psychiatric Nurses, Association of Nurses in AIDS Care, National Gerontological Nursing Organization, and International Association of Forensic Nurses. Specialty organizations provide additional opportunities for student nurses to network with other student nurses, as well as with registered nurses and noted leaders in the specialty field. Students who have a particular interest in a subfield of nursing may benefit greatly from early exposure to organizations and individuals with a shared interest, and may become more motivated through the positive role modeling, mentoring, and active encouragement by nursing professionals with similar specialty interests and goals. Ethnic nursing organizations, such as the National Black Nurses Association, and religious nursing organizations, such as the Nurses Christian Fellowship, provide opportunities for students to network with other student nurses and registered nurses with whom they closely identify in identity, background, ideals, and/or concerns. The positive influence of role models as mentors can greatly promote professional integration, satisfaction, stress reduction, self-efficacy, motivation, persistence behaviors, and retention.

Unfortunately, many nurse educators and nursing students undervalue and underestimate the significance of student memberships. Chapter 11 will describe strategies for enhancing professional integration and socialization via memberships.

PROFESSIONAL EVENTS

Professional events are nursing conferences, workshops, meetings, volunteer services, or social activities that have specific goals relevant for nursing education, practice, research, or theory. They are often sponsored by professional organizations or associations that actively encourage student participation and/or membership. Participation in professional events is valuable because it encourages interaction with other nursing students and nurses within a professional context (Joel & Kelly, 2002; Spickerman, 1988). Such events offer unique opportunities for students to engage in socialization activities and networking while expanding professional knowledge and skills. Nursing conferences and workshops exemplify a professional commitment to lifelong learning that can be motivating and uplifting to students. Professional nurses can serve as role models through their commitment to learning and the nursing profession. Positive role models can enhance self-efficacy and motivation, in turn enhancing persistence and retention.

Events that encourage active participation either through discussion or implementation of specific nursing roles offer students validation for their achievements thus far in their professional development and their educational process. For example, students who volunteer to assist a nursing organization with blood pressure screening at a community wellness fair gain personal and professional validation from nurses and peers and from members of the community as well. Validation is especially important for nontraditional students (older, commuter, and/or minority) and has been positively linked with persistence behaviors and retention (Rendon, 1994; Rendon, Jalomo, & Nora, 2000). Students who are recognized and thanked by members of the professional and lay community for their nursing knowledge, skill, and time are receiving positive feedback for their professional nursing actions.

It is proposed within the NURS model that positive experiences in professional event participation positively affect retention by enhancing self-efficacy and motivation, promoting professional integration, and facilitating positive psychological outcomes. Individual students may view the importance of professional events differently, necessitating individual appraisal on the part of the nurse educator. For example, if a nursing student views attendance at a professional conference as unimportant or fears feeling out of place, the student may never elect to attend a conference. His or her professional integration will be limited without the extra opportunities for peer interaction, faculty interaction outside the classroom, networking with nursing professionals, and/or exposure to the other benefits of professional nursing conferences. The use of network systems has been positively linked to enhanced persistence (Calder & Gordon, 1999). Strategies that enhance opportunities to participate in various professional integration factors will ultimately benefit students. Chapter 11 will discuss such creative strategies.

ENCOURAGEMENT BY FRIENDS IN CLASS

The higher education literature supports the idea that encouragement by friends in class has the potential to positively influence students' academic and psychological outcomes, persistence behaviors, and retention (Antonio, 2001; Braxton, 2000; Calder & Gordon, 1999; Kuh, 2001; Olenchak & Hebert, 2002; Skahill, 2002). The nursing education literature similarly acknowledges the significance of class friendships, especially among groups underrepresented in nursing (Ramsey et al., 2000; Tucker-Allen & Long, 1999; Weaver, 2001; Yurkovich, 2001). Accordingly, encouragement by friends in class is included as a component of the NURS model. It is proposed that encouragement by friends in class will actively promote positive psychological outcomes, self-efficacy, professional socialization, persistence, and retention. Lack of class friends will adversely affect retention through social isolation, dissatisfaction, stress, low self-efficacy, and decreased motivation.

Friends in class are peers who interact positively with each other by establishing and maintaining friendships in class that are continued within the context of the college learning environment. (Required off-campus clinical placement sites are considered to be part of the college learning environment.) Friends in class do not include family members. They are mutually bonded in career goals, expectations, and stage of educational and professional development. The main focus of in-class friends is on the common goal of successfully completing course require-ments and becoming a registered nurse. Friends in class may also elect to participate in outside social events; however, this element is secondary.

Encouragement by friends in class is the active emotional involvement of class friends in relation to the student's academic endeavors and career goals. Positive encouragement is manifested by supporting realistic career and educational goals, promoting positive feelings of self-worth, believing in the student's ability to succeed, listening to problems and concerns, showing interest in academic progress, expressing optimism, offering assistance, and presence. Mutual assistance or reciprocation of academic and nonacademic (emotional) supports by class friends can enhance confidence and independence. Friendships that encourage mutu-al reciprocation and individual independence, rather than dependence, can help with professional integration, growth, and development.

Pressure by friends to participate in outside activities (such as social engagements) that conflict with the student's ability to successfully com-plete academic and career goals is incongruent with positive encourage-ment behaviors. Becoming overly dependent on another student or attempting to cause dependence by others is equally incongruent. Positive encouragement behaviors recognize the unique contributions of the other class friend and facilitate mutual collaboration, with valued contri-butions from each individual, while promoting independent behaviors. An unequal balance between class friends is counterproductive to pro-fessional development and integration. Difficulty setting limits on friends and social activities negatively influences academic performance and retention (Campbell & Davis, 1996).

Nursing faculty and students alike may underestimate the potential influence of class friends on academic achievement, professional devel-opment, satisfaction, stress, and retention. Student perceptions about friendships, learning, education, and peers can be influenced by student profile characteristics, affective factors, and environmental factors. Among several samples of nontraditional associate degree students, approximately 80% of subjects perceived encouragement from friends in class as supporting retention. Most of the students were older (over 25) and were perhaps more experienced in maintaining friendships with people who provided encouragement (Jeffreys, 1993, 1998, 2001, 2002). Nurse educators may wish to further explore and consider the impact of class friends in relation to the student's age.

Although encouragement by in-class friends offers many unique advantages (see chapter 12), there are some limitations. One barrier to the potential benefits is that students may be reluctant to join new groups and make new friends. They may elect to band together with students of similar academic ability or background. Such banding together limits the diversity of ideas, views, and strategies that can enhance academic achievement and professional development. For example, weaker students may attempt to cluster together. Nurse educators have the unique opportunity to encourage the development of diverse, positive friendships in class through learning activities within the classroom, clinical work, and outside class assignments. Chapter 12 discusses strategies to promote positive peer interactions and maximize desired outcomes from in-class friendships.

Another limitation is that friends in class may be unable to see the whole picture, the rationale for prerequisites or sequencing of courses, benefits of course assignments within the whole scope of the educational process, preparation for the RN licensing exam, the next course, employment as a RN, or continued education. Class friends are at the same point in the educational process, so that their view of the interconnectedness between courses along the path to professional development is myopic, sometimes unknown, and prospective. In contrast, previous experience and retrospective appraisal can lead to a broader insight. Partnership connections with peer mentor-tutors who are further advanced in the educational process can assist in minimizing this limitation.

PEER MENTORING AND TUTORING

In the NURS model, peer mentoring and tutoring is a formalized, structured, collaborative partnership in learning and professional development between a peer mentor-tutor (PMT) and one or more students (protégé). A PMT is a student who is at a more advanced level of the educational process and who has demonstrated academic and professional excellence. Usually this means that the student is enrolled in a more advanced nursing course; however, an academically strong and caring peer-colleague could serve as a peer mentor-tutor. With a peer-colleague, the role of tutor would probably be more dominant than the mentor role because both students would be at the same point in the educational process; therefore, the experience of connecting pieces along the educational journey would be limited.

The NURS model proposes that peer mentoring and tutoring offers the utmost possibility in professional integration and socialization. Although mentoring alone can have positive effects on professional integration and socialization, it is presumed that tutoring alone does not have this effect. Peer tutoring focuses solely on the learning of cognitive knowledge and/or psychomotor skills, rather than affective learning; therefore, it may do little in the realm of professional integration and socialization. As conceptualized here, tutoring is not interchangeable with remediation, but instead emphasizes enrichment and enhancement. Remediation focuses on fixing deficits in students who have not mastered basic skills and knowledge, whereas the tutoring component in the NURS model focuses on realistic self-appraisal of strengths and weaknesses, maximizing strengths, addressing weaknesses, and assisting students in achieving their optimal academic potential. Peer tutoring without mentoring, however, does not enhance professional integration and socialization to any great degree.

In mentoring, professional nursing values, beliefs, practices, expectations, and attitudes can be nurtured. The "mentor connection is a developmental, empowering, and nurturing relationship extending over time in which mutual sharing, learning, and growth occur in an atmosphere of respect, collegiality, and affirmation" (Vance & Olson, 1998, p. 5). Both the mentor and the mentee will benefit from their interactions, thus enhancing their professional integration, socialization, and acculturation into the nursing student role and future RN role. Furthermore, the opportunity to share experiences and watch role models and peers struggle with similar academic and nonacademic challenges can help increase self-efficacy and motivation to persist (Bandura, 1986; Zimmerman, 1995).

"Mentoring is complex and elusive—difficult to define and to measure. It cannot be seen, but is a powerful, enriching phenomenon that can be described by those who experience it" (Vance & Olson, 1998, p. 5). For example, quantitative results from students participating in study groups led by peer mentor-tutors indicated that participants were greatly satisfied with their interactions. Respondents indicated that their tutoring experience enhanced retention. Qualitative comments from student participants substantiated and added richness to the quantitative data by describing the positive emotional and academic outcomes from their experience with their PMTs. Several students who were mentored then became PMTs, further enriching their opportunities for professional growth and development. Many students reported that they now aimed for a higher level of academic and professional excellence, rather than merely settling for minimal achievement levels or passing standards. Furthermore, many students were motivated to persist in their nursing courses beyond the associate degree because of the influence of their PMTs, who were RNs enrolled in the RN-to-BSN program (Jeffreys, 2001, 2002).

In the NURS model, peer mentoring and tutoring enhance professional integration and socialization. They can maximize academic achievement, promote positive psychological outcomes, encourage self-efficacy and motivation, facilitate persistence behaviors, and enhance retention, assisting students maximally in achieving positive outcomes. Nurse educators can develop creative strategies for fostering peer mentoring and tutoring partnerships individually or as a component of an enrichment program (EP). Chapters 12 and 13 will provide examples.

ENRICHMENT PROGRAMS

An enrichment program (EP) is a formally designed multiservice program that aims to enrich the total nursing student experience by maximizing strengths, remedying weaknesses, promoting positive psychological outcomes, facilitating positive academic outcomes, and nurturing professional growth and development. Services may include several of the following: orientation, mentoring, tutoring, newsletters, career advisement and guidance, workshops, study groups, networking, transitional support, financial stipends, and referral. Services are best facilitated through a collaborative partnership in learning and professional development between nursing faculty, other professional nurses, and students. Enrichment programs are different than remedial programs; however, students and faculty alike often do not distinguish between the two. Misperceptions about enrichment programs create barriers. Because remedial programs are often criticized and stigmatized, students may be reluctant to participate in EPs. Similarly, nursing faculty may not appropriately advocate and support enrichment programs. Assuming that EPs are only appropriate for the academically weak or struggling student limits the immense possibilities that a well-designed EP can offer. Nurse educators should recognize that all students benefit from various forms of academic and emotional support throughout all stages of the educational process, especially during key transitional phases (Courage & Godbey, 1992; Schön, 1987).

The most successful EPs offer a coordinated integration of proactive, ongoing, and transitional interventions that are free and available to all nursing students throughout the educational process. Proactive interventions are implemented before the beginning of the semester and aim to prepare students academically, psychologically, and practically for the new semester, and focus on enhanced performance, satisfaction, and success. Ongoing interventions aim to maximize success by the early identification of strengths and weaknesses before academic difficulties, role conflicts, or stresses arise. Early identification of the at-risk student can prevent failure or withdrawal. Often students do not seek help until difficulty arises, and then it can be too late to improve an academically precarious situation. Therefore, nurse educators should be actively involved on an ongoing basis to assist students, especially because at-risk students often do not initiate adaptive and active help-seeking behaviors (Alexitch, 2002).

As students move from one phase of the educational process to the next, transitional interventions should be implemented (Schon, 1987). Transition from preprofessional to professional education (first nursing course) and from one nursing course to the next level nursing course challenges students to embark on a new, unknown path in their journey toward becoming a registered nurse. Guidance at these transitional stages is crucial for self-efficacy, motivation, satisfaction, stress reduction, academic achievement, and retention. It is proposed that students who actively engage in EP services throughout the educational process will be exposed to more opportunities to interact with peers, students in various stages of the educational process, faculty, nurses, and college staff. This increased interaction has the potential to enhance professional integration. Additionally, it has the potential to positively influence self-efficacy and motivation. Students who perceive such interaction as beneficial will have more positive psychological outcomes (satisfaction and stress reduction) and maximized potential for positive academic outcomes. Consequently, persistence behaviors and retention will be enhanced.

The results of several studies using samples of EP study group participants indicated that the intervention (EP) group had lower failure rates, lower withdrawal rates, higher course success rates, and positive psychological outcomes (satisfaction). Social integration variables, such as faculty advisement and helpfulness, tutoring, and the EP, were perceived as highly supportive (Jeffreys, 2001, 2002). High student satisfaction with the EP and perceptions that the EP supported retention emphasize the ongoing need for innovative strategies that enrich the nursing student experience. Additionally, the nursing and higher education literature strongly advocates retention programs that incorporate academic and nonacademic components. Enrichment program design, implementation, and evaluation should be a systematic and well-planned process. Chapter 13 presents the eleven-step process that can guide EP development; a case exemplar is also provided.

KEY POINTS SUMMARY

- Professional integration factors are those that enhance students' interaction with the social system of the college environment within the context of professional socialization and career development. These factors include nursing faculty advisement and helpfulness, memberships in professional organizations, professional events, encouragement by friends in class, enrichment programs, and peer mentoring and tutoring.
- Professional integration factors are at the center of the NURS model because it is believed that they are at the crossroads of the decision to persist, drop out, or stop out.
- Lack of professional integration increases the risk of attrition, whereas strong professional integration increases commitment, persistence behaviors, and retention.
- Faculty advisement and helpfulness means the active involvement of nursing faculty in the student's academic endeavors, career goals, and professional socialization.
- Memberships refer to affiliation or participation in nursing organizations or associations as a member, as prescribed by the respective bylaws.
- Professional events are nursing conferences, workshops, meetings, volunteer services, or social activities that have specific goals relevant for nursing education, practice, research, or theory.
- Encouragement by friends in class is the active emotional involvement of class friends in relation to the student's academic endeavors and career goals. Positive encouragement is manifested by supporting realistic career and educational goals, promoting positive feelings of self-worth, believing in the student's ability to succeed, listening to problems and concerns, showing interest in academic progress, expressing optimism, offering assistance, and presence.
- Peer mentoring and tutoring is a formalized, structured, collaborative partnership in learning and professional development between a peer mentor-tutor (PMT) and one or more students (protégé).
- An enrichment program (EP) is a formally designed multiservice program that aims to enrich the total nursing student experience by

maximizing strengths, remedying weaknesses, promoting positive psychological outcomes, facilitating positive academic outcomes, and nurturing professional growth and development. Services may include several of the following: orientation, mentoring, tutoring, newsletters, career advisement and guidance, workshops, study groups, networking, transitional support, financial stipends, and referral.

- Nurse educators are the key initiators and advocates of professional integration because they have the power to actively promote enrichment programs, professional events, memberships, encouragement by friends in class, and peer mentoring-tutoring.

EDUCATOR-IN-ACTION

After teaching for one year in an undergraduate nursing program, Professor Change concludes that student opportunities for professional integration and socialization are few, disconnected, and virtually invisible within the existing curriculum. Nursing program retention rates have declined; NCLEX pass rates on the first attempt have also decreased. During the curriculum committee meeting, Professor Change proposes that faculty work together to carefully plan and coordinate strategies to enhance professional integration and socialization throughout the curriculum. Furthermore, she suggests that strategies be purposely designed to complement each other so that professional integration, socialization, and development are visible vertical threads that creatively combine cognitive, affective, and practical dimensions. Consider the following faculty responses:

Professor Always: "We have always had the curriculum this way. We have always had some students who either pass, fail, stop out, drop out, or graduate. It will always happen no matter what we do."

Professor Solo: "We all work individually on our own courses. Every teacher is responsible for including a professional development objective in the course outline."

Professor Waver: "Well, maybe we should think about doing something different, but maybe we should just leave things the way they are."

Professor Sloth: "That sounds like a lot of work. If students just worked harder, they would be more successful. We shouldn't be the ones doing extra work."

Professor Challenger: "What proof do you have that professional integration and socialization is insufficient? How do you know that more opportunities would make a difference?"

Fortunately, two other nursing faculty members support Professor Change's idea and suggest that further exploration of this topic is warranted. Although Professor Change suggests a faculty development workshop with a featured guest speaker knowledgeable in this area, some faculty members are reluctant to allocate funds and their personal time to this event. Professor Change offers to provide faculty with several key articles and chapters concerning this topic prior to the next meeting. At the next meeting, she distributes a handout summarizing key points, a select bibliography of relevant nursing and higher education literature, and two books and three articles for quick reference. Additionally, she introduces two nursing students who were invited to discuss issues related to opportunities for professional integration and socialization within the curriculum. Students report:

Donna: "I am in my last semester of nursing. This is the first semester I was ever invited to attend a nursing conference by my instructor. I didn't even know there were so many nursing conferences available for students to attend. Professor Change arranged for me and two other students to attend free in return for helping with the registration. Nurses were so friendly and treated us like part of the profession. It motivated me to try harder. I wish I had had other opportunities earlier in nursing."

Jerry: "Last semester I was thinking about dropping out of school. There are no other men in my clinical group and there were no male nurses on the hospital unit so I really felt out of place. Then I saw a male student in the library reading a nursing textbook so I asked him if he liked nursing. He was in his last semester and told me about some positive experiences and about dealing effectively with negative experiences. I decided not to drop out. Now I try to encourage other nursing students in the library whenever I see them."

Later, faculty agree that curricular concept mapping and strategy mapping will be conducted after attending a three-hour faculty development workshop on "Promoting Achievement and Retention by Enhancing Opportunities for Professional Integration and Socialization in the Curriculum."

REFERENCES AND BIBLIOGRAPHY

Alexitch, L. R. (2002). The role of help-seeking attitudes and tendencies in students' preferences for academic advising. *Journal of College Student Development, 43*(1), 5–19.

Alvarez, A., & Abriam-Yago, K. (1993). Mentoring undergraduate ethnic-minority students: A strategy for retention. *Journal of Nursing Education, 32*(5), 230–232.

Antonio, A. L. (2001). Diversity and the influence of friendship groups in college. *Review of Higher Education, 25*(1), 63–89.

Baldwin, D., & Wold, J. (1993). Students from disadvantaged backgrounds: Satisfaction with a mentor-protégé relationship. *Journal of Nursing Education, 32*(5), 225–226.

Bandura, A. (1986). *Social foundations of thought and action: A social cognitive theory.* Englewood Cliffs, NJ: Prentice-Hall.

Bean, J. P., & Metzner, B. (1985). A conceptual model of nontraditional undergraduate student attrition. *Review of Educational Research, 55*, 485–540.

Bessent, H. (Ed.). (1997). *Strategies for recruitment, retention, and graduation of minority nurses in colleges of nursing.* Washington, DC: American Nurses Publishing.

Betts, V. T., & Cherry, B. (2002). Health policy and politics. In B. Cherry & S. R. Jacob (Eds.), *Contemporary nursing: Issues, trends, and management* (2nd ed., pp. 219–235). Philadelphia: Mosby.

Braxton, J. M. (Ed.). (2000). *Reworking the student departure puzzle.* Nashville, TN: Vanderbilt University Press.

Braxton, J. M., & McClendon, S. A. (2001). The fostering of social integration and retention through institutional practice. *Journal of College Student Retention: Research, Theory, & Practice, 3*(1), 57–72.

Braxton, J. M., & Mundy, M. E. (2001). Powerful institutional levers to reduce college student departure. *Journal of College Student Retention: Research, Theory, & Practice, 3*(1), 91–118.

Brockopp, D., Schooler, M., Welsh, D., Cassidy, K., Ryan, P. Y., Mueggenberg, K., & Orr Chlebowy, D. (2003). Sponsored professional seminars: Enhancing professionalism among baccalaureate nursing students. *Journal of Nursing Education, 42*(12), 562–564.

Calder, W. B., & Gordon, W. (1999). Institutionalizing college networks for student success. *Journal of College Student Retention: Research, Theory, and Practice, 1*(4), 323–333.

Cameron-Buccheri, R., & Trygstad, L. (1989). Retaining freshman nursing students. *Nursing and Health Care, 10*(7), 389–393.

Campbell, A. R., & Davis, S. M. (1996). Faculty commitment: Retaining minority nursing students in majority institutions. *Journal of Nursing Education, 35*(7), 298–303.

Campbell, T. A., & Campbell, D. E. (1997). Faculty/student mentor program: Effects on academic performance and retention. *Research in Higher Education, 38*(6), 727–742.

Chaney, B., Muraskin, L. D., Cahalan, M. W., & Goodwin, D. (1998). Helping the progress of disadvantaged students in higher education: The federal student support services program. *Educational Evaluation and Policy Analysis, 20*(3), 197–215.

Christman, L. (1997). Socialization to professional nursing roles. In B. Kozier, G. Erb, & K. Blais (Eds.), *Professional nursing practice: Concepts and perspectives* (p. 127). New York: Addison-Wesley.

Cook, T. H., Gilmer, M. J., & Bess, C. J. (2003). Beginning students' definitions of nursing: An inductive framework of professional identity. *Journal of Nursing Education, 42*(7), 311–317.

Courage, M. M., & Godbey, K. L. (1992). Student retention: Policies and services to enhance persistence to graduation. *Nurse Educator, 17*(2), 29–32.

Davis, J. E. (1995). College in black and white: Campus environment and academic achievement of African American males. *Journal of Negro Education, 63*(4), 620–633.

Diekelmann, N. (1993). Spending time with students: Keeping my door open. *Journal of Nursing Education, 32*(4), 149–150.

Fleming, J. (2002). Who will succeed in college? When the SAT predicts black students' performance. *Review of Higher Education, 25*(3), 281–296.

Hernandez, J. C. (2000). Understanding the retention of Latino college students. *Journal of College Student Development, 41*(6), 575–588.

Herndon, J. B., Kaiser, J., & Creamer, D. G. (1996). Student preferences for advising style in community college environments. *Journal of College Student Development, 37*(6), 637–647.

Hesser, A., Pond, E., Lewis, L., & Abbott, B. (1996). Evaluation of a supplementary retention program for African-American baccalaureate nursing students. *Journal of Nursing Education, 35*(7), 304–309.

Hinderlie, H. H., & Kenny, M. (2002). Attachment, social support, and college adjustment among black students at predominantly white universities. *Journal of College Student Development, 43*(3), 327–340.

Hoffman, M., Richmond, J., Morrow, J., & Salomone, K. (2002). Investigating "sense of belonging" in first-year college students. *Journal of College Student Retention: Research, Theory, & Practice, 4*(3), 227–256.

Jeffreys, M. R. (1993). *The relationship of self-efficacy and select academic and environmental variables on academic achievement and retention.* Unpublished doctoral dissertation, Teachers College, Columbia University, New York.

Jeffreys, M. R. (1998). Predicting nontraditional student retention and academic achievement. *Nurse Educator, 23*(1), 42–48.

Jeffreys, M. R. (2001). Evaluating enrichment program study groups: Academic outcomes, psychological outcomes, and variables influencing retention. *Nurse Educator, 26*(3), 142–149.

Jeffreys, M. R. (2002). Students' perceptions of variables influencing retention: A pretest and post-test approach. *Nurse Educator, 27*(1), 16–19 [Erratum, 2002, 27(2), 64].

Joel, L. A., & Kelly, L. Y. (2002). *The nursing experience: Trends, challenges, and transitions.* New York: McGraw-Hill.

Kirkpatrick, M. K., & Koldjeski, D. (1997). Career planning: The nurse educator as facilitator and career counselor. *Nurse Educator, 27*(3), 17–20.

Kozier, B., Erb, G., & Blais, K. (1997). *Professional nursing practice: Concepts and perspectives.* New York: Addison-Wesley.

Kraemer, B. A. (1997). The academic and social integration of Hispanic students into college. *Review of Higher Education, 20*(2), 163–179.

Kuh, G. D. (2001). Organizational culture and student persistence: Prospects and puzzles. *Journal of College Student Retention: Research, Theory, & Practice, 3*(1), 23–40.

Lehna, C., Jackonen, S., & Wilson, L. (1996). Navigating a nursing curriculum: Bridges and barriers. *Association for Black Nursing Faculty Journal, 7*(July/August), 98–103.

Leininger, M. M. (1995). *Transcultural nursing: Concepts, theories, research and practice.* Blacklick, OH: McGraw-Hill College Custom Services.

Leininger, M. M., & McFarland, M. R. (2002). *Transcultural nursing: Concepts, theories, research, and practice* (3rd ed.). New York: McGraw-Hill.

Mancuso, S. (2001). Adult-centered practices: Benchmarking study in higher education. *Innovative Higher Education, 25*(3), 165–181.

Mayo, J. R., Murguia, E., & Padilla, R. V. (1995). Social integration and academic performance among minority university students. *Journal of College Student Development, 36*(6), 542–552.

Merrill, E. B. (1998). Culturally diverse students enrolled in nursing: Barriers influencing success. *Journal of Cultural Diversity, 5*(2), 58–67.

Milem, J. F., & Berger, J. B. (1997). A modified model of college student persistence: Exploring the relationship between Astin's theory of involvement and Tinto's theory of student departure. *Journal of College Student Development, 38*(4), 387–400.

Metzner, B. (1989). Perceived quality of academic advising: The effect on freshman attrition. *American Educational Research Journal, 26,* 422–442.

Metzner, B., & Bean, J. P. (1987). The estimation of a conceptual model of non-traditional undergraduate student attrition. *Research in Higher Education, 27,* 15–38.

Mohr, J. J., Eiche, K. D., & Sedlacek, W. E. (1998). So close, yet so far: Predictors of attrition in college seniors. *Journal of College Student Development, 39*(4), 343–354.

Mozingo, J., Thomas, S., & Brooks, E. (1995). Factors associated with perceived competency levels of graduating seniors in a baccalaureate nursing program. *Journal of Nursing Education, 34*(3), 115–122.

Myton, C. L., Allen, J. K., & Baldwin, J. A. (1992). Students in transition: Services for retention and outplacement. *Nursing Outlook, 35*(1), 227–230.

Nora, A. (1987). Determinants of retention among Chicano college students: A structural model. *Research in Higher Education, 26,* 31–60.

Nora, A. (2001). The depiction of significant others in Tinto's "Rites of Passage": A reconceptualization of the influence of family and community in the persistence process. *Journal of College Student Retention: Research, Theory, & Practice, 3*(1), 41–56.

Nora, A., & Cabrera, A. F. (1996). The role of perceptions of prejudice and discrimination on the adjustment of minority students to college. *Journal of Higher Education, 67*(2), 119–148.

Olenchak, F. R., & Hebert, T. P. (2002). Endangered academic talent: Lessons learned from gifted first-generation college males. *Journal of College Student Development, 43*(2), 195–212.

Pascarella, E. T., & Chapman, D. W. (1983). Validation of a theoretical model of college withdrawal: Interaction effects in a multi-institutional sample. *Research in Higher Education, 19,* 25–47.

Perry, L. (1997). The Bridge Program: An overview. *Association of Black Nursing Faculty Journal, 8*(1), 4–7.

Poorman, S. G., Webb, C. A., & Mastorovich, M. L. (2002). Students' stories: How faculty help and hinder students at risk. *Nurse Educator, 27*(3), 126–131.

Ramsey, P., Blowers, S., Merriman, C., Glenn, L. L., & Terry, L. (2000). The NURSE Center: A peer mentor-tutor project for disadvantaged nursing students in Appalachia. *Nurse Educator, 25*(6), 277–281.

Reed, S. B., & Hudepohl, N. C. (1985). High-risk nursing students, part 3: Evaluating a student retention program. *Nurse Educator, 10*(5), 32–38.

Rendon, L. I. (1994). Validating culturally diverse students: Toward a new model of learning and student development. *Innovative Higher Education, 19*(1), 23–32.

Rendon, L. I., Jalomo, R. E., & Nora, A. (2000). Theoretical considerations in the study of minority student retention in higher education. In J. M. Braxton (Ed.), *Reworking the student departure puzzle* (pp. 127–156). Nashville, TN: Vanderbilt University Press.

Rew, L. (1996). Affirming cultural diversity: A pathways model for nursing faculty. *Journal of Nursing Education, 35*(7), 310–314.

Schön, D. (1987). *Educating the reflective practitioner.* San Francisco: Jossey-Bass.

Schultz, E. D. (1998). Academic advising from a nursing theory perspective. *Nurse Educator, 22*(2), 22–25.

Schwitzer, A., & Thomas, C. (1998). Implementation, utilization, and outcomes of a minority freshman peer mentor program at a predominantly white university. *Journal of the Freshman Year Experience, 10*(1), 31–50.

Sherrod, R. A., & Harrison, L. (1994). Evaluation of a comprehensive advisement program designed to enhance student retention. *Nurse Educator, 19*(6), 29–33.

Skaggs, B. J., & deVries, C. M. (1998). You and your professional organization. In D. J. Mason & J. K. Leavitt (Eds.), *Policy and politics in nursing and health care* (pp. 535–542). New York: W. B. Saunders.

Skahill, M. P. (2002). The role of social support network in college persistence among freshman students. *Journal of College Student Retention: Research, Theory, & Practice, 4*(1), 39–52.

Spady, W. (1970). Dropouts from higher education: Toward an empirical model. *Interchange, 2,* 38–62.

Spickerman, S. (1988). Enhancing the socialization process. *Nurse Educator, 13*(6), 10–14.

Tayebi, K., Moore-Jazayeri, M., & Maynard, T. (1998). From the borders: Reforming the curriculum for the at-risk student. *Journal of Cultural Diversity, 5,* 101–109.

Terenzini, P. T., Pascarella, E. T., & Blimling, G. S. (1996). Students' out-of-class experiences and their influence on learning and cognitive development: A literature review. *Journal of College Student Development, 37*(2), 149–162.

Thurber, F., Hollingsworth, A., Brown, L., & Whitaker, S. (1989). The faculty advisor role: An imperative for student retention. *Nurse Educator, 13*(3), 27–33.

Tinto, V. (1975). Dropout from higher education: A theoretical synthesis of recent research. *Review of Educational Research, 45,* 89–125.

Tinto, V. (1997). Classrooms as communities. *Journal of Higher Education, 68*(6), 599–623.

Tinto, V. (2000). Linking learning and leaving: Exploring the role of the college classroom in student departure. In J. M. Braxton (Ed.), *Reworking the student departure puzzle* (pp. 81–94). Nashville, TN: Vanderbilt University Press.

Trent, B. A. (1997). Student perceptions of academic advising in an RN-to-BSN program. *Journal of Continuing Education in Nursing, 28*(6), 276–283.

Tucker-Allen, S., & Long, E. (1999). *Recruitment and retention of minority students: Stories of success.* Lisle, IL: Tucker.

Vance, C., & Olson, R. K. (1998). *The mentor connection in nursing.* New York: Springer.

Villaruel, A. M., Canales, M., & Torres, S. (2001). Bridges and barriers: Educational mobility of Hispanic nurses. *Journal of Nursing Education, 40*(6), 245–251.

Wang, H., & Grimes, J. W. (2000). A systematic approach to assessing retention programs: Identifying critical points for meaningful interventions and validating outcomes assessment. *Journal of College Student Retention: Research, Theory, & Practice, 2*(1), 59–68.

Weaver, H. N. (2001). Indigenous nurses and professional education: Friends or foes? *Journal of Nursing Education, 40*(6), 252–258.

Wilson, S. B., Mason, T. W., & Ewing, M. J. M. (1997). Evaluating the impact of receiving university-based counseling services on student retention. *Journal of Counseling Psychology, 44*(3), 316–320.

Winters, C. E. (1990). Excellence in advisement: A strategy for declining nursing enrollments. *Journal of Nursing Education, 29*(5), 233–234.

Wolahan, C. G., & Wieczorek, R. R. (1991). Enrichment education: Key to NCLEX success. *Nursing and Health Care, 12*(5), 234–239.

Yurkovich, E. E. (2001). Working with American Indians toward educational success. *Journal of Nursing Education, 40*(6), 259–269.

Zimmerman, B. J. (1995). Self-efficacy and educational development. In A. Bandura (Ed.), *Self-efficacy in changing societies* (pp. 202–231). New York: Cambridge University Press.

Chapter 7

Academic and Psychological Outcomes

The general college experience involves multiple psychological and developmental opportunities and outcomes, beyond course grades or GPA. The complex nursing educational experience offers unique professional, discipline-specific, psychological and developmental opportunities and outcomes beyond course grades or GPA. Outcome expectations include learning, personal growth, and satisfaction. Students anticipate gaining more benefits than knowledge alone; therefore, any analysis of student outcomes should recognize various dimensions (Toutkoushian & Smart, 2001). Occasionally, academic outcome is the *only* variable considered in achievement and retention studies, thereby omitting nonacademic outcomes that may greatly influence both achievement and retention.

As presented in the NURS model, student profile characteristics, student affective factors, academic factors, environmental factors, and professional integration factors interact and result in a range of academic and psychological outcomes. Outside and surrounding factors may also impact on academic and psychological outcomes. Academic outcomes are represented by the student's nursing course grade, cumulative GPA for nursing courses, and overall GPA. Psychological outcomes include satisfaction and stress. Both academic and psychological outcomes influence persistence and retention (Bean & Eaton, 2000). Furthermore, academic and psychological outcomes interact and impact upon self-efficacy, motivation, persistence, and retention.

As originally proposed by Bean and Metzner (1985), nonacademic factors may compensate for low levels of academic success, and yet high levels of academic success result in persistence and continued enrollment only when accompanied by positive psychological outcomes. For nursing students, good academic performance results in retention only when accompanied by positive psychological outcomes for the nursing program and profession. In the NURS model, positive psychological outcomes include satisfaction and low (manageable) stress. In contrast, negative psychological outcomes include dissatisfaction and high stress. Although the constructs of satisfaction and stress seem dichotomous, in reality they are not. Even the use of a continuum of satisfaction or stress is insufficient in capturing the multidimensional and intertwining phenomenon of satisfaction and stress. This chapter will address pertinent issues surrounding academic outcomes and psychological outcomes (satisfaction and stress), present proposed relationships with other variables in the NURS model, and suggest implications for nurse educators.

ACADEMIC OUTCOMES

The academic outcome most frequently measured in persistence and retention studies is GPA. Unfortunately, retention studies in higher education may not differentiate between majors, thereby confounding results. For example, a student may fail a course, yet still have a GPA high enough to avoid probation or dismissal from the college or nursing program. The NURS model proposes that persistence and attrition decisions occur during and after each individual nursing course, and so course grade is included as an essential academic outcome measure. Looking at GPA alone is insufficient in determining progression within the nursing curriculum. Conducting discipline-specific retention studies allows for assessment of the particular nuances of a discipline.

Generalization in attrition research is difficult because institutional and program differences present extraneous variables (Eaton & Bean, 1995). Whereas the big picture may be college (institutional) retention, the NURS model allows for investigation at the course and program level. For this reason, course grade is included. Nursing course grade certainly impacts upon nursing major GPA and overall college GPA, which in turn influence attrition. For example, a student may successfully complete a nursing course yet still be dismissed from the college if other non-nursing courses lower overall GPA. Consequently, nursing course grade, nursing GPA, and overall GPA are all important academic measures to assess when seeking to identify at-risk students. Any low or failed academic outcome measure places a student at risk for attrition.

Established policies concerning progression in the nursing curriculum require minimum standards for nursing courses, non-nursing required courses, nursing GPA, overall GPA, minimum course grades for repeated courses, and progression in the curriculum. Whether nursing program retention policies are the same as or different from general college policies can skew retention rate results for nursing when contrasted with other majors or the college in general. Such policy differences should be considered when comparing data. Policy differences may also affect retention indirectly through satisfaction and stress.

Course grades and GPA may seem to allow for direct comparison from course to course; however, methods of evaluation differ between courses and instructors, skewing a seemingly straightforward quantitative measure (calculation). Comparisons will always contain some degree of error. Because error is often overlooked when using academic outcome measures, further scrutiny and data analysis are warranted. Academic outcomes (course grades) may sometimes be collapsed into categories for the purpose of data analysis and descriptive statistics. For example, academic outcomes may be divided into pass, fail, or withdrawal. Theoretically, any student who achieves a passing grade can progress in the curriculum as expected. Students who withdraw or fail are at risk for nursing program attrition, either involuntarily or voluntarily, and are greatly influenced by nursing program progression policies. For example, a policy that requires students who withdraw or fail to reapply or file an appeal to continue in the nursing program discourages program retention. However, the need to assure client safety and maintain professional standards outweighs the risks of lenient retention policies. Screening reapplicants offers nurse educators an opportunity to proactively assist such at-risk students through the individual appraisal of their strengths and weaknesses and through the design of diagnostic-prescriptive support strategies for them. For some students, counseling and guidance recommending delayed continuation in the nursing program or alternate career options may be indicated (Myton, Allen, & Baldwin, 1992).

Advantages of pass rate calculations include the ability to compare from year to year and to notice changes after intervention strategies are initiated. Even a moderate improvement in retention (course pass rates), with other variables kept constant, supports continuation of the retention strategies. Examining trends over time, as strategies are continued and/or expanded lends support for ongoing interventions. Frequently, academic outcome measures are the yardstick that funding agencies and institutions use to determine continued or canceled support. Therefore, it behooves nurse educators to exercise great care in determining what academic outcome measures will be appraised and to control for extraneous variables that might skew results, making them invalid or impractical. A rise in course pass rates needs to be viewed in relation to achievement in subsequent courses, graduation, and RN licensing exam pass rate. In other words, high course pass rates as a result of low standards defeats the desired outcome of the NURS model, which addresses not only retention but emphasizes program success. Program success includes the desired outcomes of graduation, passing the RN licensing exam, obtaining employment as a registered nurse, and/or enrolling in an advanced educational nursing program.

Academic outcomes are complex beyond a mere numerical calculation. A calculation does not tell educators if minimum or maximum effort was expended or if there were other factors that influenced academic outcomes. Furthermore, the course grade or GPA may have a different meaning to the nurse educator and the academic institution than to the individual student. The same academic outcome (nursing course grade, nursing GPA, or cumulative GPA) may hold different meanings for different students. For example, to the nurse educator and the academic institution, a B grade in nursing may mean "above average," "program retention," and "continued enrollment;" however, an "A" student who exerted much energy, time, and commitment toward a course may be dissatisfied or distressed over a "B" grade. Another student who works full-time and is a single parent may feel satisfaction and (stress) relief after earning a "B" grade.

Table 7.1 contrasts student responses to several positive academic outcomes. To the institutional researcher, nurse educator, or college administrator, all of the academic outcomes would appear to lead to retention. Using just an academic outcome criterion measure, students would be viewed as low attrition risk; however, this conclusion is incorrect. Clearly, academic outcomes cannot be viewed without the understanding and exploration of psychological outcomes.

PSYCHOLOGICAL OUTCOMES

Satisfaction

Student satisfaction strongly influences persistence and retention. Unmet expectations and unrealistic assumptions put the nursing student at risk for dissatisfaction and attrition (Yoder & Saylor, 2002). In this book, dissatisfaction refers to the emotional discontent that arises from the discrepancy between expected academic, developmental, personal, and/or professional outcomes from the nursing educational process, and what actually occurs. Satisfaction refers to the emotional gratification that arises from the congruency between expected academic, developmental, personal, and/or professional outcomes from the nursing educational process and what actually occurs.

TABLE 7.1   Student Psychological Outcome Responses to Positive Academic Outcomes

Positive Academic Outcome	Positive Psychological Outcomes (High satisfaction or satisfaction, low stress, manageable stress, or stress relief)	Negative Psychological Outcomes (Low satisfaction or dissatisfaction, high stress or unmanageable stress)
B+ grade in nursing course	"Between working full-time, taking care of the kids, and going to school, I am so happy and relieved to get a B+ grade."	"I can't believe this B+ grade messes up my 4.0 GPA. I'm really dissatisfied and distressed."
75 (passing) grade in first nursing course	"After this first class, I know nursing is the career for me. I was stressed out in the beginning because I wasn't sure, but now I'm sure. I'll try to get higher grades next semester."	"I really thought nursing was different. I don't like it at all. I almost wish I failed so I would have an excuse to change my major. I feel more stressed now than if I failed."
A- grade in nursing course	"I got the grade I deserved and I'm so relieved."	"It's too much stress, between work, school, and family responsibilities."
"Pass" grade in clinical component	"I really worked hard in clinical and learned a lot. The instructor made some good comments and suggestions."	"All that work, time, and stress in clinical and all I get is a Pass. What difference do the instructor's comments make?"

Positive Academic Outcome	Positive Psychological Outcomes (High satisfaction or satisfaction, low stress, manageable stress, or stress relief)	Negative Psychological Outcomes (Low satisfaction or dissatisfaction, high stress or unmanageable stress)
2.9 nursing course GPA	"I wish my nursing course GPA was higher. I tried my best so I just have to be satisfied."	"Only a 2.9. All I ever wanted to be was a pediatric nurse practitioner. I'll never get into a NP program now."
3.7 nursing course GPA	"Great, I made the dean's list this time. I can't wait to start critical care next semester."	"Now everyone will always expect me to excel. I feel so much pressure."
3.0 overall cumulative GPA	"Nursing really is different than other courses I've taken. My GPA dropped with nursing courses, but I love nursing. I'm learning so much so it's OK."	"Why does nursing have to be so different from other courses? My friends in other majors have higher GPAs and don't work half as hard as me."
3.2 overall cumulative GPA	"I really like going to this college. Everyone is so helpful. I feel welcome and included in many of the college and professional events."	"I hate this college. It's so hard to get help around here. I have never felt so out of place."

The nursing educational experience results in varying degrees of satisfying and/or dissatisfying outcomes. Perceived satisfaction varies among students and within students at different times. The impact of satisfaction on intent to persist, persistence behaviors, and retention may affect various student subgroups differently. Similarly, the impact of dissatisfaction on withdrawal cognitions (thoughts of withdrawal), dropout behavior, and attrition varies accordingly. The higher education literature addresses the impact of satisfaction on various student subgroups. Studies on retention have typically targeted beginning students, because of high attrition rates; however, retention among other student populations must be considered as well. Studies among senior baccalaureate students have shown that dissatisfaction was a statistically significant predictor of attrition (Mohr, Eiche, & Sedlacek, 1998). Studies of minority student attrition and retention note the significance of satisfaction as a variable influencing academic achievement, persistence, and retention (Constantine & Watt, 2002; Mayo, Murguia, & Padilla, 1995; Solis, 1995). Despite high levels of academic performance, minority students with low levels of satisfaction were at greater attrition risk than non-minority students. Satisfaction is believed to be more important for female college students than for males (Bean & Bradley, 1986). However, this finding may not be generalizable to nursing. In a predominantly female profession, more studies on male students' satisfaction and retention are needed.

The overall college, individual departments, and specific academic programs influence student satisfaction, which in turn influences academic outcomes, persistence, and retention. Satisfaction with faculty, peers, and facilities affects overall college satisfaction (Liegler, 1997). Satisfaction with particular student services, such as academic advisement or the mentor–protégé relationship, can also impact on the overall college experience, thereby affecting academic outcomes, persistence, and retention (Baldwin & Wold, 1993; Cameron-Buccheri & Trygstad, 1989; Metzner, 1989; Mohr et al., 1998).

Satisfying and rewarding interactions in college lead to greater integration and persistence. Unpleasant or limited interactions lead to decreased persistence. Psychosocial outcomes, such as satisfaction, mediate academic and persistence outcomes (Napoli & Wortman, 1998). Working backwards in the NURS model, persistence or departure behavior is directly influenced by two dimensions of outcomes: academic and psychological. Satisfaction is also influenced by self-efficacy through self-perceptions of ability and effort expenditure (Greene & Miller, 1996).

Through their psychological model of attrition, Eaton and Bean (1995) propose that students who take an active approach and responsibility for learning are more satisfied. Students satisfied with their academic performance become more academically integrated, and self-perceptions of future academic integration are positively influenced. In contrast, those who avoid responsibility for learning are more dissatisfied, often with the result of poor academic outcomes and lowered self-efficacy, whereby students envision a bleak academic future. This proposition has been empirically supported in nursing. Nursing students who participated consistently in enrichment program study groups led by peer mentor/tutors reported high satisfaction with nursing as a career choice, nursing courses, overall learning opportunities at the college, and specific enrichment program components. Such students took an active approach and responsibility for learning and self-selected participation in study groups; more positive academic outcomes (course pass rates) were noted among study group participants in comparison with nonparticipants (Jeffreys, 2001, 2002a, 2003).

Satisfaction measures help identify responsiveness to student needs of the institution, program, or strategy. Student satisfaction is a complex, multidimensional construct. Because both general satisfaction and specific satisfaction variables can influence retention, it is helpful to assess both dimensions. General satisfaction in nursing includes (1) nursing as a career, (2) nursing courses, and (3) learning opportunities at the college. Specific satisfaction items include the evaluation of specific retention strategy components or services. Despite positive academic outcomes, dissatisfaction with nursing as a career, nursing courses, and/or learning opportunities at the college adversely influences retention. If a student is truly dissatisfied with nursing as a career choice, then career guidance and referral to other programs is warranted. Nurse educators must recognize that not all students will or should be retained in nursing programs. Satisfaction with career choice but dissatisfaction with nursing courses presents a different case scenario, speaking to the need to view satisfaction on an individual item level, and not just use an aggregate measure of satisfaction.

Some of the purposes of a satisfaction scale are to provide a meaningful quantitative comparison over time and to identify differences between student subgroups. Each response category represents a different point on the satisfaction continuum; however, it must be remembered that satisfaction surveys provide ordinal data. Furthermore, positively packed scales can affect the quality of student responses (Beltyukova & Fox, 2002), therefore adversely impacting on reliability and validity. Appendix C and Appendix D present two satisfaction surveys used to assess general and specific satisfaction. Among several student samples, student responses were consistently diverse, suggesting that respondents were discriminating between items, lending support to the instruments' validity and reliability (Jeffreys, 2001, 2002a, 2002b). Student responses in each of the general satisfaction items should be viewed both separately and together with other item responses. Specific satisfaction items delineating specific interventions or student services provide valuable information for guiding future strategies. Another benefit of administering a satisfaction survey is that students may perceive that faculty care enough to find out if they are satisfied. This benefit is nullified if students do not perceive that faculty responded to their needs; students may even become dissatisfied. Therefore it behooves nurse educators to carefully consider the direct and indirect impact or consequences of each survey item.

Nurse educators are in a powerful position to maximize satisfaction and minimize dissatisfaction. The NURS model can be used to systematically consider each factor as potentially influencing satisfaction. Student profile characteristics, student affective factors, academic factors, environmental factors, professional integration factors, and outside and surrounding factors can all affect and be affected by satisfaction. Satisfaction must be viewed in context with academic outcomes and the other psychological outcome of the NURS model: stress. An ongoing bidirectional relationship exists between the two psychological outcomes in the NURS model: satisfaction and stress.

Stress

The process of college is challenging and stressful. All college students experience stress to some degree as a result of the many developmental and life changes (Bean & Eaton, 2000). The perception of an event or situation as stressful varies among students and within an individual student at different times. Through cognitive appraisal, a student perceives something to be stressful if its demands exceed the perceived ability to cope with the stressor. Coping is the process of managing the demands of the perceived stressful event or situation and the ensuing emotions (Lazarus & Folkman, 1984). Ineffective coping places a student at risk for negative academic achievement, dissatisfaction, decreased persistence, and attrition. Perceived confidence for college-related tasks is a critical component in cognitive appraisal and coping; self-efficacy is a mediator of stress (Solberg & Villarreal, 1997). (See chapter 3.)

Stress may range in degree from mild to high and may also have positive or negative effects. There is a marked difference between manageable (positive) stress and unmanageable (negative) stress. A mild degree of stress is stimulating, impressing upon students the need for preparation, attentiveness, detail, and preciseness. Undoubtedly, high levels of stress negatively affect academic achievement, performance, and outcomes, thus adversely affecting student persistence and retention. Anticipatory efforts to manage and reduce stress are urgently needed.

Although the general college experience commonly produces some degree of stress, the nursing student is particularly at risk. It is well documented that the nursing educational process is highly stressful. Citations in the literature purport that nursing students experience greater stress throughout their educational process than do college students in general or even college students enrolled in other health professional programs (Beck, Hackett, Srivastava, McKim, & Rockwell, 1997; Courage & Godbey, 1992; Kirkland, 1998; Lambert & Nugent, 1994; Meadows, 1998). Enculturation into nursing is a developmental process (Leininger, 2002) that presents new challenges that are especially stressful for beginning students. Nurse educators can play a significant role in recognizing sources of stress, anticipating stress, implementing prophylactic measures to prevent stress, assessing for stressors and stress levels, implementing strategies to reduce or manage stress, and evaluating outcomes.

The educational process of nursing students is unique and different from other types of educational experiences; there are specific stressors prevalent within the nursing educational experience. The rigors of nursing education include difficult courses, didactic courses, diversity within coursework, and clinical components (Burris, 2001). Unlike most college courses, nursing courses may include theoretical, skills laboratory, and clinical laboratory components. More academic credits per course and more course contact hours may be an added stressor, especially to beginning nursing students. Additionally, more stress has been observed among students enrolled in an accelerated track (Youssef & Goodrich, 1996) and among evening students (O'Connor & Bevil, 1996) in comparison to students enrolled in traditional and day programs. Lengthy commutes to clinical sites, long hours, and nontraditional class schedules are added stressors to nontraditional students, especially those with dependent children (Burris, 2001). Lengthy clinical hours require both physical and emotional endurance that puts increased demands on students.

If the numerous uncertainties that prevail in clinical settings are stressful for registered professional nurses, the uncertainty surrounding the nursing student clinical experience is often overwhelming. In a "human lab," variables are not easily controlled; situations are dynamic, intense, and frequently unpredictable. Moreover, nursing students deal with the added demands of assuming responsibility for client safety, where inadequate preparation and performance can lead to serious outcomes and even death (Kirkland, 1998). Beginning students may lack the appropriate resources and effective coping strategies needed to deal with complex human experiences such as the pain and suffering of others (Meadows, 1998). Mozingo, Thomas, and Brooks (1995) discovered that stress and anxiety also affected the perceived competency levels of graduating baccalaureate seniors. Conclusively, stress is encountered throughout all stages of the nursing educational process.

Encountering new clinical rotations is another perceived stressor for nursing students. The uncertainty of a new site, experiences, peers, nursing skills, nursing staff, and instructor can all be stressful. For example, the community health experience may be stressful as a student ventures out of the somewhat familiar hospital environment into the unknown territory of a client's home; the home is the client's domain and the student lacks on-site professional support (Shipton, 2002). Yonge, Myrick, and Hoase (2002) noted nursing student stress associated with the preceptorship experience. Certain clinical rotations may be increasingly stressful for particular student subgroups. Empirical evidence documents high stress levels among male nursing students during the obstetrical or maternal-child clinical rotation (Patterson & Morin, 2002). Awareness of the transitional stress experienced as students encounter new clinical rotations should be acknowledged and addressed sensitively.

Other stressors that may affect specific subgroups of nursing students include perceived cultural incongruence, perceived (or fear of) discrimination and bias, acculturation stress, student role incongruence (lack of fit between self and student role in comparison with peer norm reference role models), maternal role stress, perceived multiple role stress, and gender role identity stress. Perceived cultural incongruence and perceived (or fear of) discrimination and bias are most prevalent among minority students in predominantly white institutions. Acculturation stress is more exacerbated by the new (challenging yet stressful) college experience; recent immigrants will experience higher levels of acculturation stress (Fuertes & Westbrook, 1996; Smart & Smart, 1995). Academically weak students and/or low efficacious students are especially at risk for student role incongruence. Obviously maternal role stress targets individuals who assume both the maternal and student roles, whereas perceived multiple role stress includes both men and women, particularly nontraditional students who may assume roles as caregiver, financial provider, employee, and student. Stress related to gender role identity may affect both female and male nursing students, however differently. Pressures to abandon traditional female roles and to embrace a "womanist" or "feminist" identity can be perceived as a stressor (Constantine, Robinson, Wilton, & Caldwell, 2002). In contrast, male nursing students may experience stress related to conflict between traditional male role and nontraditional career choice (Baker, 2001; Patterson & Morin, 2002; Streubert, 1994). Any single stressor or combination of stressors adversely influences student satisfaction with the learning environment and academic achievement, thus increasing attrition risk.

Minimal passing grades, fear of failure, academic uncertainty, high academic demands, overwhelming academic workload, test anxiety, and poor academic performance are all potential academic stressors that can result in even higher stress levels when compounded by unmet expectations and/or poor academic outcomes (Brown, 1987; Courage & Godbey, 1992; Kirkland, 1998). High levels of test anxiety may adversely affect academic performance and poor academic performance may intensify test anxiety. Among nursing students, test anxiety may be exacerbated by a rigorous nursing educational program that emphasizes test scores such as preadmission exams and the RN licensing exam (Gallagher, Bomba, & Crane, 2001; Siktberg & Dillard, 2001; Waltman, 1997). Even in controlled environments (such as a nursing skills laboratory) that aim to enhance learning opportunities in a nonthreatening environment, the testing and retesting of nursing skills can greatly increase stress, thereby decreasing learning and satisfaction (Delgado & Mack, 2002). Test anxiety and other related academic stressors interact, adversely affecting academic achievement and retention.

Nurse educators are in a key position to recognize, reduce, and sometimes eliminate known stressors. The NURS model can be used to systematically appraise each factor as a potential stressor. Student profile characteristics, student affective factors, academic factors, environmental factors, professional integration factors, and outside and surrounding factors can all be potential stressors. Promoting stress management strategies for stressors that cannot be eliminated is equally important. Empirical studies of nursing students' process of seeking stress care to facilitate effective coping has been limited; however the unpredictability of clinical faculty can be a barrier to seeking stress care and help (Shipton, 2002). Because help-seeking behaviors differ and may be influenced by cultural values and beliefs, nurse educators should anticipate stress surrounding help-seeking behaviors and actively offer stress management solutions (for example, teaching relaxation techniques such as guided imagery, deep breathing, visualization, and music therapy for use before an exam can help manage the stress associated with exams, or by assisting a student who is a single parent to develop acceptable time management strategies, task prioritization, and task delegation in order to manage multiple role conflict [maternal role stress]).

INTERACTION BETWEEN ACADEMIC AND PSYCHOLOGICAL OUTCOMES

There is an ongoing, complex, and multidimensional interaction between academic and psychological outcomes in the NURS model that influences persistence, retention, and other factors. Entry into the nursing educational process assures an academic outcome, at least minimally, at the course level. That is, all students who begin a course will pass, fail, or withdraw. Incomplete grades are excluded because most colleges have policies that predetermine progression of incomplete (I) grades to either a passing or a failing grade. Nursing major GPA and overall GPA will be affected by pass and fail grades; official withdrawals are invisible in GPA calculations. All nursing students will experience some degree of stress; however, not all students may experience satisfaction. Academic and psychological outcomes are a complex, multidimensional component of the nursing student retention process. Outcome factors continually interact with each other and with the other factors in the NURS model.

KEY POINTS SUMMARY

- Two dimensions of outcomes directly influence student persistence, retention, and departure: academic and psychological.
- Academic outcomes are represented by the student's nursing course grade, cumulative GPA for nursing courses, and overall GPA.
- Good academic performance results in retention only when accompanied by positive psychological outcomes.
- Positive psychological outcomes include satisfaction and low (manageable) stress.
- Negative psychological outcomes include dissatisfaction and high stress.
- Outcome factors continually interact with each other and with the other factors in the NURS model, influencing persistence.
- Nurse educators are in a strategic position to promote nursing student retention through anticipatory and ongoing efforts aimed at maximizing satisfaction, minimizing stress, and optimizing academic outcomes.

EDUCATOR-IN-ACTION

As part of the Writing-Across-the-Curriculum (WAC) initiative, Professor Glass continues with the low stakes written "reflection" component in the first introductory nursing fundamentals and medical-surgical nursing course. After mid-semester, she asks students to first reflect and then write about "How have your perceptions about nursing changed since the beginning of the semester? (Or how they have remained the same?)." Although students respond diversely, Professor Glass identifies several students with varying levels of satisfaction and stress. She sees this as an important opportunity to intervene and promote positive psychological and academic outcomes. Professor Glass returns the written assignment the next week with constructive comments written for each student. Common themes will be addressed generally in class. Select written excerpts and instructor written responses and actions follow:

Marilyn: "I realize now that nursing is a profession. Nurses have great responsibility for patients' health status. Most of my patients in clinical were so appreciative of the care I provided. I know for sure that nursing is the right career for me."

Analysis: Marilyn has a high level of satisfaction for nursing.

Professor Glass writes, "Yes, nurses have much responsibility and make quite a difference in patients' lives. Keep up your positive attitude, commitment, motivation, and hard work." Intermittently Professor Glass asks Marilyn about her perceived progress in clinical and continues to encourage her diligent efforts, recognizing that all students can benefit from encouragement and sincere interest.

Derrick: "I didn't think nurses had so many responsibilities and so many patients. In the beginning I thought that nurses just carried out doctors' orders. I learned that nurses perform physical assessments, plan patient care, make important decisions, and are under a lot of stress. Nursing is not at all what I expected. The nursing program involves more study time and is very stressful."

Analysis: Derrick mentions stress both in the nursing profession and in his student role. There is a mismatch between his previous expectations and current perceptions. Derrick may be at risk for undesirable academic and psychological outcomes (unmanageable stress and dissatisfaction).

Professor Glass writes, "Nursing is more complex than many people initially realize; however it can be quite a rewarding profession. I would like to talk with you about the nursing profession and share some ideas for maximizing study strategies and reducing stress."

Professor Glass meets with Derrick. He is appreciative of strategies for enhancing time management, study skills, and stress management. Derrick reports being "somewhat satisfied" with nursing as a career choice although he sometimes "feels like an outsider." He admits that he had been thinking about dropping out of the nursing program, despite his B+ course average. Professor Glass links him with a nursing program alumnus who has volunteered to mentor a student. As the alumnus describes satisfying professional experiences, vast opportunities in nursing, and past struggles, Derrick views nursing in a different light and becomes more satisfied with his career choice.

REFERENCES AND BIBLIOGRAPHY

Ansari, W. E. (2002a). Student nurse satisfaction levels with their courses: Part 1—Effects of demographic variables. *Nurse Education Today, 22*(2), 159–170.

Ansari, W. E. (2002b). Student nurse satisfaction levels with their courses: Part II—Effects of academic variables. *Nurse Education Today, 22*(2), 171–180.

Baker, C. R. (2001). Role strain in male diploma nursing students: A descriptive quantitative study. *Journal of Nursing Education, 40*(8), 378–380.

Baldwin, D., & Wold, J. (1993). Students from disadvantaged backgrounds: Satisfaction with a mentor-protégé relationship. *Journal of Nursing Education, 32,* 225–226.

Bean, J. P., & Bradley, R. K. (1986). Untangling the satisfaction-performance relationship for college students. *Journal of Higher Education, 57*(4), 393–412.

Bean, J. P., & Eaton, S. B. (2000). A psychological model of student retention. In J. Braxton (Ed.), *Reworking the student departure puzzle* (pp. 48–61). Nashville, TN: Vanderbilt University Press.

Bean, J. P., & Eaton, S. B. (2001). The psychology underlying successful retention practices. *Journal of College Student Retention: Research, Theory, & Practice, 3*(1), 73–90.

Bean, J. P., & Metzner, B. (1985). A conceptual model of nontraditional undergraduate student attrition. *Review of Educational Research, 55,* 485–540.

Beck, D. L., Hackett, M. B., Srivastava, R., McKim, E., & Rockwell, B. (1997). Perceived level and sources of stress in university professional schools. *Journal of Nursing Education, 36*(4), 180–186.

Beltyukova, S. A., & Fox, C. M. (2002). Student satisfaction as a measure of student development: Towards a universal metric. *Journal of College Student Development, 43*(2), 161–172.

Bessent, H. (Ed.). (1997). *Strategies for recruitment, retention, and graduation of minority nurses in colleges of nursing.* Washington, DC: American Nurses Publishing.

Braxton, J. M. (Ed.). (2000). *Reworking the student departure puzzle.* Nashville, TN: Vanderbilt University Press.

Brown, M. L. (1987). The effects of a support group on student attrition due to academic failure. *Journal of Nursing Education, 26*(8), 324–327.

Burris, R. F. (2001). Teaching student parents. *Nurse Educator, 26*(2), 64–65, 98.

Callister, L. C., Khalaf, I., & Keller, D. (2000). Cross-cultural comparison of the concerns of beginning baccalaureate nursing students. *Nurse Educator, 25*(6), 267–271.

Cameron-Buccheri, R., & Trygstad, L. (1989). Retaining freshman nursing students. *Nursing and Health Care, 10*(7), 389–393.

Chartrand, J. M. (1990). A causal analysis to predict the personal and academic adjustment of nontraditional students. *Journal of Counseling Psychology, 37*(1), 65–73.

Coffman, D. L., & Gilligan, T. D. (2002). Social support, stress, and self-efficacy: Effects on students' satisfaction. *Journal of College Student Retention: Research, Theory, & Practice, 4*(1), 53–66.

Constantine, M. G., Robinson, J. S., Wilton, L., & Caldwell, L. D. (2002). Collective self-esteem and perceived social support as predictors of cultural congruity among black and Latino college students. *Journal of College Student Development, 43*(3), 307–316.

Constantine, M. G., & Watt, S. K. (2002). Cultural congruity, womanist identity attitudes, and life satisfaction among African American college women attending historically black and predominantly white institutions. *Journal of College Student Development, 43*(2), 184–193.

Courage, M. M., & Godbey, K. L. (1992). Student retention: Policies and services to enhance persistence to graduation. *Nurse Educator, 17*(2), 29–32.

Crawford, L. A., & Olinger, B. H. (1988). Recruitment and retention of nursing students from diverse cultural backgrounds. *Journal of Nursing Education, 27*(8), 379–381.

Delgado, C., & Mack, B. (2002). A peer-reviewed program for senior proficiencies. *Nurse Educator, 27*(5), 212–213.

Eaton, S. B., & Bean, J. P. (1995). An approach/avoidance behavioral model of college student attrition. *Research in Higher Education, 36*, 617–645.

Eimers, M. T., & Pike, G. R. (1997). Minority and nonminority adjustment to college: Differences or similarities? *Research in Higher Education, 38*(1), 77–97.

Elliott, K. M. (2002). Key determinants of student satisfaction. *Journal of College Student Retention: Research, Theory, & Practice, 4*(3), 271–280.

Fuertes, J. N., & Westbrook, F. D. (1996). Using the social, attitudinal, familial, and environmental (S.A.F.E.) acculturation stress scale to assess the adjustment needs of Hispanic college students. *Measurement and Evaluation in Counseling and Development, 29*, 67–76.

Gallagher, P. A., Bomba, C., & Crane, L. R. (2001). Using an admissions exam to predict student success in an ADN program. *Nurse Educator, 26*(3), 132–135.

Gigliotti, E. (1999). Women's multiple role stress: Testing Neuman's flexible line of defense. *Nursing Science Quarterly, 12*(1), 36–44.

Gigliotti, E. (2001). Development of the perceived multiple role stress scale (PMRS). *Journal of Nursing Measurement, 9*(2), 163–180.

Greene, B. A., & Miller, R. B. (1996). Influences on achievement: Goals, perceived ability, and cognitive engagement. *Contemporary Educational Psychology, 21,* 181–192.

Greenhaus, J. H., & Beutell, N. J. (1985). Sources of conflict between work and family roles. *Academy of Management Review, 10,* 76–88.

Jeffreys, M. R. (1993). *The relationship of self-efficacy and select academic and environmental variables on academic achievement and retention.* Unpublished doctoral dissertation, Teachers College, Columbia University, New York.

Jeffreys, M. R. (1998). Predicting nontraditional student retention and academic achievement. *Nurse Educator, 23*(1), 42–48.

Jeffreys, M. R. (2001). Evaluating enrichment program study groups: Academic outcomes, psychological outcomes, and variables influencing retention. *Nurse Educator, 26*(3), 142–149.

Jeffreys, M. R. (2002a). Students' perceptions of variables influencing retention: A pretest and post-test approach. *Nurse Educator, 27*(1), 16–19 [Erratum, 2002, *27*(2), 64].

Jeffreys, M. R. (2000b). *Nursing student withdrawal data.* Unpublished material.

Jeffreys, M. R. (2003). Strategies for promoting nontraditional student retention and success. In M. Oermann & K. Heinrich (Eds.), *Annual review of nursing education: Volume I* (pp. 61–90). New York: Springer.

Kirkland, M. L. S. (1998). Stressors and coping strategies among successful female African American baccalaureate nursing students. *Journal of Nursing Education, 37*(1), 5–12.

Lambert, V. A., & Nugent, K. E. (1994). Addressing the academic progression of students encountering mental health problems. *Nurse Educator, 19*(5), 33–39.

Lazarus, R. S., & Folkman, S. (1984). *Stress, appraisal, and coping.* New York: Springer.

Leininger, M. M. (2002). Essential transcultural nursing care concepts, principles, examples, and policy statements. In M. M. Leininger & M. R. McFarland (Eds.), *Transcultural nursing: Concepts, theories, research, and practice* (3rd ed., pp. 45–69). New York: McGraw-Hill.

Leininger, M. M., & McFarland, M. R. (2002). *Transcultural nursing: Concepts, theories, research, and practice* (3rd ed.). New York: McGraw-Hill.

Liegler, R. M. (1997). Predicting student satisfaction in baccalaureate nursing programs: Testing a causal model. *Journal of Nursing Education, 36*(8), 357–364.

Loerch, K. J., Russell, J. E. A., & Rush, M. C. (1989). The relationships among family domain variables and work-family conflict for men and women. *Journal of Vocational Behavior, 35,* 288–308.

Mason, D. J., & Leavitt, J. K. (1998). *Policy and politics in nursing and health care* (3rd ed.). New York: Saunders.

Maville, J., & Huerta, C. G. (1997). Stress and social support among Hispanic student nurses: Implications for academic achievement. *Journal of Cultural Diversity, 4*(1), 18–25.

Mayo, J. R., Murguia, E., & Padilla, R. V. (1995). Social integration and academic performance among minority university students. *Journal of College Student Development, 36*(6), 542–552.

Meadows, L. C. (1998). Integrating self-care into nursing education. *Journal of Nursing Education, 37*(5), 225–227.

Metzner, B. S. (1989). Perceived quality of academic advising: The effect on freshman attrition. *American Educational Research Journal, 26,* 422–442.

Metzner, B., & Bean, J. P. (1987). The estimation of a conceptual model of nontraditional undergraduate student attrition. *Research in Higher Education, 27,* 15–38.

Mohr, J. J., Eiche, K. D., & Sedlacek, W. E. (1998). So close, yet so far: Predictors of attrition in college seniors. *Journal of College Student Development, 39*(4), 343–354.

Mozingo, J., Thomas, S., & Brooks, E. (1995). Factors associated with perceived competency levels of graduating seniors in a baccalaureate nursing program. *Journal of Nursing Education, 34*(3), 115–122.

Myton, C. L., Allen, J. K., & Baldwin, J. A. (1992). Students in transition: Services for retention and outplacement. *Nursing Outlook, 35*(1), 227–230.

Napoli, A. R., & Wortman, P. M. (1998). Psychosocial factors related to retention and early departure of two-year community college students. *Research in Higher Education, 39*(4), 419–455.

O'Connor, P. C., & Bevil, C. A. (1996). Academic outcomes and stress in full-time day and part-time evening baccalaureate nursing students. *Journal of Nursing Education, 35*(6), 245–251.

Patterson, B. J., & Morin, K. H. (2002). Perceptions of the maternal-child clinical rotation: The male student nurse experience. *Journal of Nursing Education, 41*(6), 266–272.

Robins, L. S., Gruppen, L. D., Alexander, G. L., Fantone, J. C., & Davis, W. K. (1997). A predictive model of student satisfaction with the medical school learning environment. *Academic Medicine, 72*(2), 134–139.

Ryan, M. P., & Glenn, P. A. (2002). Increasing one-year retention rates by focusing on academic competence: An empirical odyssey. *Journal of College Student Retention: Research, Theory, & Practice, 4*(3), 297–324.

Shipton, S. P. (2002). The process of seeking stress-care: Coping as experienced by senior baccalaureate nursing students in response to appraised clinical stress. *Journal of Nursing Education, 41*(6), 243–256.

Siktberg, L. L., & Dillard, N. L. (2001). Assisting at-risk students in preparing for NCLEX-RN. *Nurse Educator, 26*(3), 150–152.

Smart, J. F., & Smart, D. W. (1995). Acculturative stress: The experience of the Hispanic immigrant. *The Counseling Psychologist, 23,* 25–42.

Solberg, V. S., & Villarreal, P. (1997). Examination of self-efficacy, social support, and stress as predictors of psychological and physical distress among Hispanic college students. *Hispanic Journal of Behavioral Sciences, 19*(2), 182–201.

Solis, E. (1995). Regression and path analysis models of Hispanic community college students' intent to persist. *Community College Review, 23*(3), 3–15.

Streubert, H. J. (1994). Male nursing students' perceptions of clinical experience. *Nurse Educator, 19*(5), 28–32.

Sullivan, E. (2002). In a woman's world. *Reflections on Nursing Leadership, 28*(3), 10–17.

Tinto, V. (1975). Dropout from higher education: A theoretical synthesis of recent research. *Review of Educational Research, 10,* 259–271.

Toutkoushian, R. K., & Smart, J. C. (2001). Do institutional characteristics affect student gains from college? *Review of Higher Education, 25*(1), 39–61.

Tucker-Allen, S., & Long, E. (1999). *Recruitment and retention of minority students: Stories of success.* Lisle, IL: Tucker.

Turner, A. L., & Berry, T. R. (2000). Counseling center contributions to student retention and graduation: A longitudinal assessment. *Journal of College Student Development, 41*(6), 627–636.

Umbach, P. D., & Porter, S. R. (2002). How do academic departments impact student satisfaction? Understanding the contextual effects of departments. *Research in Higher Education, 43*(2), 209–233.

Waltman, P. A. (1997). Comparison of traditional and non-traditional baccalaureate nursing students on selected components of Meichenbaum and Butler's model of test anxiety. *Journal of Nursing Education, 36*(4), 171–179.

Wilson, S. B., Mason, T. W., & Ewing, M. J. M. (1997). Evaluating the impact of receiving university-based counseling services on student retention. *Journal of Counseling Psychology, 44*(3), 316–320.

Yoder, M. K., & Saylor, C. (2002). Student and teacher roles: Mismatched expectations. *Nurse Educator, 27*(5), 201–203.

Yonge, O., Myrick, F., & Haase, M. (2002). Student nurse stress in the preceptorship experience. *Nurse Educator, 27*(2), 84–88.

Youssef, F. A., & Goodrich, N. (1996). Accelerated versus traditional nursing students: A comparison of stress, critical thinking ability and performance. *International Journal of Nursing Studies, 33*(1), 76–82.

Chapter **8**

The Outside Climate: Forecast, Impact, and Action

Despite students' positive academic and psychological outcomes, and despite other background, affective, academic, environmental, and professional integration factors favorable for student success, students may still drop out or stop out. Models proposed to explain attrition in higher education have generally focused on variables (or interventions) within the specific domain of the academic institution. Frequently, models incorporated student background characteristics and/or student personal environmental factors in an attempt to identify at-risk students prospectively or to explain failed retention efforts retrospectively. It has been important to examine these factors in student persistence research, theory, and practice; however, a different explanation for attrition and variation in persistence behaviors must also be considered. Outside surrounding factors (OSF) exist that can exert great influence on student persistence. The NURS model seeks to acknowledge the importance of these factors with specific application for nursing student retention.

Outside surrounding factors exist outside the academic setting and the individual student's personal environment and can influence retention. They include world, national, and local events; politics and economics; the health care system; nursing professional issues; and job certainty. Together, OSF interact to create an outside climate that has the power to influence student persistence, retention, and success. These factors may affect students at any point in the model and may be unpredictable. They may affect student retention positively or negatively. In the NURS model, a cloud illustration is used to signify the possible uncertainties that continually exist and surround nursing student persistence, retention, and success. The peeking sun represents a favorable climate conducive for retention, and the lightning represents adverse climate conditions. Students' motivation to overcome hardships and obstacles and persist in the program may be heightened when OSF are more favorable or appealing. In contrast, it may be lessened when OSF are perceived to be overwhelming obstacles to success.

OSF have the power to affect all undergraduate nursing students, but in potentially different ways. Some OSF may result in a wide range of voluntary student choices whereas others may lead to a predetermined involuntary result. Nurse educators are in a key position to survey the existing outside surrounding climate, to forecast climate conditions favorable or unfavorable to student persistence, to evaluate the impact of select factors on student subgroups, and to determine appropriate actions. The purpose of this chapter is to enhance awareness of OSF on student retention, highlight the potential significance of select factors, stimulate further inquiry, and suggest implications for nurse educators.

WORLD, NATIONAL, AND LOCAL EVENTS

World, national, and local events usually happen unpredictably and can have a positive or negative effect on nursing student persistence, retention, and success. Local events occur near the student's nursing program residence, such as neighborhood, town, city, county, state, province, or region. Local events may become national or world events if they are either publicized nationally and globally or if they have an effect on a nation or the world. Such effects may include changes in policy, resource allocation, government, priorities, and philosophy. National events occur within the student's country of residence/attendance while in the nursing program, and world events are those occurrences outside of the student's country of residence/attendance while in the nursing program.

Some events, such as natural disasters, are beyond human control, yet can have tremendous impact on nursing student retention. For example, a local flood, tornado, hurricane, earthquake, or other natural disaster may result in financial loss, homelessness, stress, and other losses, requiring nursing students to withdraw from school. Other local accidental disasters such as fires, explosions, train derailments, plane crashes, building collapses, or partial bridge collapses can also result in losses or obstacles that necessitate student withdrawal. Nonaccidental tragic events resulting from terrorist or other criminal acts may have local, national, and world-wide impact both directly and indirectly. Reallocation of local and national funds to assist in the aftermath of disasters and tragedies may necessitate smaller budget allocation for public higher education, scholarships, student stipends, or financial aid, thus potentially creating adverse effects on future student persistence and retention.

War, threats of war, or impending war can result in drafting or activation of soldiers in reserve units. A student in the military or military reserve may be required to stop out if called into active duty during a time of national crisis. Recent immigrants, refugees, or asylees may be personally affected by wars or civil unrest in their former residence or place of origin. For example, a nursing student whose family is missing after a war incident in another country may need to return and search for lost family members. Similarly, students may withdraw from school following a natural disaster, accidental disaster, or other world event that directly or indirectly affects them emotionally.

Positive local events can exert great positive influence on nursing student retention, and may have direct and immediate effects or indirect and delayed effects. Additionally, the effects may be instrumental (concrete) or motivational (abstract). A substantial donation to the nursing school for resources and scholarships, new grant funding for nursing student stipends, or tuition-work exchange programs at the local hospital present favorable conditions that can cause direct, immediate, and positive effects on student retention. Both instrumental and motivational support would result through the enhancement of the surrounding climate favorable for optimizing student success. The addition of a new hospital wing, a local hospital reaching the prestigious "Magnet" status, or worldwide recognition of a local hospital's expertise are examples of events leading to possible direct and indirect positive effects. Motivation to persist would be enhanced with the indirect, long-term focus on locally enhanced opportunities for highly satisfying, rewarding careers in nursing.

Local, national, and world events that involve nurses are yet another indication of how nursing student persistence can be influenced. News media publicity showcasing the heroic acts of nurses rendering assistance during times of crisis is one example. Reporting the positive difference a nurse made in the life of a local "everyday" person, a national celebrity, or a world-respected leader may altruistically motivate current nursing students to persist. On the other hand, nurses may also gain local, national, or worldwide attention when guilty of malpractice, drug abuse, insurance fraud, abandonment, or murder. A publicized local event involving a patient death and an impaired nurse does much damage to the nursing image. A nurse shot to death in an emergency room or other acts of violence against nurses at the workplace are disturbing and frightening, thus potentially influencing nursing student retention through decreased motivation, ambivalence over career selection, and fear.

Threat of a nursing strike or an actual nursing strike at a local hospital shows discontent over professional issues ranging from unsafe working conditions, patient overcrowding, unsafe staffing, poor salary and benefits, lack of nursing governance, dissatisfaction, and/or lack of professional respect. A favorable outcome settlement for nurses may represent hope and professional unity to undergraduate nursing students, thus favorably influencing persistence. On the other hand, some students may become discouraged by the dissatisfaction experienced by many working nurses. The manner in which news media coverage portrays the event and the outcome can greatly skew the event in the eyes of nursing students and the public.

Consequently, nurse educators are challenged to keep actively informed of current events, forecast the potential impact of events on nursing student retention (professional nursing and the public), and demonstrate visionary leadership actions in context with the event(s). Proactive action rather than retrospective reaction is the recommended approach for obtaining the best results. Openly discussing the event, encouraging students to reflect on it, presenting alternative perspectives, and offering constructive suggestions for effectively dealing with an event empowers students to take appropriate actions that facilitate persistence behaviors.

POLITICS AND ECONOMICS

Politics refers to the process of influence used for decision making and allocation of resources (Mason & Leavitt, 1998). Economics refers to the financial investment in specific resources used for particular purposes. Both politics and economics critically impact upon nursing student retention. In the NURS model, politics and economics are labeled as one OSF so as to recognize the virtually inseparable relationship between them, as specifically pertinent to nursing student retention. Politics and economics foster the development of policies that can directly or indirectly influence nursing student persistence and retention.

Most definitely, national policies that support the growing need for nurses are an impetus for nursing student recruitment and retention. The Nurse Reinvestment Act (United States House of Representatives, 2002) is one example of a legislative measure aimed at resolving the severe nursing shortage crisis. The "Nurse Education, Practice, and Retention Grants" and the "Loan Repayment and Scholarship Program" will provide both financial and motivational incentives for nursing student persistence. The Nurse Faculty Loan Program aims to increase the number of prepared nursing faculty, thus providing an indirect and more distant effect on student retention. However, in the future the program could have potentially more impact on nursing student persistence, retention, and success by having more full-time and well-prepared nursing faculty.

Current financial aid policies and scholarship incentives for disadvantaged students usually stipulate full-time enrollment and demonstrated financial need. Frequently, older students with family and employment responsibilities are unable to pursue educational endeavors full time, and have substantial financial strain. Similarly, middle-class full-time students also report severe financial strain, which discourages persistence (Nora, Cabrera, Hegedorn, & Pascarella, 1996; Padilla, Trevino, Gonzalez, & Trevino, 1997). Publicly supported career ladder programs offer an incentive to those employed within health care agencies; however, second-career students employed elsewhere are excluded. The current nursing applicant pool reflects a great number of nontraditional, second-career students who may not be able to meet the criteria for full-time student status and/or financial need requirements, yet still experience financial strain. The perception that one is excluded from incentive measures could be construed as an obstacle for student persistence. Therefore, new policies that accommodate the part-time, nontraditional college student are urgently needed to promote persistence. Current financial aid policies, loans, and other financial incentives must be transformed to enhance college access and success.

Visionary nurse educators must remain updated about politics, policy, and economics; forecast the potential impact of proposed policies on nursing student retention; evaluate the actual and potential impact on student subgroups; and demonstrate commitment to active political involvement. Commitment may range from philosophical support of a nursing organization's position on current and/or proposed policies to more personal political action initiatives such as running for political office. The danger of inaction is the assumption that the status quo is acceptable. Silence and inactivity often assume support whereas action demands sincere thought, commitment, effort, ingenuity, energy, enthusiasm, and deliberate activity.

HEALTH CARE SYSTEM

The health care system is the combination of resources, financing, organization, and management that results in the delivery of health services (Barton, 1999; Roemer, 1991). The health care system presents favorable and unfavorable conditions within the current and future outside surrounding climate. The existence (or nonexistence) of national health insurance, socialized medicine, private health insurance, no health insurance, and/or government-subsidized health benefits for all (or select) citizens and residents offers different types of environments for current nursing student education and later nursing student employment. Additionally, the emphasis (or lack of emphasis) of the health care system on primary preventive care (health promotion and illness prevention) helps shape the present and future of nursing practice and societal health. A health care system that is truly consistent with the World Health Organization's (WHO) position that health is not merely the absence of disease but the state of physical, mental, and social well-being and that health care is a human right, not a privilege (World Health Organization, 1947) must emphasize primary health care. Such a health care system demands qualified nurses in sufficient numbers and must provide incentives for current and future nurses.

Whether the health care system embraces the full scope of professional nursing practice or restricts it is an important consideration. For example, a health care system that favors replacing registered nurse positions with unlicensed assistive personnel devalues or minimizes the scope of nursing practice. Such an action would be detrimental to societal health overall, let alone the severe long-term effects on cost and quality of health care. Similarly, a health care system that favors downsizing by eliminating positions held by experienced nurses and/or advanced practice nurses is counterproductive to patient and employee satisfaction, and adversely impacts on nursing student retention through decreased motivation and morale.

In contrast, a health care system that embraces professional nursing practice seeks to provide quality patient care by maximizing the quality of nursing practice, thereby enhancing positive client outcomes, patient satisfaction, and nurse-employee satisfaction (Kimball & O'Neill, 2002). For example, a health care system promoting nurses as CEOs or facilitating the development of Magnet hospitals presents a favorable outside climate that can motivate nursing student persistence. A health care system that directly reimburses nurses acknowledges that nurses have provided unique, valuable services to society; nursing services that are not directly reimbursed or itemized on a bill make professional nursing invisible. Direct reimbursement to advanced practice nurses through Medicare is a beginning step for the recognition of nursing services (Wong, 1999).

Nurse educators must not only be astutely aware of the political and economic dynamics that shape the health care system but recognize how the current and projected health care system will potentially impact on nursing students, nursing practice, and societal health care needs of the future. The changing health care system can influence the popularity or desirability of becoming a nurse, and hence influence persistence and retention. Addressing nursing students' concerns, questions, dissatisfaction, confusion, and/or ambivalence regarding the health care system proactively opens discussion and acknowledges the favorable and unfavorable conditions within the health care system environment. Candid dialogue directed toward stimulating creative nursing student involvement in the development, implementation, and evaluation of strategies to improve the health care system acknowledges the imperfections of any health care system yet offers the option for change through active and committed involvement.

NURSING PROFESSIONAL ISSUES

Nursing professional issues are numerous and can be any topic or matter that is directly relevant to the nursing profession. They include entry into practice, credentialing, nursing image, nursing shortage, professional self-image, public nursing image, burnout, reality shock, salaries, workplace conditions, malpractice, educational mobility, career advancement, satisfaction, and organizations. Several of these topics will be highlighted and relationships to actual and/or potential impact on nursing student retention in the United States will be proposed.

Continued controversy over entry into practice is often confusing to students, nurses, and the public (Joel & Kelly, 2002; Kimball & O'Neill, 2002; Neal, 2003). Academically well prepared college-bound high school students may be discouraged from nursing as a career because it appears that it is unnecessary for nurses to pursue a full, four-year college education. The availability of various nearby nursing educational programs may influence student selection or consideration of nursing as a career option. For example, an academically well prepared high school student may never consider nursing as a career option if the only nearby program is offered in a community college. Nursing student retention is affected through a less academically prepared and a more academically diverse nursing student applicant pool.

Positive images of nurses on local, national, or worldwide levels can be motivating to potential and currently enrolled nursing students, especially if the nurses portrayed are similar to students in age, cultural identity, and/or gender. Some examples include movie releases or TV shows featuring nurses in a positive way. Nursing recruitment advertisements and commercials targeting diverse student populations and portraying vast career opportunities broaden the applicant pool but also motivate currently enrolled nursing students.

Nursing students are greatly influenced by nursing professional self-image. Nurse educators, nurses in affiliating agencies, and preceptors all have the potential to make a positive or negative impact on nursing student retention. Statements to students by nurses on the clinical unit such as "I'm just a nurse so I don't know . . . ," "Don't become a nurse . . . ," or "You're too smart to be a nurse . . ." all have potentially adverse effects on nursing student retention and the nursing profession. Diplomatically confronting nurses with poor professional self-image may be an unpopular nurse educator task; however, it is important. Seeking continual opportunities for student exposure to outstanding nurse role models of different gender, age, and cultural backgrounds is an equally important nurse educator responsibility.

The nursing shortage has been well publicized and can have various impacts on nursing student retention (Kimball & O'Neill, 2002). Patient safety issues, mandatory overtime, lack of whistleblower legislation, nurse dissatisfaction, low nurse morale, unsafe work environments, lack of respect, complexity of health care needs, high patient acuity levels, the aging patient population, the aging practicing nurse population, low nurse retention rate, high dropout of new nurses from nursing, and poor salary and job benefits all contribute to the nursing shortage. Certainly many of these issues present an unfavorable outside climate unless students are mainly motivated by altruistic reasons (to help humanity) or if unfavorable conditions are outweighed by the high probability of employment following graduation and licensure.

Nurse educators must recognize the challenges facing the nursing profession today and be able to forecast the impact of these challenges on future nursing practice and nursing student retention. Ongoing dialogue, coursework on professional issues, and strategies to promote positive professional integration provide students with opportunities to explore the nursing profession from various perspectives. Such guided opportunities should encourage active involvement in strategy design, implementation, and evaluation aimed at advancement of the nursing profession. Active involvement in the nursing profession throughout the nursing educational experience is strongly recommended (Fitzpatrick, 2000).

JOB CERTAINTY

Job certainty has been included as a variable within other conceptual models of college student attrition (Bean & Metzner, 1985). Proponents of adult learning theory attest to the marked influence of educational endeavors, motivation, and commitment in relation to immediate career goals (Brookfield, 1986; Knowles, 1984). Historically, nursing enrollment has fluctuated according to nursing shortages, supply, and demand. Recent welfare-to-work initiatives, displaced homemakers, high divorce rates, increasing single-parent families, prevalence of mid-life career changes, large employee layoffs, and a fluctuating world economy contribute to a greater emphasis on job certainty. Loan repayment initiatives, financed career ladder programs, and full tuition for post-graduation work agreements offer incentives that promote post-graduation job certainty. The NURS model acknowledges the powerful influence of job certainty on nursing student retention due to both practical and motivational effects. It is proposed that a high degree of job certainty correlates with higher student motivation and effort expenditure to overcome obstacles; therefore, nursing student persistence, retention, and success will be enhanced. Many students will be driven by practical reasons such as economic advancement, financial independence, employee health benefits, or even escape from unwanted domestic/family relationships. During periods of nursing shortages, especially when there is an economic recession and job cuts in the corporate world, there may be an increased motivation to persist and complete the nursing program swiftly.

Although nursing students today and in the near future may be certain that nursing jobs exist, students may be overwhelmed by the diversity of job opportunities and choices. Recognizing that graduating nursing students who become licensed then become part of the outside surrounding factors, nurse educators must focus efforts on a smooth transition into the nursing work force. Collaborative partnerships with employers of nurses can assist in this process (Kimball & O'Neill, 2002). Preparing students at the onset of their first nursing course and subsequently reinforcing and expanding on professional nursing job issues in other courses will help.

KEY POINTS SUMMARY

- Outside surrounding factors exist that can exert great influence on student persistence.
- Outside surrounding factors (OSF) exist outside the academic setting and the individual student's personal environment and can influence retention. They include world, national, and local events; politics and economics; the health care system; nursing professional issues; and job certainty.

- Together, OSF interact to create an outside climate that has the power to positively or negatively influence student persistence, retention, and success.
- Nurse educators are in a key position to survey the existing outside surrounding climate, to forecast climate conditions favorable or unfavorable to student persistence, to evaluate the impact of select factors on student subgroups, and to determine appropriate actions.

EDUCATOR-IN-ACTION

During a post-clinical conference, Professor Change notices that two students (Veronica and Jamie) who usually are quite talkative, energetic, enthusiastic, and conscientious seem distracted and do not participate in the group discussion. She asks them if they have anything to add to the group discussion topic or if they would like to discuss another topic. At first, neither student answers. Then Veronica says, "When Jamie and I gave our report about our patients to the nurse, we felt rather discouraged." When Professor Change asks for further elaboration, Jamie says, "I asked the nurse whether the patient had any difficulty with or questions about her new medications yesterday. The nurse said to me 'I'm just a nurse here for eight hours, so I don't know about medications given yesterday. My advice is—don't become a nurse. Get out while you can. This is the most horrible job. You must be smart enough to do something else.'" Veronica adds, "The same nurse said something similar to me. When I said I liked nursing, she said I would quickly change my mind when I got my first job. I now wonder if I'm really wasting my time, money, energy, and college degree on nursing." Several other students report positive experiences and interactions with other nurses and yet several students confirm having had similar negative experiences in the past.

Professor Change clarifies the issues of concern, writes them on the chalkboard, and invites further discussion from the whole group. The group's main issues are quality patient care, nursing self-image, satisfaction, motivation, and opportunities in professional nursing. Professor Change assists students in identifying ways to prioritize issues and develop strategies accordingly. The students collaborate and plan strategies to promote and publicize positive nursing image and opportunities in professional nursing—especially to motivate students. Additionally, they discuss and plan strategies for predicting, preventing, and dealing effectively with negative nursing image. Several student comments/ideas and educator actions are presented below:

Hilda: "We should tell the nurse how her comments make us feel. With such a nursing shortage, shouldn't nurses be happy that there are nursing students interested in providing quality patient care? Why isn't she happy?"

Action: Professor Change institutes a role play in which students take turns expressing their feelings after a nurse makes inappropriate remarks. Her constructive comments assist students in developing assertive, professional communication techniques. Professor Change offers to meet with the nurse privately to explore issues related to her negative behavior and to offer strategies for promoting a satisfying and rewarding professional nursing practice.

Jamie: "Maybe it would be a good idea to post positive stories about professional nursing practice on the Nursing Student Club (NSC) bulletin board and webpage. We could feature a new story every month."

Action: Professor Change assists NSC officers to select stories from professional nursing publications. Stories are posted on the bulletin board and are accessible via a website link on the NSC webpage. At the monthly NSC meeting, students are invited to discuss the motivational stories.

Veronica: "I guess I focused on the negative today and felt discouraged. There isn't time to hear positive stories from the nurses while we're on the unit. Other nurses before were encouraging and nice to me but right now I need more positive stories and feelings to keep going."

Action: Professor Change invites several local nursing alumni to share motivational stories and participate in a roundtable luncheon discussion with students.

REFERENCES AND BIBLIOGRAPHY

Baum, S. (2003a). *The financial aid partnership: Strengthening the federal government's leadership role.* Retrieved February 27, 2003, from http://www.collegeboard.com

Baum, S. (2003b). *The role of student loans in college access.* Retrieved February 27, 2003 from http://www.collegeboard.com

Barton, P. L. (1999). *Understanding the U. S. health services system.* Chicago: Health Administration Press.

Bean, J. P., & Metzner, B. (1985). A conceptual model of nontraditional undergraduate student attrition. *Review of Educational Research, 55,* 485–540.

Brookfield, S. D. (1986). *Understanding and facilitating adult learning.* San Francisco: Jossey-Bass.

Campbell, S. L. (2003). Cultivating empowerment in nursing today for a strong profession tomorrow. *Journal of Nursing Education, 42*(9), 423–426.

College Board. (2003). *Challenging times, clear choices: An action agenda for college access and success.* Retrieved February 27, 2003, from http://www.collegeboard.com

Crawford, L. A., & Olinger, B. H. (1988). Recruitment and retention of nursing students from diverse cultural backgrounds. *Journal of Nursing Education, 27*(8), 379–381.

Fitzpatrick, J. J. (2000). 2000: The millennium of the student. *Nursing and Health Care Perspectives, 21*(1), 3.

Heller, D. E. (2003). *State financial aid and college access.* Retrieved February 27, 2003, from http://www.collegeboard.com

Joel, L. A., & Kelly, L. Y. (2002). *The nursing experience: Trends, challenges, and transitions.* New York: McGraw-Hill.

Johnstone, D. B. (2003). *Fundamental assumptions and aims underlying the principles and policies of federal financial aid to students.* Retrieved February 27, 2003, from http://www.collegeboard.com

Kimball, B., & O'Neill, E. (2002). *Health care's human crisis: The American nursing shortage.* Princeton, NJ: Robert Wood Johnson.

Knowles, M. (1984). *The adult learner: A neglected species.* Houston, TX: Gulf.

Malveaux, J. (2003). *What's at stake: The social and economic benefits of higher education.* Retrieved February 27, 2003, from http://www.collegeboard.com

Mason, D. J., & Leavitt, J. K. (1998). *Policy and politics in nursing and health care* (3rd ed.). New York: Saunders.

McPherson, M. S., & Schapiro, M. O. (2003). *Getting the most out of federal student aid spending—encouraging colleges and universities to promote the common good.* Retrieved February 27, 2003, from http://www.collegeboard.com

Metzner, B., & Bean, J. P. (1987). The estimation of a conceptual model of nontraditional undergraduate student attrition. *Research in Higher Education, 27,* 15–38.

Neal, L. J. (2003). Elder RNs' perspectives on nursing education: Lessons learned. *Nurse Educator, 28*(1), 18–22.

Nora, A., Cabrera, A., Hagedorn, L. S., & Pascarella, E. (1996). Differential impacts of academic and social experiences on college-related behavioral outcomes across different ethnic and gender groups at four-year institutions. *Research in Higher Education, 37*(4), 427–451.

Padilla, R. V., Trevino, J., Gonzalez, K., & Trevino, J. (1997). Developing local models of minority student success in college. *Journal of College Student Development, 38*(2), 125–135.

Roemer, M. I. (1991). *National health systems of the world, Vol. I.* New York: Oxford University Press.

United States House of Representatives. (2002). *H.R. 3487—Nurse Reinvestment Act.* Retrieved April 6, 2003, from http://thomas.loc.gov

Wong, S. T. (1999). Reimbursement to advanced practice nurses (APNs) through Medicare. *Image: Journal of Nursing Scholarship, 31*(2), 167–172.

World Health Organization. (1947). *Constitution.* Geneva: Author.

Chapter 9

Dropout, Stopout, or Go On?

Attrition may be voluntary or involuntary; however, retention is strictly voluntary. The decision to remain in a course, persist in the nursing program, graduate, take the RN licensing exam, and enter the nursing work force and/or begin a more advanced nursing program occurs during and at the conclusion of each nursing course. Engaging in activities associated with course progress, remaining in a course past the college withdrawal date, and registering for a subsequent course all involve a decision to persist. Student profile characteristics, student affective factors, academic factors, environmental factors, professional integration factors, academic outcomes, psychological outcomes, and outside surrounding factors interact and influence retention decisions (see Figure 1.1).

Retention decisions are the determined resolution to persist in the nursing curriculum and educational pathway toward becoming a registered nurse. Ideally, they should be made after careful consideration, purposeful deliberation, and thoughtful weighing of benefits and costs. To ensure retention, the values or benefits of pursuing nursing education, graduation, licensing, and entry into professional nursing practice and/or advanced nursing program must outweigh the costs of nursing program attendance. Careful consideration of factors supporting or restricting success must be realistically appraised. Unfortunately, student expectations and perceptions may be unrealistic, thus increasing the risk for limited option appraisal, myopic views, and misguided decisions. Additionally, students are frequently indecisive and ambivalent, vacillating between persistence, stopout, or dropout.

Nurse educators are in a strategic position to make a difference by facilitating the process of systematic decision making and enhancing opportunities for retention and success. Awareness of the intricate complexities of retention decisions is a necessary precursor for taking effective action. This chapter will briefly introduce select background information and main concepts surrounding retention decisions. Implications for nurse educators will be proposed.

BACKGROUND

Attempts to understand decisions about persistence and voluntary attrition has mainly centered on students' perceived reasons for withdrawal via post-hoc studies. Data from autopsy attrition studies, however, should be viewed cautiously for several reasons. First, students are called upon to account for their attrition but may be unaware of the underlying reasons that may have contributed to their decision. Second, students may feel the need to cope with their dropout decision by rationalizing it and providing the most socially acceptable response. Moreover, they may be reluctant to criticize the institution (Braxton, Brier, & Hossler, 1988). With time, students' perceptions about their withdrawal decisions may become clouded and assume less importance, therefore adversely affecting validity.

Several valuable benefits concerning autopsy attrition data should be noted nonetheless. First, it is important to differentiate between voluntary and involuntary attrition, especially when evaluating the impact of specific retention strategies on attrition rates. Students who withdraw for nonacademic reasons can be considered separately in data analysis when evaluating postintervention attrition rates. For example, a student who withdraws due to an unplanned pregnancy does not provide valid data on the effectiveness of an educational support intervention to prevent attrition. The decision to withdraw was not influenced by the nursing program, educational support intervention, or academic institution. Including this student in the evaluation of the intervention would incorrectly lower the intervention's success rate.

Second, data can provide additional and valuable insight into the student's overall learning experience. For example, students who withdrew from a nursing course were surveyed to gain insight into why students withdraw. The questionnaire (Appendix E) was mailed after the end of the semester and asked students to respond anonymously. Consistent with other autopsy attrition studies and mailed questionnaires, the response rate was poor. Data was not robust enough to conduct statistical analyses;

however, respondents did provide interesting information. Most cited several academic and nonacademic underlying factors (see Appendix E) that influenced withdrawal decisions, with the most influential factor usually nonacademic.

The comment section added richness to the data. Several students indicated that after settling other interfering life situations, they would return to the nursing program and expected to be successful. Students who consider themselves as stopping out are different from dropouts, who have no intention of reentering the nursing program. Notably, several students wrote that they thanked faculty for their concern; others wrote that they felt encouraged about reenrolling because they believed that faculty "cared" enough to send a letter and questionnaire (Jeffreys, 2000). However, as mentioned above, autopsy attrition data do need to be interpreted cautiously, especially with small samples.

Several researchers proposed a psychological approach to understanding attrition decisions. Mashburn (2000) suggested that dropout decisions are preceded by a psychological process that involves level of student satisfaction and withdrawal cognitions, which include thoughts of quitting, intentions to search for other options (transfer), and dropout intentions. Low satisfaction combined with high withdrawal cognitions resulted in higher dropout rates. In contrast, students with low satisfaction but low withdrawal cognitions demonstrated lower dropout rates. Eaton and Bean (1995) purported a relationship among attitudes, intentions, and behaviors. Stress, coping, self-efficacy, avoidance/approach behaviors, satisfaction, and intent to leave were all important contributors to attrition decisions. (See chapter 7 for more details on satisfaction).

Although asking students why they decided to discontinue their education provides valuable information, it does not explain why other students decide to persist. Optimally, it is advantageous to examine closely the factors perceived as supportive or restrictive among students who persist. In one study, persisters were surveyed at the end of the semester and asked to rate the supportiveness or restrictiveness of select variables on their retention in a nursing course that semester (Jeffreys, 2002). As a group, students perceived faculty advisement and helpfulness, the enrichment program, tutoring, personal study skills, and friends in class as "greatly supportive." The most restrictive variables included family responsibilities, family crises, financial status, family financial support for school, family emotional support, financial aid, and child care arrangements. Conclusively, environmental variables greatly influenced retention, with professional integration variables perceived as greatly supportive.

CROSSROADS IN DECISION MAKING

As presented in the NURS model, professional integration factors are at the crossroads of the decision to persist, drop out, or stop out. Here, "crossroads" means a critical turning point in the student's decision-making process. Professional integration factors can enhance students' interaction with the social system of the college environment within the context of professional socialization and career development (see chapter 6). These factors include nursing faculty advisement and helpfulness, professional events, memberships in professional organizations, encouragement by friends in class, peer mentoring and tutoring, and enrichment programs. Such factors offer many advantages, resources, and support for students in the decision-making process. Lack of professional integration factors isolates students, hinders realistic option appraisal, and limits thoughtful decision making.

Although nurse educators have a legal responsibility for communicating nursing program policies concerning course withdrawals and progression criteria, they also have an ethical responsibility to assist students in the decision-making process. Proactive interventions that take into account cultural and other individual differences in decision making will be most effective (Brown & Kurpius, 1997; Nora, Cabrera, Hagedorn, & Pascarella, 1996) (see chapters 3 and 10). Nurse educators may need to initiate dialogue before misperceptions arise, before students are confronted with overwhelming obstacles, and before they make haphazard decisions. Figure 9.1 presents a systematic approach to the decision-making process that can serve as a beginning guide for student self-reflection, proactive group discussion, family/significant other consideration, and nurse educator intervention. Appraisal of options, strengths, supports, weaknesses, obstacles, benefits, costs, and expectations should be systematically considered before arriving at a decision.

Good academic performance results in retention decisions only when accompanied by positive psychological outcomes for the nursing program and profession. Additionally, academic strengths cannot compensate for weak environmental factors, although strong environmental supports may compensate for weak academic factors (Bean & Metzner, 1985; Metzner & Bean, 1987). Students with weak environmental supports are increasingly at risk for attrition, despite academic strengths and past successes. Professional integration factors have the power to tip the scale in favor of retention and success because of their unique potential for enhancing academic outcomes, satisfaction, and stress management via a holistic and integrated approach. Nurse educators can make a tremendous positive difference in the overall student experience and thus enhance retention. Part II presents several strategies for making a difference.

KEY POINTS SUMMARY

- The decision to remain in a course, persist in the nursing program, graduate, take the RN licensing exam, and enter the nursing work

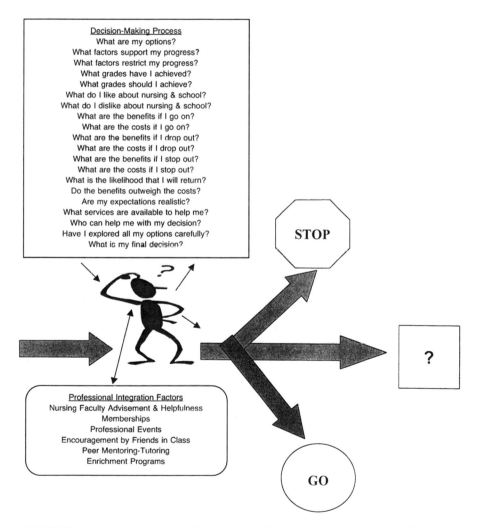

FIGURE 9.1   Crossroads in decision making: A systematic approach.

force and/or begin a more advanced nursing program occurs during and at the conclusion of each nursing course.

- Student profile characteristics, student affective factors, academic
  factors, environmental factors, professional integration factors, academic outcomes, psychological outcomes, and outside surrounding
  factors interact and influence retention decisions.
- Retention decisions are the determined resolution to persist in the
  nursing curriculum and educational pathway toward becoming a
  registered nurse.
- Professional integration factors are at the crossroads of the decision
  to persist, drop out, or stop out.
- Options, strengths, supports, weaknesses, obstacles, benefits, costs,
  and expectations should be systematically considered before arriving at a decision.
- Nurse educators have an ethical responsibility to assist students in
  the decision-making process.

EDUCATOR-IN-ACTION

Nurse educators are in a strategic position to facilitate the process of
systematic decision making and enhancing opportunities for retention
and success. After the second exam, three students (Cindy, Paolina, and
Maxine) have averages below 70 in the nursing course; a minimum 75
grade is required for passing. The nonpenalty course withdrawal date is
next week. Two additional exams, two quizzes, and a final exam remain.
Professor Bridges asks to meet with each failing student privately. As
another reminder to previous announcements, she offers to meet with
students to discuss course progress and career decision making. Rosita
schedules a meeting with Professor Bridges. Another student, Dawn, stops
in during office hours. Professor Bridges asks each student to review the
steps of the decision-making process (Figure 9.1). Excerpts of student
responses, educator actions, and resulting decisions follow below:

Cindy: "I know I haven't been keeping up with the reading or studying
the way I should. My grades reflect the amount of time I've been putting
into nursing. I will need to get at least an 80 on all of the exams and at least
a 78 on the quizzes in order to pass the course. If I withdraw now, I will
have to repeat all of the coursework and clinical completed so far. It's better that I stay in the course and work hard. I really want to be a nurse."

Professor Bridges discusses positive study and time management strategies with Cindy. Together, they develop a weekly schedule for reading,

review, and study. Cindy is referred to the Nursing Student Resource Center for additional support.

Decision: Continue.

Paolina: "I will need to get at least a 90 on all of the exams and at least an 86 on the quizzes in order to pass the course. I'm taking two advanced chemistry courses, Spanish, and art history. Those courses require a lot of time and I'm struggling to pass them too. All I do is study or go to class. If I withdraw from any class, I will not be a full-time student so I will lose my financial aid and health insurance. I can't afford to withdraw."

Professor Bridges encourages Paolina to discuss her future career goals. Paolina admits that she is really interested in being a pharmacist but thinks that pharmacy school will be too expensive. She indicates that her parents think it is more appropriate for her to become an associate degree nurse and start earning money in two years to help support her seven younger brothers and sisters. She dislikes nursing, especially the clinical component. Professor Bridges arranges for Paolina to meet with a career counselor individually and then with her parents present.

Decision: Drop out (of nursing). Paolina changes her major and applies for a student loan and on-campus work.

Maxine: "I do not work or have other responsibilities. I only need at least a 76 on all of my future exams and quizzes. I've always wanted to be a nurse. When I study in my group and with my tutor, I know everything. My anxiety gets in the way and I change many of my answers. I'm so close to passing that I don't want to drop out but I'm afraid of failing."

Professor Bridges determines, after some discussion, that Maxine does comprehend course material. She further explores the issue of test anxiety, suggests several strategies to reduce it, and refers Maxine to test anxiety reduction workshops.

Decision. Continue.

Rosita: "My second test grade dropped by 30 points. I really like nursing and I'm usually a good student. My husband was just diagnosed with terminal cancer with a six months prognosis. I am devastated. I feel that I want to spend every moment with him, yet I don't know what will happen if I drop the course."

Professor Bridges offers emotional support and invites Rosita to talk more about her feelings. Rosita appreciates the opportunity to talk about her husband. Professor Bridges provides her with information concerning readmission into the nursing program and counseling services.

Decision: Stopout.

Dawn: "I don't want to mess up my 4.0 average. My last grade was only an 86. I was thinking about withdrawing and taking the class next semester, but I don't want to be behind my classmates. Tell me what to do."

Professor Bridges assists Dawn to appraise her academic situation, goals, and career progress by going through each step of the decision-making process. She asks Dawn to write "Pros and Cons" for each step on the dry erase board. Together they compare and contrast reasons for stopping out or continuing. Professor Bridges does not make the decisions, but patiently guides Dawn through the process.

Decision: Continue.

Professor Bridges actively seeks to promote persistence and retention by meeting with the at-risk enrolled nursing students periodically. Follow-up correspondence via e-mails, letters, and phone calls are conducted with students who stopout.

REFERENCES AND BIBLIOGRAPHY

Bean, J. P. (1986). Assessing and reducing attrition. In D. Hossler (Ed.), *Managing college enrollments* (pp. 47–61). New Directions for Higher Education, 53. San Francisco: Jossey-Bass.

Bean, J. P., & Eaton, S. B. (2001). The psychology underlying successful retention practices. *Journal of College Student Retention: Research, Theory, & Practice, 3*(1), 73–90.

Bean, J. P., & Metzner, B. (1985). A conceptual model of nontraditional undergraduate student attrition. *Review of Educational Research, 55,* 485–540.

Braxton, J. M. (Ed.) (2000). *Reworking the student departure puzzle.* Nashville, TN: Vanderbilt University Press.

Braxton, J. M., Brier, E. M., & Hossler, D. (1988). The influence of student problems on student withdrawal decisions: An autopsy on "autopsy" studies. *Research in Higher Education, 28*(3), 241–253.

Brown, L. L., & Kurpius, S. E. R. (1997). Psychosocial factors influencing academic persistence of American Indian college students. *Journal of College Student Development, 38*(1), 3–12.

DesJardins, S. L., Kim, D-O., & Rzonca, C. S. (2002). A nested analysis of factors affecting bachelor's degree completion. *Journal of College Student Retention: Reseach, Theory, & Practice, 4*(4), 407–435.

Eaton, S. B., & Bean, J. P. (1995). An approach/avoidance behavioral model of college student attrition. *Research in Higher Education, 36,* 617–645.

Jeffreys, M. R. (2000). *Nursing student withdrawal data.* Unpublished material.

Jeffreys, M. R. (2002). Students' perceptions of variables influencing retention: A pretest and post-test approach. *Nurse Educator, 27*(1), 16–19 [Erratum, 2002, 27*(2), 64].

Knowles, M. (1984). *The adult learner: A neglected species.* Houston, TX: Gulf.

LeSure-Lester, G. E. (2003). Effects of coping styles on college persistence decisions among Latino students in two year colleges. *Journal of College Student Retention, Research, Theory, & Practice, 5*(1), 11–22.

Mashburn, A. J. (2000). A psychological process of student dropout. *Journal of College Student Retention, Research, Theory, & Practice, 2*(3), 173–190.

Metzner, B., & Bean, J. P. (1987). The estimation of a conceptual model of nontraditional undergraduate student attrition. *Research in Higher Education, 27,* 15–38.

Nora, A., Cabrera, A., Hagedorn, L. S., & Pascarella, E. (1996). Differential impacts of academic and social experiences on college-related behavioral outcomes across different ethnic and gender groups at four-year institutions. *Research in Higher Education, 37*(4), 427–451.

Polinsky, T. L. (2002). Understanding student retention through a look at student goals, intentions, and behavior. *Journal of College Student Retention: Research, Theory, & Practice, 4*(4), 361–376.

Porter, S. R. (2003). Understanding retention outcomes: Using multiple data sources to distinguish between dropouts, stopouts, and transfer-outs. *Journal of College Student Retention: Research, Theory, & Practice, 5*(1), 53–70.

PART II

Making a Difference: Promoting Retention and Success

P art II presents strategies for promoting retention and success. Chapters describe the process of designing, implementing, and evaluating specific strategies. Topics include culturally congruent nursing faculty advisement and helpfulness, expanding the web of inclusion through professional events and memberships, promoting positive and productive peer partnerships, enrichment programs, and nursing student resource centers. Case exemplars, illustrations, and tables are included to assist in creatively adapting described strategies. Consistent with Part I, practical application is further emphasized in the "Educator-in-Action" vignettes that follow the chapter summaries.

The main purpose of chapter 10 is to describe the process of developing a culturally congruent approach to faculty advisement and helpfulness. The process includes self-assessment, literature review, consultation and collaboration, student assessment, analysis, plan, communication, and interaction. Culturally congruent and culturally incongruent faculty actions, student perspectives and their influence on academic outcomes, psychological outcomes, and retention are examined.

Chapter 11 discusses creative strategies for expanding the web of inclusion by enhancing student opportunities for participation in professional events and memberships. Barrier recognition, solutions, strategies, and incentives are proposed.

Chapter 12 describes strategies for promoting positive and productive peer partnerships (purposeful affiliations, alliances, and connections among peers that result in constructive, generative, creative, and desirable outcomes). Carefully patterned and interwoven student-centered interactive experiences throughout the nursing curriculum can be structured to promote positive and productive peer partnerships. Recommendations for barrier recognition, solutions, strategies, and incentives are presented.

Nurse educators can make a difference in nursing student retention and success through a carefully designed enrichment program (EP). Chapter 13 describes the process of designing, implementing, and evaluating such a program. An illustrative case exemplar, using the Prenursing Enrichment Program (PEP), complements each step of the process.

The well-designed Nursing Student Resource Center (NSRC) offers a place for effectively linking multiple strategies. The main purpose of chapter 14 is to describe the process of designing, operating, and evaluating a NSRC. Key definitions, concepts, decisions, and considerations are discussed. Several checklists are provided to assist in planning and practical application.

Current and future enrollment trends predict a more academically and culturally diverse nursing student population, suggesting that nursing student persistence, retention, and success will be even more complex in the future. Nurse educators will always be in the most strategic position to influence retention positively. Unfortunately, the predicted nursing faculty shortage; the declining number of nurses who will be adequately prepared for the educator role; the growing need to defend, define, and redefine the "scholarship of teaching," compounded by the substantial gaps in nursing student retention research impose grave obstacles for the future. Chapter 15 proposes future directions and suggests a positive vision for tomorrow.

Several appendices provide valuable supplementary resources for educators and graduate students, including evaluation tools (questionnaires) designed to measure various dimensions of the retention process, with prestrategy and poststrategy evaluation. Additionally, the extensive "References and Bibliography" section after each chapter identifies contributive resources in the nursing and higher education literature.

Chapter **10**

Nursing Faculty Advisement and Helpfulness: A Culturally Congruent Approach

aculty advisement and helpfulness is the active involvement of nursing faculty in the student's academic endeavors, career goals, and professional socialization (see chapter 6). It is manifested through such actions as encouraging realistic educational and career goals, promoting positive feelings of self-worth, verbalizing belief in the student's ability to succeed, listening to problems and concerns, expressing interest in academic progress, showing optimism, offering assistance, and presence. Presence means caring about the student as a whole person, being available as a resource person, and making appropriate referrals when needed.

Consideration of the student as a whole person demands a culturally congruent approach to advisement and helpfulness. The inclusion of cultural values and beliefs (CVB) in the NURS model recognizes that a student's cultural values and beliefs unconsciously and consciously guide thinking, decisions, and actions that ultimately affect nursing student retention. The NURS model proposes that high levels of cultural congruence will serve as a bridge to promoting positive academic and psychological outcomes, thus enhancing persistence behaviors and retention (see chapter 3). Cultural congruence is the degree of fit between students' values and beliefs and those of their surrounding environment, that is,

nursing education within the educational institution and the nursing profession. The term "cultural congruent nursing care" was first coined and
defined by Leininger (1991) to describe nursing care with clients that is
meaningful, beneficial, and satisfying; however, the definition can be adapted to the educational setting. In this book, a culturally congruent approach
to faculty advisement and helpfulness refers to those faculty actions that
are tailored to fit with the student's CVB in order to promote, facilitate, or
support academic endeavors, career goals, and professional socialization.

A culturally congruent approach to faculty advisement and helpfulness requires faculty commitment and active engagement in the ongoing
process of developing cultural congruence and becoming "culturally
competent" faculty advisors and helpful teachers. The concept of cultural
competence as a process is prevalent in the nursing literature (Campinha-
Bacote, 1998a, 1998b; Davidhizar, Dowd, & Giger, 1998; Leininger, 1991;
Leininger & McFarland, 2002; Purnell, 2003). The main purpose of this
chapter is to describe the process of developing a culturally congruent
approach to faculty advisement and helpfulness. The process includes
self-assessment, literature review, consultation and collaboration, student
assessment, analysis, plan, communication, and interaction.

SELF-ASSESSMENT

Because faculty may be "unconsciously incompetent" in providing nursing advisement and help, the first step is self-assessment. According to
Purnell (2003), one is unconsciously incompetent when one is unaware
of cultural differences or when one unknowingly carries out actions that
are not culturally congruent. Cultural blindness, cultural imposition
and culturally incongruent actions can cause cultural pain to others
(Leininger & McFarland, 2002). The major aim of self-assessment is raising consciousness and self-awareness.

Self-assessment is a process in which the nurse educator systematically appraises various factors that can impact upon the achievement of culturally congruent advisement and helpfulness. A systematic assessment
can be initiated using the dimensions described in chapter 3, listed in
Table 3.1, and illustrated in Figure 10.1. The realization that there are
multidimensional variables influencing student–faculty interaction can
be overwhelming; yet these variables are essential to evaluate before
developing a culturally congruent approach. In addition to raising consciousness and self-awareness, self-assessment can help identify areas
of strengths and weaknesses and should be compared with students'
self-assessments and expectations.

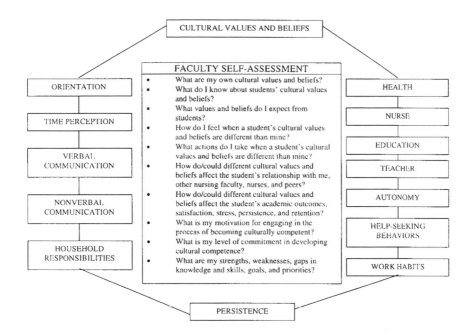

FIGURE 10.1   Cultural values and beliefs: Faculty self-assessment.

Note: Multidimensional cultural values and beliefs (CVB) surround and encompass all aspects of a systematic faculty self-assessment. See Table 3.1 for CVB category examples.

Although the faculty member may be immersed within the "culture" of nursing education and be familiar with long-held nursing education CVB, it is important to be aware that unconscious and conscious CVB in nursing education and in one's own values and belief systems, many of which were developed long before entering the nursing culture, may influence practices, behaviors, and actions. For example, a nursing faculty member whose traditional cultural values favor direct eye contact for all communication and who views lack of eye contact suspiciously will need to be consciously aware of his or her underlying values and beliefs and aim to consciously avoid distrusting students based solely on this nonverbal cue.

Awareness of one's knowledge about different CVB, especially those that most directly affect nursing student retention (through academic and psychological outcomes) must be explored. Although Table 3.1 presents a snapshot approach of selected CVB that may impact upon nursing student retention, it does allow for a quick comparison of different CVB. One benefit of this approach is that it evokes the awareness that there may be CVB in various cultures that the nurse educator is unaware of. The realization that one is not and cannot be "culturally competent" all of the time is often a powerful awakening. Becoming conscious of one's incompetence can be a humbling experience but frequently sparks a desire for obtaining cultural knowledge. Cultural awareness, desire, and knowledge are essential for the process of cultural competence (Campinha-Bacote, 2003).

Cultural knowledge is a thorough educational foundation about various CVB with the goal of comprehending and empathizing with others' perspectives. The nurse educator must assess his or her desire or motivation for becoming culturally competent. Reflecting on the feelings one experiences and the actions one takes when students' CVB are different from one's own can further one's insight. Because the process of cultural competence is ongoing, nurse educators should examine their commitment toward achieving this goal. True commitment requires time, energy, persistence, extra effort to overcome obstacles, and willingness to learn from mistakes. Commitment is essential in achieving positive outcomes in student retention (Campbell & Davis, 1996).

Nurse educators must appraise the multidimensional factors influencing undergraduate nursing student achievement, retention, and success, or full understanding will not truly be achieved. Furthermore, they need to evaluate how CVB can influence persistence behaviors (Kuh & Love, 2000). Nurse educators should reflect on the last time an updated review of the literature, workshop, or conference on student retention and success was completed. Again, appraisal of one's desire for updated knowledge and commitment in relation to other faculty responsibilities and available time should be critically determined.

Similarly, self-expectations of the advisor role and helpfulness to students should be examined. Faculty often overlook the significant role that their attitudes and behaviors can have on student satisfaction and retention (Lundquist, Spalding, & Landrum, 2002). Student perceptions and expectations about the faculty advisement role are often different from those of the faculty. Expectations about "helpfulness" can differ as well (Poorman, Webb, & Mastorovich, 2002). The mismatch between student and faculty expectations and perceptions creates another barrier whereby students can become disappointed and dissatisfied; poor psychological outcomes for the nursing program increase the risk for attrition.

Consequently, faculty members should appraise their knowledge about student expectations and perceptions. Lack of knowledge or limited knowledge in this area identifies targets for further self-development. However, one must have the desire to obtain such knowledge and be committed to its pursuit amidst other faculty responsibilities. Finally, self-assessment should conclude with a listing of strengths, weaknesses, gaps in knowledge, goals, commitment, and priorities.

LITERATURE REVIEW

Next, a review of the nursing and higher education literature should be conducted. The literature in psychology, anthropology, and sociology may also prove fruitful. Materials should be reviewed for gathering background information or updating previously gathered information about CVB, cultural competence, student retention, advisement, faculty helpfulness, help-seeking behaviors, and faculty–student interactions. Priority areas, weaknesses, or gaps in knowledge previously identified in the self-assessment can guide the review. Choice of a relevant conceptual framework can be instrumental to an organized review. For example, the NURS model can structure a systematic approach to the review and organization of retention literature. After gathering general background information, it may be appropriate to begin targeting specific student cultural groups, especially those with whom there is frequent interaction. The dimensions targeted in chapter 3 (Table 3.1) and Figure 10.1 can provide a guide for organizing specific information; however, it is vital to appraise each student individually and avoid stereotypical assumptions.

CONSULTATION AND COLLABORATION

Once sufficient background information has been reviewed and integrated, collaboration with others should be initiated. Sufficient background knowledge is a precursor for successfully optimizing consultation and collaboration. The nurse educator will now have a shared conceptual and empirical knowledge base with colleagues and experts that will promote deeper dialogue and added benefits. Consultation with experts in specific cultures, cultural competency, advisement, and student retention is helpful. Collaboration with colleagues (other nursing faculty) can help coordinate efforts and avoid unnecessary duplication. Consultation and collaboration can occur formally and informally via conferences, e-mail, telephone, and meetings.

A major benefit of collaboration among faculty is that nurse educators can become aware of each other's expertise and interests. Other goals include learning from others, avoiding pitfalls, and gaining insight into special program-specific considerations. Still another plus is broadening information sources and soliciting conceptual and/or instrumental support from others.

STUDENT ASSESSMENT

The ability to gather relevant and valid cultural information is an essential component in the development of cultural competence (Campinha-Bacote, 1998a). Moreover, a systematic appraisal of CVB is a precursor to determining the needs and priorities within a cultural context (Leininger, 1978). Promoting student self-assessment of cultural values and beliefs must be initiated in a positive, supportive environment that embraces diversity. Students will need to feel comfortable exploring their own CVB in the context of the nursing educational setting and sharing them with others, especially faculty. The literature suggests that students of different cultural backgrounds than faculty often feel isolated and reluctant to share differences for fear of reprimand, discrimination, or misunderstanding (Labun, 2002; Manifold & Rambur, 2001; Villaruel, Canales, & Torres, 2001; Weaver, 2001; Yurkovich, 2001).

Encouraging students to explore their own CVB concerning such dimensions as listed in Table 3.1 will enhance awareness of cultural similarities and differences with peers, clients, and faculty. This awareness will aid in the development of cultural competence in professional settings with clients, peers, other health care professionals, and ancillary workers. Asking about students' expectations of faculty advisement and helpfulness in the classroom, clinical setting, college skills laboratory, and informal settings will publicize and emphasize the fact that faculty care and have the desire to help. Students' perception that an instructor or advisor is concerned about their needs is helpful in and of itself and creates a caring environment. Perceptions that faculty sincerely care about students and openly apologize for (cultural) mistakes is more important than flawless, superficial, and distant interactions.

Student assessment may be done formally through the use of survey tools; however the development of valid and reliable tools that are free of cultural bias and social desirability response bias is a complicated and lengthy process. A previous review of literature may reveal already existing survey tools with adequate estimates of reliability and validity that can be used or adapted with permission. Use of a survey tool that has not been tested for validity and reliability not only provides questionable results but can impact adversely on student perceptions if items are offensive, misinterpreted, unclear, or culturally inappropriate. Such unwanted outcomes create dissatisfaction, add stress, and negatively influence retention.

Another formalized assessment approach is the use of focus groups consisting of select small groups of students (Yearwood, Brown, & Karlik, 2001). Dialogue with students, using a set of predetermined questions to guide the discussion and allow for comparison between student groups, will allow for unsolicited and solicited comments and qualitative data that can add a richness not achievable via quantitative or close-ended survey questioning. Focus groups that are guided by peer mentors or faculty who are not in a teaching role may ease fear of penalty or adverse consequences. A systematic assessment can be initiated using the dimensions listed in Table 3.1 and illustrated in Figure 10.2. Student responses can then be compared with those of faculty.

In the classroom, clinical setting, or college laboratory, a simple technique is to survey students anonymously on the first day. After an introduction, the instructor can express interest in meeting student needs through advisement and helpfulness and can ask students to write several ways that they believe the instructor can be helpful during the semester. It may also be beneficial to ask students to write anything that they experienced in the past that was not helpful or anything that they would perceive to be inappropriate or not helpful. This strategy can also be adapted to ask questions about faculty helpfulness in an informal setting.

Advisement and helpfulness should be developmental, that is, changing over time as student needs and expectations change, and so student assessment should be ongoing throughout the course and throughout the program at regularly scheduled intervals. For example, mid-semester, a classroom instructor may want to ask students to write comments again as before and compare them with the group's previous responses. Over time, common trends or themes may emerge, especially in a particular clinical setting or classroom course component. A systematic program appraisal can provide an overview of successful strategies and outcomes (Padilla, 1999).

ANALYSIS

Insight into students' perceptions is important in meeting needs of adult learners (Knowles, 1984). A systematic analysis of students' self-assessment should identify realistic versus unrealistic expectations, areas of untapped or underutilized advisor role, trends among the students surveyed, group similarities, individual differences, and perceived student needs. A thorough

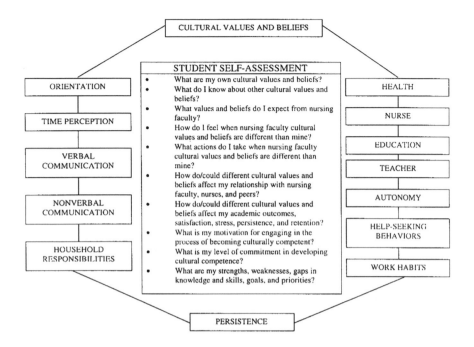

FIGURE 10.2   Cultural values and beliefs: Student self-assessment.

Note: Multidimensional cultural values and beliefs (CVB) surround and encompass all aspects of a systematic student self-assessment. See Table 3.1 for CVB category examples.

and objective analysis to determine the gap between student and faculty expectations, perceptions of what is important, and level of cultural congruence should be conducted. Mismatches need priority attention. The analysis should list strengths and congruency as well as weaknesses, gaps, and incongruency. Analysis of findings may be enhanced through the review of relevant literature to explain findings, elaborate major points, and offer suggestions.

PLAN

Next, a written action plan is developed. Individual faculty can review student comments for areas of unrealistic or unclear expectations and then plan to address them in a group setting to clarify advisor and faculty role. Similarly, faculty can verbally and positively respond to realistic, clear, and important expectations in faculty–student interactions. Relevant issues reported in the literature and/or uncovered through consultation and collaboration should be incorporated.

A plan for a faculty development workshop or series of workshops in enhancing culturally congruent advisement and helpfulness is central to promoting retention through positive psychological outcomes. Inadequate planning of effective advisement strategies appropriate for various students throughout the educational process supports the need for faculty development workshops (Braxton & Mundy, 2001; Sherrod & Harrison, 1994; Tucker-Allen & Long, 1999; Yoder, 2001). Nursing education goes beyond a single nurse educator. It is the whole nursing educational experience that impacts positively or negatively in the minds of students. One experience of cultural pain can do much to undermine the efforts of other faculty members who strongly advocate and consciously implement culturally congruent approaches.

The plan for faculty development should recognize that some faculty may fail to recognize the need for a workshop or may demonstrate reluctance to participate. Even if a workshop or series of workshops is mandatory, this does not necessarily mean that faculty will change values, beliefs, and traditions in favor of culturally congruent advisement and helpfulness. However, it is important to remember that all faculty members and students have CVB that may potentially be congruent or incongruent with each other and/or traditional nursing education values (Table 3.1). Both faculty and students may belong to multiple cultural groups, and the boundaries between cultural groups and affiliations is often unclear (Kuh & Love, 2000; Phinney, 1996). Therefore, formalized educational experiences concerning culture are necessary for all individuals, regardless of age, ethnicity, gender, sexual orientation, lifestyle, religion, socioeconomic status, or geographic location (Andrews, 1995; Jeffreys, 2000; Leininger, 1995b).

Tables 10.1, 10.2, and 10.3 provide case examples contrasting culturally incongruent and culturally congruent student–faculty interactions and the resulting outcomes. These case examples can be incorporated into a plan to initiate discussion with faculty and students. Such dialogue may help promote inner reflection or self-awareness of one's CVB, cultural imposition, ethnocentric tendencies, and potential impact of cultural pain on nursing student retention. Using case examples can point out that despite the intent to help, one's actions may not always be helpful. In fact, they may be counterproductive, causing pain, conflict, dissatisfaction, and stress for the student. Planning communication strategies to convey faculty commitment and holistic caring about culturally diverse students is necessary to avoid misunderstandings and to enhance the quality of faculty-student interactions.

TABLE 10.1 Examples of Culturally Incongruent and Culturally Congruent Advisement Approaches

Advisement Situation	Culturally Incongruent	Culturally Congruent
Shari arrives for academic course advisement accompanied by her husband. She states that she prefers having her husband with her. Shari's husband asks several questions concerning the nursing curriculum. Her CVB view decision making as a process involving her husband. Nonverbal communication cues (relaxed facial expression and relaxed body posture) suggest comfort with each other's presence during the advisement session.	Professor ignores student's CVB and does not actively explore preferred advisement style. Professor imposes her own CVB by stating, "I will be glad to answer any questions that Shari has. Shari, if you want to be a professional nurse, you must learn to be assertive, speak for yourself, and make decisions on your own." *Result:* Shari and her husband experience cultural pain and feel embarrassed. Because they view the professor as an authority figure, they do not want to confront her. Instead, they remain quiet. Later, Shari and her husband decide that she should drop out of the nursing program.	Professor recognizes the importance of Shari's CVB. Professor states, "It is nice to see such strong family support. I hope that I will be able to answer your questions. If you would like to move your chairs into a more comfortable arrangement please feel free to do so. I want to help you in the best way possible, so please let me know if something I say or do makes you uncomfortable or is unclear." *Result:* Shari and her husband feel that the professor genuinely cares about Shari holistically and is sincerely interested in accommodating their needs.

Advisement Situation	Culturally Incongruent	Culturally Congruent
Dana, a 25 year-old unmarried, part-time student visits the nursing advisor for registration. She has her three small children with her. She expresses concern over getting daytime courses that coincide with the college child care services. Her CVB place family responsibilities over all other responsibilities. Single parenting is not viewed negatively in her culture.	Professor holds traditional nursing values and beliefs as well as CVB that are congruent with nursing CVB. Professor states, "When I went to school, we weren't concerned about things like that. None of us were married and none of us had children. School was the priority. Nursing is hard work and should be a priority." *Result:* Dana feels discouraged and experiences hurt, anger, and pain.	Professor acknowledges the importance of Dana's concerns, and compliments her beautiful children and her motivation to pursue her nursing degree. Professor offers to call the child care guidance counselor to assist her with the child care aspect. *Result:* Dana feels satisfied that the advisor respects and understands her values and beliefs.
Iris experiences a personal crisis during the last semester before graduation. The stress associated with the crisis situation interferes with her ability to complete assignments and tests successfully. Iris's CVB stigmatize psychological stress. Talking about one's personal feelings is taboo. Indirect verbal communication and periods of silence for reflection are the preferred communication patterns. Iris asks the advisor for help in improving her grades.	Professor values a direct approach that aims to encourage verbalization of feelings. Professor states, "You obviously are under a lot of emotional stress. I think you should talk about your feelings with me or a college counselor." *Result:* Iris experiences cultural pain and distress because her emotional stress is outwardly recognizable. She feels stigmatized and reluctant to talk about feelings. This results in negative psychological feelings associated with school.	Professor recognizes that students may view stress differently and that different advisement approaches may be needed. Professor states, "Last month I had a student whose grades dropped following a personal crisis. Sometimes students experience stress related to outside issues or events. Some students have benefited from speaking with a counselor about their feelings." (pause) *Result:* Iris does not feel stigmatized and is satisfied with the advisor's approach.

TABLE 10.2   Faculty Helpfulness in the Classroom, Clinical Setting, and Nursing Skills Laboratory: Examples of Culturally Incongruent and Culturally Congruent Approaches

Situation	Culturally Incongruent	Culturally Congruent
Classroom Lou performed excellently on an exam, achieving the highest grade. Lou has group orientation rather than individual orientation, therefore is uncomfortable with individual praise.	Professor intends to be helpful, acknowledge strong performance, and motivate other students. Professor verbally praises Lou's performance in the classroom, announcing her name and exceptional performance. *Result:* Lou is embarrassed and feels ashamed over being singled out in the class.	Professor intends to be helpful and acknowledges strong performance and motivate other students, yet is aware of CVB that impact upon a cultural congruent approach. Professor verbally acknowledges the outstanding performance demonstrated by several students without mentioning their names. *Result:* Lou feels satisfied and comfortable with the knowledge that her performance and that of others in the group have been appreciated.
Clinical During clinical post-conference, one student (Jane) assertively questions the clinical instructor's statement about a medication. Jane's CVB openly encourage assertiveness and equally view teachers and learners as co-participants in the teaching–learning process. Several students with different CVB are obviously uncomfortable by the perceived confrontation.	Professor's CVB consider the preservation of group harmony and "saving face" as a priority. She sees the discomfort of two other students in the group and aims to help the group avoid conflict. Professor's response is to avoid answering Jane's question and dismiss the post-conference early. *Result:* Jane is still confused and feels stressed about the medication. She is dissatisfied with the professor's actions.	Professor recognizes differences between individual versus group orientation. Although her own CVB are group orientation, Professor realizes that Jane's behavior is appropriate. Professor answers Jane's question and uses this opportunity to discuss various differences in communication patterns, values, and beliefs among different cultures. *Result:* Jane and the other students receive clarification about the statement and receive new information about culture and values clarification, enhancing academic outcomes and promoting positive psychological outcomes.

Situation	Culturally Incongruent	Culturally Congruent
Nursing Skills Laboratory After a detailed skills laboratory class on injections, it is now Lee's turn to administer an intramuscular injection into the skill's laboratory mannequin for the first time. Lee's CVB view the teacher as an authority figure. Less than perfect performance would poorly reflect on the teacher and cause embarrassment for the teacher in front of the other students. Lee is fearful that she will not demonstrate the skill perfectly and feels that she must "save face," yet Lee does not want to refuse the professor's request to inject. Anxiously, she asks if she can first practice with her peers.	Professor wants to help all students equally and aims to "treat all students alike." Professor insists that Lee administer the injection. *Result:* Lee feels increasingly anxious and pressured that she must perform the injection perfectly. Additionally, she feels cultural pain because she believes that she initiated conflict with an authority figure. Lee attempts the injection but when she forgets to aspirate, she becomes even more anxious and experiences cultural pain because she has now "embarrassed her teacher." Lee feels much dissatisfaction and stress; she questions her ability to complete the nursing program.	Professor recognizes that Lee's anxiety may not be related to lack of academic readiness, but due to underlying CVB. Professor reassures Lee that she does not expect perfection on the first attempt; however she still notes nonverbal cues of anxiety (facial tension, shaking hands, flushed appearance). Professor pairs Lee with a strong student who has already performed the injection and allows privacy for several practice injections. *Result:* Lee does not feel pressured to "save face" and can relax enough with her peer to perfect her skill prior to observation by the instructor. After demonstrating the injection to the professor accurately, Lee experiences satisfaction.

TABLE 10.3   Faculty Helpfulness Beyond Class: Examples of Culturally Incongruent and Culturally Congruent Approaches

Situation	Culturally Incongruent	Culturally Congruent
Outside Maria is walking across the campus with her father and encounters her former nursing instructor. Maria's CVB place parents, elders, teachers, and nurses as a highly respected individuals. Family and traditions are priorities; education is secondary. She formally introduces her father and the instructor.	Professor values casual, informal interaction with students, thinking that this is helpful for all students. She states, "Oh, just call me Cathy. There's no need to be so formal." *Result:* Maria and her father experience cultural pain and embarrassment. Maria's father is concerned that Maria will abandon her traditional CVB. Maria feels pulled between her traditional CVB and pursuit of a nursing career.	Professor is comfortable with casual, informal interaction with students, yet respects alternative values. Professor does not attempt to impose her values; rather she graciously thanks Maria for the formal introduction and responds formally. *Result:* Maria and her father experience positive psychological outcomes (satisfaction).
Office Hours During office hours, several students asked the instructor's help for completing a written paper assignment. Pat does not understand how to complete a written paper assignment; however his CVB are not congruent with self-initiated, actively help-seeking behaviors.	Professor holds CVB that value assertiveness, active help-seeking behaviors, and confrontation with authority. Professor states to her colleague, "I keep my office door open so students can stop by and ask for help. If students don't ask for help, they deserve the grade they get." *Result:* Pat still does not understand the assignment, fails the paper, resulting in poor academic and psychological outcomes.	Professor recognizes that help-seeking behaviors vary culturally and consciously makes an effort to follow up on students who do not seek help. Professor requests that Pat meet during office hours to discuss the written paper assignment, stating, "When students share their questions and feedback concerning papers and the class, it helps me a great deal. Could you please help me by stopping by to talk about the paper?" *Result:* Pat receives the necessary help needed and passes the assignment. Positive academic and psychological outcomes occur.

COMMUNICATION

Communicating that culture matters and that students matter requires an integrated, well-planned approach. Multimedia strategies to promote open communication, clarify misperceptions about the faculty advisor role, convey caring and helpfulness, and develop student–faculty partnerships in achieving cultural congruency should be proactive and ongoing. For example, communication can be initiated in new student orientations, on initial assignment to an advisor, on the first day of class/clinical via verbal, written, and other media format. Slides, PowerPoint presentations, videos, case examples, and other multimedia approaches can be used to supplement previous information and initiate discussions in large groups, small groups, or individual settings with students. The faculty advisor role, teacher's role, and student rights and responsibilities can be delineated and described in student newsletters, handout materials, student handbook, welcome letters to new students, course outlines, bulletin board postings, e-mail list serves, and Web pages. Messages that openly celebrate diversity encourage others to appreciate and embrace the diversity among students, faculty, clients, and society in general. Such messages permit the open sharing and exchange of cultural information that is a necessary precursor to mutually satisfying interactions with culturally different individuals.

INTERACTION

It is not sufficient for educators to have read about cultures, attended workshops, professed commitment to cultural competence, or surveyed students; faculty must take action and enter a new phase in achieving cultural competence. Campinha-Bacote (1998a) calls this interaction phase "cultural encounter." Leininger (2002), however, defines cultural encounter as a situation in which someone meets or briefly interacts with a culturally different individual. Such a brief encounter does not allow deep understanding or insight into the culture. In this book, cultural interaction refers to the ongoing, planned and unplanned situations in which faculty and students with various CVB have shared experiences or interactions. The faculty member committed to the goal of developing cultural competence and providing culturally congruent advisement and helpfulness will make a concerted effort to actively initiate and engage in cultural interactions throughout the educational process and possibly beyond graduation and into the student's entry into the nursing profession.

Cultural interaction leads to greater insight into the student's culture on the individual level. Interactions offer the opportunity to recognize the cultural variations among individuals, families, and groups (Leininger, 2002). Through ongoing interactions, the discovery that cultural variations exist and impact differently on faculty–student interactions, persistence, and all dimensions of culture helps prevent stereotyping of individuals based on perceived cultural group affiliation. Cultural interaction fosters the exchange of CVB, thus facilitating personal growth, professional growth, and the development of cultural competence for educators and students. An initial interaction that values, appreciates, and embraces diversity will do much to encourage the further exchange of information, values, beliefs, and ideas as well as promote positive psychological outcomes (satisfaction and decreased stress) associated with the educational experience.

Entering a culturally different or unknown world can be intimidating or stressful for fear of making a mistake or inadvertently doing something "wrong." Such fears are a barrier to initiating and engaging in substantive cultural interactions with students. Acknowledging ahead of time that mistakes may occur is important; however, learning from one's mistakes and moving forward is even more important. A "cultural mistake" can make one more consciously competent next time when encountering a similar or even different situation.

Cultural competency must never be taken for granted. One cannot ever be totally culturally competent, but one can exert conscious effort into achieving cultural congruence. Insight can be enhanced by self-reflection and reflection-in-action (Schon, 1987). Reflection calls for ongoing self-assessment, updated knowledge, consultation, collaboration, student assessment, analysis, plan, communication, and cultural interactions.

KEY POINTS SUMMARY

- Faculty advisement and helpfulness is manifested through such actions as encouraging realistic educational and career goals, promoting positive feelings of self-worth, verbalizing belief in the student's ability to succeed, listening to problems and concerns, expressing interest in academic progress, showing optimism, offering assistance, and presence.
- A culturally congruent approach to faculty advisement and helpfulness refers to those faculty actions that are tailored to fit with the student's cultural values and beliefs (CVB) in order to promote, facilitate, or support meaningful, beneficial, and satisfying academic endeavors, career goals, and professional socialization.

- A culturally congruent approach to faculty advisement and help-fulness requires faculty commitment and active engagement in the ongoing process of developing cultural congruence and becoming "culturally competent" faculty advisors and helpful teachers. The process includes self-assessment, literature review, consultation and collaboration, student assessment, analysis, plan, communication, and interaction.
- Self-assessment is a process in which the nurse educator systematically appraises various factors that can impact upon the achievement of culturally congruent advisement and helpfulness.
- Promoting student self-assessment of cultural values and beliefs must be initiated in a positive, supportive environment that embraces diversity.
- A plan for a faculty development workshop or series of workshops in enhancing culturally congruent advisement and helpfulness is central to promoting retention through positive psychological outcomes.
- Multimedia strategies to promote open communication, clarify misperceptions about the faculty advisor role, convey caring and helpfulness, and develop student–faculty partnerships in achieving cultural congruency should be proactive and ongoing.
- Cultural interaction refers to the ongoing, planned and unplanned situations in which faculty and students with various CVB have shared experiences.
- High levels of cultural congruence will serve as a bridge to promoting positive academic and psychological outcomes, thus enhancing persistence behaviors and retention.

EDUCATOR-IN-ACTION

At a nursing faculty meeting, Professor Glass introduces the topic of "Culturally Congruent Faculty Advisement and Helpfulness" by sharing a personal experience. "I used to think of myself as being a helpful advisor to all students; however this opinion changed recently. I realized that I made a cultural mistake with one of my students. This mistake set up obstacles for future communication and caused her obvious stress. I apologized immediately but later I always felt a gap was present. I realized that the increased number of new immigrant nursing students from diverse countries meant that I could not use the same approach with all students. I was also concerned that I may have offended others unintentionally. The next week in class, I asked students to reflect on their experiences with nursing faculty so far and anonymously write down helpful faculty actions, unhelpful faculty actions, student expectations about faculty advisement and helpfulness, and any cultural customs relevant to faculty–student interactions. Responses were amazing."

Professor Glass read several student comments that contrasted student perceptions, cultural values and beliefs, and student experiences with faculty.

1. "My advisor always stares right into my eyes during the registration advisement session. I get so uncomfortable that I feel as though I can't even speak."
2. "My advisor hardly ever looks me in the eye so I don't think she even sees me as a person."
3. "When nursing faculty greet me in the hall or library and offer to help me during office hours, it makes me feel like they care."
4. "My advisor was right behind me in the cafeteria line and didn't even acknowledge my greeting or say hello."
5. "When my advisor changed her office hours to Friday afternoons, she offered to set an alternate meeting time with me instead of making me change advisors. That made me feel as though she really cared about me and respected my religious beliefs."
6. "Thank you for asking about our (students') feelings, experiences, and concerns. Even if you do something other than what I expect, I will now feel as though you are trying to treat us as individuals and respect our cultural values and beliefs."

Other faculty members relate similar experiences and concerns about providing culturally congruent advisement and helpfulness. Faculty decide that the annual faculty development workshop topic will be "Culturally Congruent Advisement and Helpfulness: Strategies to Enhance Nursing Student Retention and Success." Subsequent plans are made to have a two-day faculty retreat to critique the curriculum, recruitment and retention strategies, and advisement approaches for culturally sensitive approaches that embrace diverse cultures.

REFERENCES AND BIBLIOGRAPHY

Alexitch, L. R. (2002). The role of help-seeking attitudes and tendencies in students' preferences for academic advising. *Journal of College Student Development, 43*(1), 5–19.
Andrews, M. (1995). Transcultural nursing: Transforming the curriculum. *Journal of Transcultural Nursing, 6* (2), 4–9.

Andrews, M., & Boyle, J. (1999). *Transcultural concepts in nursing* (3rd ed.). Philadelphia: Lippincott.

Baldwin, D., & Wold, J. (1993). Students from disadvantaged backgrounds: Satisfaction with a mentor-protégé relationship. *Journal of Nursing Education, 32*(5), 225–226.

Barbee, E. L., & Gibson, S. E. (2001). Our dismal progress: The recruitment of non-whites into nursing. *Journal of Nursing Education, 40*(6), 243–244.

Bessent, H. (Ed.). (1997). *Strategies for recruitment, retention, and graduation of minority nurses in colleges of nursing.* Washington, DC: American Nurses Publishing.

Braxton, J. M. (Ed.). (2000). *Reworking the student departure puzzle.* Nashville, TN: Vanderbilt University Press.

Braxton, J. M., & Mundy, M. E. (2001). Powerful institutional levers to reduce college student departure. *Journal of College Student Retention: Research, Theory, & Practice, 3* (1), 91–118.

Campbell, A. R., & Davis, S. M. (1996). Faculty commitment: Retaining minority nursing students in majority institutions. *Journal of Nursing Education, 35* (7), 298–303.

Campinha-Bacote, J. (1998a). *The process of cultural competence in the delivery of healthcare services: A culturally competent model of care* (3rd ed.). Cincinnati, OH: Transcultural C.A.R.E. Associates.

Campinha-Bacote, J. (1998b). Cultural diversity in nursing education: Issues and concerns. *Journal of Nursing Education, 37*(1), 3–4.

Campinha-Bacote, J. (2003). *The process of cultural competence in the delivery of healthcare services: A culturally competent model of care* (4th ed.). Cincinnati, OH: Transcultural C.A.R.E. Associates.

Davidhizar, R., Dowd, S. B., & Giger, J. N. (1998). Educating the culturally diverse healthcare student. *Nurse Educator, 23*(2), 38–42.

Davidhizar, R., & Giger, J. N. (2001). Teaching culture within the nursing curriculum using the Giger-Davidhizar model of transcultural nursing assessment. *Journal of Nursing Education, 40*(6), 282–288.

Hammond, P. V., Davis, B. L., Hodges, G., & Warfield, M. (1997). Increasing retention rates of disadvantaged students through a faculty development program. *The Association of Black Nursing Faculty Journal, 8*(3), 51–53.

Herndorn, J. B., Kaiser, J.,& Creamer, D. G. (1996). Student preferences for advising style in community college environments. *Journal of College Student Development, 37*(6), 637–647.

Hesser, A., Pond, E., Lewis, L., & Abbott, B. (1996). Evaluation of a supplementary retention program for African-American baccalaureate nursing students. *Journal of Nursing Education, 35*(7), 304–309.

Jeffreys, M. R. (2000). Development and psychometric evaluation of the Transcultural Self-Efficacy Tool: A synthesis of findings. *Journal of Transcultural Nursing, 11*(2), 127–136.

Jeffreys, M. R. (2001). Evaluating enrichment program study groups: Academic outcomes, psychological outcomes, and variables influencing retention. *Nurse Educator, 26*(3), 142–149.

Jeffreys, M.R. (2002). Students' perceptions of variables influencing retention: A pretest and post-test approach. *Nurse Educator, 27*(1), 16–19 [Erratum, 2002, *27*(2), 64].

Jeffreys, M. R., & Smodlaka, I. (1996). Steps of the instrument-design process: An illustrative approach for nurse educators. *Nurse Educator, 21*(6), 47–52; (erratum, 1997, 22(1), 49).

Kirkland, M. L. S. (1998). Stressors and coping strategies among successful female African American baccalaureate nursing students. *Journal of Nursing Education, 37*(1), 5–12.

Kirkpatrick, M. K., & Koldjeski, D. (1997). Career planning: The nurse educator as facilitator and career counselor. *Nurse Educator, 27*(3), 17–20.

Knowles, M. (1984). *The adult learner: A neglected species.* Houston, TX: Gulf.

Kuh, G. D., & Hu, S. (2001). The effects of student–faculty interaction in the 1990's. *The Review of Higher Education, 24*(3), 309–332.

Kuh, G. D., & Love, P. G. (2000). A cultural perspective on student departure. In J. M. Braxton (Ed.), *Reworking the student departure puzzle* (pp. 196–212). Nashville, TN: Vanderbilt University Press.

Labun, E. (2002). The Red River College Model: Enhancing success for native Canadian and other nursing students from disenfranchised groups. *Journal of Transcultural Nursing, 13*(4), 311–317.

Lehna, C., Jackonen, S., & Wilson, L. (1996). Navigating a nursing curriculum: Bridges and barriers. *Association for Black Nursing Faculty Journal, 7*(July/August), 98–103.

Leininger, M. M. (1978). *Transcultural nursing: Theories, concepts, and practices.* New York: Wiley.

Leininger, M. M. (1991). *Culture care diversity and universality: A theory of nursing.* New York: National League for Nursing.

Leininger, M. M. (1995). Teaching transcultural nursing in undergraduate and graduate programs. *Journal of Transcultural Nursing, 6*(2), 10–26.

Leininger, M. M. (2002). Essential transcultural nursing care concepts, principles, examples, and policy statements. In M. M. Leininger & M. R. McFarland (Eds.), *Transcultural nursing: Concepts, theories, research, and practice* (3rd ed., pp. 45–69). New York: McGraw-Hill.

Leininger, M. M., & McFarland, M. R. (2002). *Transcultural nursing: Concepts, theories, research, and practice* (3rd ed.). New York: McGraw-Hill.

Lundquist, C., Spalding, R. J., & Landrum, R. E. (2002). College student's thoughts about leaving the university: The impact of faculty attitudes and behaviors. *Journal of College Student Retention: Research, Theory, and Practice, 4*(2), 123–134.

Manifold, C., & Rambur, B. (2001). Predictors of attrition in American Indian nursing students. *Journal of Nursing Education, 40*(6), 279–281.

Nora, A. (2001). The depiction of significant others in Tinto's "Rites of Passage": A reconceptualization of the influence of family and community in the persistence process. *Journal of College Student Retention: Research, Theory, & Practice, 3*(1), 41–56.

Padilla, R. V. (1999). College student retention: Focus on success. *Journal of College Student Retention: Research, Theory, and Practice, 1*(2), 131–146.

Phinney, J. S. (1996). Understanding ethnic diversity. *American Behavioral Scientist, 40*(2), 143–152.

Poorman, S. G., Webb, C. A., & Mastorovich, M. L. (2002). Students' stories: How faculty help and hinder students at risk. *Nurse Educator, 27*(3), 126–131.

Purnell, L. D. (2003). Purnell's model for cultural competence. In L. D. Purnell & B. J. Paulanka (Eds.), *Transcultural health care: A culturally competent approach* (2nd ed., pp. 8–39). Philadelphia: Davis.

Purnell, L. D., & Paulanka, B. J. (2003). *Transcultural health care: A culturally competent approach* (2nd ed.). Philadelphia: Davis.

Rew, L. (1996). Affirming cultural diversity: A pathways model for nursing faculty. *Journal of Nursing Education, 35*(7), 310–314.

Schön, D. (1987). *Educating the reflective practitioner.* San Francisco: Jossey-Bass.

Schultz, E. D. (1998). Academic advising from a nursing theory perspective. *Nurse Educator, 22*(2), 22–25.

Sherrod, R. A., & Harrison, L. (1994). Evaluation of a comprehensive advisement program designed to enhance student retention. *Nurse Educator, 19*(6), 29–33.

Thurber, F., Hollingsworth, A., Brown, L., & Whitaker, S. (1989). The faculty advisor role: An imperative for student retention. *Nurse Educator, 13*(3), 27–33.

Trent, B. A. (1997). Student perceptions of academic advising in an RN-to-BSN program. *Journal of Continuing Education in Nursing, 28*(6), 276–283.

Tucker-Allen, S., & Long, E. (1999). *Recruitment and retention of minority students: Stories of success.* Lisle, IL: Tucker.

Villaruel, A. M., Canales, M., & Torres, S. (2001). Bridges and barriers: Educational mobility of Hispanic nurses. *Journal of Nursing Education, 40*(6), 245–251.

Weaver, H. N. (2001). Indigenous nurses and professional education: Friends or foes? *Journal of Nursing Education, 40*(6), 252–258.

Winters, C. E. (1990). Excellence in advisement: A strategy for declining nursing enrollments. *Journal of Nursing Education, 29*(5), 233–234.

Yearwood, E., Brown, D. L., & Karlik, E. C. (2002). Cultural diversity: Students' perspectives. *Journal of Transcultural Nursing, 13*(3), 237–240.

Yoder, M. K. (2001). The bridging approach: Effective strategies for teaching ethnically diverse nursing students. *Journal of Transcultural Nursing, 35*(7), 315–321.

Yoder, M. K., & Saylor, C. (2002). Student and teacher roles: Mismatched expectations. *Nurse Educator, 27*(5), 201–203.

Yurkovich, E. E. (2001). Working with American Indians toward educational success. *Journal of Nursing Education, 40*(6), 259–269.

Chapter **11**

Expanding the Web of Inclusion Through Professional Events and Memberships

P articipation in professional events and memberships is viewed as an essential activity for professional growth and career mobility by providing unique opportunities for professional socialization, networking, skill enhancement, knowledge expansion, and professional attitude development (Joel & Kelly, 2002). Professional events are nursing conferences, workshops, meetings, volunteer services, or social activities that have specific goals relevant for nursing education, practice, research, or theory. Memberships refer to affiliation or participation within nursing organizations or associations as a "member" prescribed by the respective bylaws (see chapter 6).

Within the NURS model, participation in professional events and memberships is viewed as an essential component for enhancing professional integration and for minimizing social isolation. Professional integration greatly enhances nursing student retention by promoting positive psychological outcomes and offering opportunities to enrich academic experiences and outcomes. It is proposed that positive experiences in professional event participation and memberships positively affect retention by enhancing self-efficacy and motivation, promoting professional integration, and facilitating positive psychological outcomes.

Although nursing students may feel a sense of cohesiveness or belonging within the classroom or clinical group, many still feel somewhat detached and disconnected from the nursing profession. This isolation is counterproductive and prevents students from achieving their optimal potential within nursing. Gaining entry and starting to feel part of the nursing professional is crucial. Nursing students must become "enculturated into nursing values, norms, and lifeways to survive, function, and become professional nurses" (Leininger & McFarland, 2002, p. 56).

Consequently, the nursing profession is challenged to include, embrace, and welcome nursing students as future valuable assets to the profession. Nurse educators are challenged to expand the web of student inclusion beyond the traditionally required educational curriculum and setting through professional events and memberships. In this book, the web of inclusion refers to an interwoven professional network that embraces students and strives to promote professional integration through participation in professional events and memberships.

Unfortunately, many nursing students (and nurse educators) undervalue and underestimate the significance of professional event participation and memberships. Visionary nurse educators are therefore challenged to develop innovative strategies and incentives to motivate students and encourage participation. Students often encounter obstacles that discourage them from professional event participation and memberships. Nurse educators can first assist students by recognizing these obstacles, removing barriers, and offering acceptable solutions. Strategies that enhance student opportunities to participate in various professional integration factors will ultimately benefit students and the nursing profession. The purpose of this chapter is to discuss creative strategies for expanding the web of inclusion by enhancing student opportunities for participation in professional events and memberships. Barrier recognition, solutions, strategies, and incentives will be proposed.

NURSE EDUCATORS AS ROLE MODELS

Participation in nursing conferences, workshops, events, meetings, and memberships exemplifies a professional commitment to lifelong learning that can be motivating and uplifting to students. Professional nurses as role models can enhance self-efficacy and motivation, thereby enhancing student persistence and retention. Because students have the most exposure to the nursing profession through faculty guidance, nurse educators can exert a powerful influence on them. If faculty do not value professional event participation and memberships for their own professional development, then it is hard to imagine that they would have a positive impact on encouraging student participation. Similarly, if nurse educators are actively involved in professional events and memberships, yet do not actively publicize their views, involvement, participation, and contribution to professional events and memberships, positive professional role modeling will not be evident to students.

Faculty self-assessment as active role models in promoting/facilitating student professional event participation and memberships is a necessary precursor for strategy development. Table 11.1 provides a guide for appraising values, beliefs, and actions, and for determining whether one is an active role model. It is proposed that the actions taken to promote/facilitate participation make one an active role model. Table 11.1 can also provide a guide for organizational self-assessment to determine if organizations are "student friendly" (inclusive) or if there are obstacles obstructing student participation, thus creating "student unfriendly" (exclusive) environments.

After self-assessment, nurse educators who have not optimally shared positive views, values, beliefs, and experiences with students should make a concerted effort to do so. However, it is not enough to profess values and beliefs to students; nurse educators must be sincerely committed and take positive actions in order to "make a difference" and enhance the "web of inclusion." In order to do this, they must recognize actual and potential barriers hindering students' participation, propose solutions, initiate strategies to remove barriers, and offer incentives to enhance participation.

Barriers may be practical or psychosocial. Practical barriers include financial cost, travel, and time (see Table 11.2). Psychosocial barriers include perceived irrelevance to immediate educational goals, perceived irrelevance to future professional goals, multiple role stress, and fear of isolation. (Table 11.3, p. 193). Often, students are faced with a combination of practical and perceptual barriers.

PRACTICAL BARRIERS: RECOGNITION, SOLUTIONS, STRATEGIES, AND INCENTIVES

Financial Cost

For many students, the financial cost of a conference, workshop, or membership is a major deterrent. Although a reduced student fee or rate may be an incentive to some, it may not be enough to attract diverse student groups. For example, an economically disadvantaged student or a nontraditional student struggling with tuition, living expenses, and child care costs may be unable to afford fees or may be unable to justify financial resource allocation to a "nonessential" expense. Even the "luxury"

TABLE 11.1   Self-Assessment: Active Role Model in
Promoting/Facilitating Student Professional Event Participation
and Memberships

Role Model	Values, Beliefs, and Actions	Role Model
Yes	Views professional event participation as important in own life *and shares beliefs with students**	No
Yes	Views memberships in nursing organizations/associations as important in own life *and shares beliefs with students*	No
Yes	Views professional event participation as important in undergraduate students' education and/or professional development and/or retention *and shares view with students*	No
Yes	Views student memberships in nursing organizations/associations as important in undergraduate students' education and/or professional development and/or retention *and shares view with students*	No
Yes	Attends professional events *and shares positive and relevant experiences with students*	No
Yes	Maintains membership(s) in nursing organizations/associations *and shares positive and relevant experiences with students*	No
Yes	Recognizes actual and potential barriers hindering students' professional event participation *and initiates strategies to remove barriers*	No
Yes	Recognizes actual and potential barriers hindering student memberships *and initiates strategies to remove barriers*	No
Yes	*Offers incentives to encourage student participation in professional events*	No
Yes	*Offers incentives to encourage student participation in memberships*	No

* Active promoter/facilitator actions are indicated by italics.

TABLE 11.2   Student Participation in Professional Events
and Memberships: Practical Barriers, Solutions, Strategies,
and Incentives

Barriers	Solutions	Strategies and Incentives
Financial cost	Waive fee Reduce fee	Sponsorship Award or scholarship Volunteer work Service exchange Group discounts Student fee
Travel	Eliminate travel Enhance ease of travel	Host event Carpools Charter bus Public transportation group travel Clear directions
Time	Eliminate extra time needed Minimize time conflicts/burden	Event corresponds with class time Sufficient advance notice Time exchange from class Schedule before or after class Readjust class assignment and test schedule Assistance with application related tasks

of a conference may not be justified for someone who is unsure of financial stability. As a strategy to increase membership participation, incorporating National Student Nurse Association (NSNA) membership as a
mandatory curricular requirement and instituting a student fee to cover
this expense may assist financially challenged students to get this expense
covered via financial aid, scholarships, and/or student loans.

Waiving of professional event fees may be a more productive option
for increasing student participation; however it may not always be feasible because of overhead costs and expenses. An alternative to fee waivers
may be soliciting sponsorship by nursing faculty, other nurses, alumni,
deans, agencies, members of professional organizations, and organizations themselves. An incentive to individuals for sponsoring a student
may be a reduction in conference or membership fees. For example:

TABLE 11.3   Student Participation in Professional Events and Memberships: Psychosocial Barriers, Solutions, Strategies, and Incentives

Barriers	Solutions	Strategies and Incentives
Perceived irrelevance to immediate educational goals	Demonstrate relevance to immediate educational goals	Link with course objectives Link with course assignments Link with test questions Provide background information Extra credit Mandatory participation Student certificates for participation
Perceived irrelevance to future professional goals	Demonstrate relevance to future professional goals	Faculty role models Student role models Professional role models Link with legal and ethical issues Link with criteria for a profession Professional portfolio and résumé Educational mobility Career mobility
Multiple role stress	Reduce role stress Demonstrate strategies to manage multiple roles effectively	Sufficient advance notice Case examples Letter to employer Written materials for significant others Extended college child care services
Fear of isolation	Eliminate fear of isolation Minimize fear of isolation Promote feelings of inclusion	Link with faculty buddy or other RN Student role models Introduction to other students Introduction to presenters and/or members Networking during lunch and break times Encourage student involvement Publicize student involvement Student outreach and welcome

"Sponsor a student, save 10%" or "sponsor one student, bring another student free." Nurse educators can actively suggest options to sponsoring agencies or organizations, such as offering an award or scholarship to student volunteers, students with the highest GPAs, or elected student nurse club (SNC) officers.

Another option may be to waive fees in exchange for volunteer services, such as assistance with workshop registration or stuffing membership renewal envelopes. Offering discounts for groups of students suggests that students are a welcome and desired audience; group discounts encourage students to attend together while also sharing costs. Offering a 20% discount for every group of five students is one such example. Other expenses associated with attending a professional event may be travel, food, parking, lodging, or child care, which can impose severe restrictions for many students. Any effort to include these expenses when approaching potential sponsors will enhance opportunities for financially challenged or financially unsure (insecure) students.

Travel

Travel costs and concerns can be minimized through the use of organized carpools, charter buses or vans, or group travel via public transportation. Ambiguous or unclear travel directions are a major deterrent. The nurse educator can facilitate the ease of travel by providing clear directions from the nursing school, and/or organizing group car travel from the familiar location of the school. Assuring that directions are provided via the various modes of transportation available from the school will serve to include more students. By offering to host a professional event sponsored by a nursing organization, nurse educators can ensure that students will have the optimal opportunity to attend a professional event on campus in a nearby, familiar setting, thus easing travel concerns.

Time

Time demands from numerous responsibilities and roles may compete with participation in professional events and memberships. Sufficient advance notice of events is particularly important to allow for work schedule requests, child care coverage, and other responsibilities that compete with the students' time in school, family, and work arenas. Nurse educators can minimize time demands by readjusting class schedules to accommodate participation in a professional event, such as shifting course topics and changing assignment due dates or test dates to avoid conflicts with the event.

Whenever possible, nurse educators should plan professional events into the class schedule in advance. This serves as a powerful incentive to students. Time exchange from class for events scheduled during the regular class meeting time is one such accommodation. For events scheduled outside the usual class session, time exchange minimizes burdens on time. Time exchange also demonstrates the nurse educator's commitment to the importance of professional event participation.

Complicated registration forms or membership application forms create additional demands to complete them and may actually discourage students. Nurse educators can facilitate the ease of registration/application by distributing forms in class, providing clear instructions, allowing for in-class completion time, and assisting with other required tasks. For example, the nurse educator can coordinate group mailings, photocopying student identification cards, and collecting student fees.

PSYCHOSOCIAL BARRIERS: RECOGNITION, SOLUTIONS, STRATEGIES, AND INCENTIVES

Perceived Irrelevance to Immediate Education Goals

The perceived irrelevance to immediate educational goals is a major obstacle to student participation. Adult learners typically place importance on tasks directly and immediately related to the achievement of educational and/or career goals (Brookfield, 1986; Knowles, 1984). Consequently, the nurse educator is challenged to change existing values and beliefs that negate or minimize the significance of professional events and memberships in achieving immediate goals. For the undergraduate student, immediate goals usually refer to successful achievement at the individual course level. Nurse educators can begin by tapping into students' motivation at the immediate course level. By specifically addressing students' immediate desired educational goals, educators can link participation in professional events with course objectives, course assignments, and test questions. For example, the course outline can clearly delineate participation in professional events as a course objective that complements other course objectives and the course description. If a professional event will take place during the usual class time, the nurse educator can schedule the event as part of class. This is especially convenient if the event is held on campus or nearby. Time off from class can help accommodate students if the event is scheduled outside of the usual class meeting time.

Mandatory participation without a link to course objectives, assignments, test questions, or other incentives may not be sufficient to change students' attitudes toward valuing professional events and developing a commitment to lifelong learning. Course assignments connected to the professional event encourage students to become active participants rather than merely attending (see chapter 4 concerning definitions of attendance). Faculty requiring students to attend events to complete assignments or participate in class discussions means that students are involved with each other outside the classroom. This intentionally brings students in ongoing contact with one another and with other resources (Kuh, 2001).

Engaging the student via written assignments, oral presentations, or class discussions should link some aspect of the professional event with course content and include a reflective component. Reflection encourages the transition from preprofessional education to professional education and is essential for affective learning (Schön, 1987). Affective learning refers to changes in attitudes, values, or beliefs. It is difficult to evaluate because it takes longer than psychomotor or cognitive learning and is difficult to measure; however it is critical for professional development (Bevis, 1989). Multiple choice, short answer, and/or essay questions based on the professional event further validate professional event participation. A written assignment grade, test item points, or test grade that directly impacts upon the course grade validates professional event participation as significant enough to award a quantitative measure that will affect the immediate course grade and progression in the nursing curriculum.

Mandatory attendance (participation) assures that all students are exposed to a professional event; however, it does not assure that students will have a positive experience, develop a lifelong commitment to professional learning, or gain positive benefits associated with professional event participation. The nurse educator has the unique opportunity to provide necessary background information about the professional event that may enhance students' experiences. It may be necessary to focus students on a particular area or feature of the professional event. Preparing and reviewing expectations concerning assignments based on a professional event may aid in focusing students on its most course-relevant topics. Assigned articles, chapters, movies, or other materials before the event serve as an advance organizer and provide essential background information to maximize the experience. Similarly, assigned reading or films after the event may support or expand upon the experience, rather than just complementing it.

Other incentives include offering extra credit for professional event participation. However this will not positively affect all individuals. In fact, this strategy may really target the most self-directed, motivated individuals or, on the other end of the continuum, attract the most desperate, failing students who view professional event participation as a last resort for passing the course. Offering certificates for attendance, free books, or other items may not be sufficient to target students who are focused on immediate goals such as successfully achieving academic outcomes. Certificates, awards, and/or oral acknowledgment of students at the professional events may, however, assist in enhancing positive psychological outcomes for nursing.

Mandatory membership in the National Nursing Student Association (NSNA) is a requirement in some nursing programs; the relevancy to immediate educational goals is evident. Writing a letter to the editor in response to an article in the NSNA journal, *Imprint,* can engage students more actively through participation rather than merely affiliation. Again, linking course objectives, assignments, course topics, and test questions with membership in NSNA will motivate students. Another incentive is to encourage active student participation in NSNA through the NSNA Leadership U program, where students can earn academic credit for their documented participation in NSNA leadership activities (National Student Nurses Association, 2002).

Perceived Irrelevance to Future Professional Goals

Frequently, students' myopic views fail to recognize the long-range benefits of professional event participation and memberships to future professional goals. This limited view is another barrier to participation. First, nurse educators can provide personal testimonies about the numerous benefits attributed to professional event participation and memberships. For example, upon return from a nursing research conference sponsored by a nursing organization, the nurse educator can distribute or display materials relevant to the course and to possible future professional goals, such as a clinical specialty area. Second, soliciting advanced students to share their positive experiences in professional events and memberships and how these experiences enhanced and facilitated achievement of their educational and future professional goals further substantiates the nurse educators' perspective. Students are most influenced by peers, with whom they most readily identify; therefore, the value of peer influence can be astounding. Third, professional role models such as clinical preceptors or invited guest speakers during class time can provide additional testimonies substantiating the significance of professional event participation and memberships for professional goal attainment. Discussing legal and ethical issues in nursing (licensure, certification, competency, and standards of practice) within the context of the "criteria for a profession" has relevance to future professional goals. Exploration of individual future goals can personalize educational and career mobility options and the relevance of professional event participation and memberships beyond the broad topic of "professional issues." Professional events and memberships as part of a professional portfolio and résumé development can be introduced as a class topic and later evolve into an actual assignment to develop a professional portfolio or résumé. Mock job interviews can also address professional event participation and membership.

Multiple Role Stress

Stress related to multiple role conflict is particularly relevant to nontraditional students with multiple role responsibilities outside the academic setting. Eliminating multiple role stress (MRS), reducing MRS, and managing MRS effectively are all appropriate goals. To accomplish this, nurse educators must identify, introduce, and demonstrate strategies for decreasing stress and effectively balancing multiple roles. Anxiety may result when students think that professional event participation and membership adversely interfere with the management of multiple roles and responsibilities. They can perceive it to be "one more responsibility" that competes for precious time. Participation in this "extra" responsibility upsets the fragile balance among an overwhelming number of responsibilities. Stress and anxiety associated with school-related tasks adversely influence persistence and retention through negative psychological outcomes (see chapter 7).

Therefore, it behooves nurse educators to develop and explore strategies to minimize stress and anxiety and assist students in managing multiple roles and responsibility. Sufficient advance notice is a primary strategy. Inadequate notice of a required or elective (extra credit) participation in an event or membership-related task increases stress and anxiety and decreases the probability that all students will be able to participate. Furthermore, the probability that students will associate positive psychological outcomes to the professional event participation is greatly reduced.

Acknowledging that students have multiple roles and busy lives, while also providing case examples of how other students have effectively balanced similar multiple roles, is helpful. Asking nontraditional students with multiple roles who successfully managed professional events and memberships and multiple role responsibilities to share experiences is a powerful incentive to students. Advance and ongoing collaboration with on-campus child care facilities to extend services beyond scheduled class sessions to allow for participation in professional events and memberships may be essential to students who rely solely on college child care services.

Letters to employers and significant others may help obtain the necessary time off, reassigned time, or redelegated tasks to allow for student participation. For example, a letter that identifies the potential benefits to a hospital agency when a student working as a nursing assistant gets a requested day off to participate in a professional conference increases the likelihood that the time off will be granted. A direct benefit may be that the knowledge learned at the conference will then be carried out in the workplace setting, potentially enhancing patient outcomes and satisfaction. Other indirect and direct benefits may include employee satisfaction, loyalty to the institution, employee retention, and the desire to continue working at the agency after licensure as a registered nurse. Similarly, written materials listing benefits can increase understanding among family members or essential support persons who may be asked to assume some additional household responsibilities or child care tasks. For example, a spouse who reads that participation at a professional workshop is required, and sees the listed benefits, may be more willing to assume additional household or child care tasks to permit attendance at this event. In contrast, an uninformed spouse may be opposed to what appears to be an unnecessary, optional event that he or she perceives will prevent the student from completing usually held household and/or child care tasks.

Fear of Isolation

Fear of isolation is an imposing barrier to many undergraduate nursing students. Ultimately, eliminating this fear and promoting feelings of inclusion are the desired goals. One effective strategy is to link student(s) with a buddy (faculty member, nursing alumni, or other RN). This may be done by assigning a buddy link at a professional event or within a nursing organization/association. It may be a one-time link for an event or may be more long term and evolve into a mentor–protégé relationship.

To enhance the web of inclusion at a professional event, nurse educators should make every effort to introduce students to professional colleagues and other students. If possible, introduction to key nursing leaders, presenters, or members can make an important impression on students through validation. Validation is especially important for nontraditional students (older, commuter, and/or minority) and has been positively linked with persistence behaviors and retention (Rendon, 1994; Rendon, Jalomo, & Nora, 2000). Encouraging students to take part in picture-taking sessions, question–answer sessions, meetings, and evaluation questionnaire completion provides a realm of diverse opportunities for student inclusion. Informal and formal networking during lunch and break times also serves to include students.

The nurse educator who is actively involved in a professional event and/or nursing organization can enhance the web of inclusion more directly by means of a welcome address, closing address, editorial, newsletter, or letter that acknowledges and embraces students. Positive feelings associated with the professional event and/or organization will be promoted. Showcasing pictures of student participants via a webpage, website, poster display, slide show, newsletter, or bulletin board illustrates student-friendly (inclusive) environments. Other students as role models are a powerful influence on student motivation, self-efficacy, and persistence.

KEY POINTS SUMMARY

- Professional events are nursing conferences, workshops, meetings, volunteer services, or social activities that have specific goals relevant for nursing education, practice, research, or theory.
- Memberships refer to affiliation or participation within nursing organizations or associations as a "member" prescribed by the respective bylaws.
- Positive experiences in professional event participation and memberships positively affect retention by enhancing self-efficacy and motivation, promoting professional integration, and facilitating positive psychological outcomes.
- The "web of inclusion" refers to a professional network that embraces students and strives to promote professional integration through participation in professional events and memberships.
- Faculty self-assessment as active role models in promoting/facilitating student professional event participation and memberships is a necessary first step.
- In order to "make a difference" and enhance the "web of inclusion," nurse educators must recognize actual and potential barriers hindering students' participation, propose solutions, initiate strategies to remove barriers, and offer incentives to enhance participation.
- Practical barriers include financial cost, travel, and time.
- Psychosocial barriers include perceived irrelevance to immediate educational goals, perceived irrelevance to future professional goals, multiple role stress, and fear of isolation.

EDUCATOR-IN-ACTION

Professor Webb teaches the first-semester nursing course and introduces the importance of professional organizations and memberships during the first class lesson. Background prerequisite reading assignments, an in-class video, and class discussion complement a brief lecture.

Heidi and several other students think, "This is nice, but it doesn't seem real."

Next, Professor Webb shares some lively yet relevant personal positive anecdotes concerning professional conferences, organizations, and networking. With student interest sparked, he invites students to attend a conference sponsored by a professional nursing specialty organization.

Heidi skeptically thinks, "It's a long way off before I'm a nurse. What does this have to do with me now?"

Professor Webb distributes a brochure to each student, pointing out that the intended audience listed in the brochure includes nursing students. The potential benefits of student attendance at the upcoming conference are highlighted and correlated with course objectives, course topics, and future professional development.

Heidi ponders, "Maybe this is relevant to me. But it's so expensive. I can't afford this. Besides, I might feel out of place."

As an added incentive, Professor Webb announces that several faculty members and college administrators volunteered to sponsor students and pay for their conference fees. Arrangements for three clinical groups to attend the conference in lieu of clinical will permit three cohorts of students to attend together during regularly scheduled class time.

Tiffany feels elated that she is in one of the groups and thinks, "Faculty must really think it's important if they took all this effort and their own money to sponsor us."

Other students interested in attending are invited to enter a college "conference fee" raffle open to all undergraduate nursing students. Faculty colleagues publicize the conference and raffle in their respective courses; announcements are placed on bulletin boards and student e-mail listservs. The raffle will be held during a Student Nursing Club (SNC) meeting featuring an outside guest speaker from the conference planning committee.

Still somewhat skeptical and pessimistic, Heidi says to another student, "I never win at raffles, why should I bother?" Optimistically, Heidi's friend Petra says, "We have nothing to lose by going. Besides, the speaker might be interesting. If not, there's always the refreshment social to look forward to."

The enthusiastic and inspirational speaker networks with students during the SNC refreshment social. Student integration in nursing is enhanced and positive feelings about nursing are nurtured. The speaker stops to chat with Petra and Heidi about nursing. Heidi now thinks, "I really would like to go to the conference." When Petra wins the raffle, Heidi is happy for her friend but disappointed that she will not be able to attend.

The next week, Professor Webb coordinates the mailing of student registration forms and fees. Several students who are not selected via the raffle decide to pay their own fees. Because the sponsoring organization offers one free student fee for every ten paid fees, additional students can attend. Heidi is thrilled that she is asked to attend but is concerned about traveling and feeling out of place.

Professor Webb organizes several carpools for students living in nearby neighborhoods. One instructor offers to meet other students at the bus stop for group travel via public transportation. Departure time, anticipated arrival time, professional dress code, and conference activity expectations are reviewed with students. Heidi and Petra join a carpool with three other students, confident that they know what to expect and what is expected of them.

Upon arrival, students are greeted by members of the sponsoring organization and by student volunteers from the sponsoring host site. Because students arrive early, they have the added opportunity to talk with other attendees, observe preconference networking in action, ask questions, become acclimated to the environment, and review conference packet materials. As a member of the nursing specialty organization, Professor Webb uses this opportunity to introduce featured speakers to students. Several of the speakers and organizational members engage in professional dialogue with students and provide encouragement for their educational and professional endeavors. Students comment that this made them feel "included," "welcome," "relaxed," and "excited about nursing." Heidi and Petra feel pleasantly surprised when the SNC guest speaker remembers them and comes over to talk with them.

Other opportunities for dialogue occur during coffee breaks, lunch, and the poster session. The welcome address, closing address, and keynote speakers direct several comments specifically to students, thus further promoting validation and professional integration. All attendees are invited to enter a raffle of select nursing items, including two memberships in the specialty nursing organization. One membership is specifically earmarked for an undergraduate nursing student and includes a subscription to the bimonthly specialty journal and quarterly newsletter. When Heidi wins the membership, she excitedly offers to share her journals and newsletters with other students in the class.

During the next class session, Professor Webb asks students to write what they most liked about attending the conference. A subsequent class discussion allows for the sharing of ideas between students. Overwhelmingly positive experiences and the desire for more opportunities to attend nursing conferences are voiced.

REFERENCES AND BIBLIOGRAPHY

Bessent, H. (Ed.). (1997). *Strategies for recruitment, retention, and graduation of minority nurses in colleges of nursing.* Washington, DC: American Nurses Publishing.

Betts, V. T., & Cherry, B. (2002). Health policy and politics. In B. Cherry & S. R. Jacob (Eds.), *Contemporary nursing: Issues, trends, and management* (2nd ed., pp. 219–235). Philadelphia: Mosby.

Bevis, E. O. (1989). *Curriculum building in nursing: A process* (2nd ed.). New York: National League for Nursing.

Brockopp, D., Schooler, M., Welsh, D., Cassidy, K., Ryan, P. Y., Mueggenberg, K., & Orr-Chlebowy, D. (2003). Sponsored professional seminars: Enhancing professionalism among baccalaureate nursing students. *Journal of Nursing Education, 42*(12), 562–564.

Brookfield, S. D. (1986). *Understanding and facilitating adult learning.* San Francisco: Jossey-Bass.

Gigliotti, E. (1999). Women's multiple role stress: Testing Neuman's flexible line of defense. *Nursing Science Quarterly, 12*(1), 36–44.

Gigliotti, E. (2001). Development of the perceived multiple role stress scale (PMRS). *Journal of Nursing Measurement, 9*(2), 163–180.

Joel, L. A., & Kelly, L. Y. (2002). *The nursing experience: Trends, challenges, and transitions.* New York: McGraw-Hill.

Knowles, M. S. (1984). *The adult learner: A neglected species* (3rd ed.). Houston, TX: Gulf.

Kuh, G. D. (2001). Organizational culture and student persistence: Prospects and puzzles. *Journal of College Student Retention: Research, Theory & Practice, 3*(1), 23–40.

Leininger, M. M., & McFarland, M. R. (2002). *Transcultural nursing: Concepts, theories, research, and practice* (3rd ed.). New York: McGraw-Hill.

National Student Nurses Association. (2002). *NSNA online.* Retrieved December 8, 2002, from http://www.nsna.org/membership/pdf/member1.pdf

Rendon, L. I. (1994). Validating culturally diverse students: Toward a new model of learning and student development. *Innovative Higher Education, 19*(1), 23–32.

Rendon, L. I., Jalomo, R. E., & Nora, A. (2000). Theoretical considerations in the study of minority student retention in higher education. In J. M. Braxton (Ed.), *Reworking the student departure puzzle* (pp. 127–156). Nashville, TN: Vanderbilt University Press.

Schön, D. (1987). *Educating the reflective practitioner.* San Francisco: Jossey-Bass.

Skaggs, B. J., & deVries, C. M. (1998). You and your professional organization. In D. J. Mason & J. K. Leavitt (Eds.), *Policy and politics in nursing and health care* (pp. 535–542). New York: Saunders.

Spickerman, S. (1988). Enhancing the socialization process. *Nurse Educator, 13*(6), 10–14.

Tinto, V. (1993). *Leaving college: Rethinking the causes and cures of student attrition.* Chicago: University of Chicago Press.

Tinto, V. (1997). Classrooms as communities. *Journal of Higher Education, 68*(6), 599–623.

Tinto, V. (1998). Colleges as communities: Taking research on student persistence seriously. *Review of Higher Education, 21,* 167–177.

Tucker-Allen, S., & Long, E. (1999). *Recruitment and retention of minority students: Stories of success.* Lisle, IL: Tucker.

Vance, C., & Olson, R. K. (1998). *The mentor connection in nursing.* New York: Springer.

Chapter 12

Promoting Positive and Productive Peer Partnerships

Interaction is instrumental for effective learning (Kennerly, 2001). The educational literature profusely advocates multidimensional strategies that enhance opportunities for student-centered interactive learning experiences (American Association of Colleges of Nursing [AACN], 1998; Brookfield, 1986; Christiaens & Baldwin, 2002; Knowles, 1984; Young & Diekelmann, 2002). Moreover, the quality of student interaction influences professional socialization, academic integration, psychological growth, self-efficacy, and motivation. In turn, such factors influence student persistence, academic outcomes, satisfaction, and levels of stress (Bean & Eaton, 2001). Therefore, nurse educators have the responsibility to structure student-centered interactive experiences that enhance the potential for quality student interactions.

High quality, rewarding, and positive student (peer) interactions may result in class friendships. Friends in class are mutually bonded in career goals, expectations, and stage of educational and professional development. The main focus of in-class friends is on the common academic goal of successfully completing course requirements and becoming a registered nurse. The NURS model proposes that encouragement by friends in class will actively promote positive psychological outcomes, self-efficacy, professional socialization, persistence, and retention (see chapter 6). In contrast, lack of class friends will adversely affect retention through social isolation, dissatisfaction, stress, low self-efficacy, and decreased motivation.

Student interactions, however, do not automatically result in friendships; nurse educator intervention can be beneficial. While nurse educators cannot "make" classmates become friends, they can make a difference or assist in the process by creating opportunities and conditions that support and nurture peer interactions. Ultimately, a series of carefully patterned and interwoven student-centered interactive experiences throughout the nursing curriculum can be structured to promote positive and productive peer partnerships. In this book, positive and productive peer partnerships are those purposeful affiliations, alliances, and connections among peers that result in constructive, generative, creative, and desirable outcomes. Desirable outcomes include both the process and product of learning; quantitative (academic) and qualitative (psychological) outcomes are expected. One desirable outcome is that positive and productive peer partnerships are valuable precursors to class friendships and to fostering encouragement by friends in class.

Desirable educational and professional outcomes can only be achieved through a faculty commitment to promoting positive and productive peer partnerships during all phases of the nursing educational process. Professional integration and partnerships must be seen as a priority and accepted as part of the mission, vision, and values of the school. Unfortunately, some nursing faculty may underestimate the potential influence of class friends in academic achievement, professional development, satisfaction, stress, and retention; student-centered activities may also be undervalued (Braxton & McClendon, 2001; Young & Diekelmann, 2002). Additionally, some nurse educators may lack prior experience with designing, implementing, and evaluating student-centered interactive learning experiences. Similarly, students may underestimate the influence of class friends and/or student-centered interactive learning activities. Student perceptions of friendships, learning, education, and peers can be influenced by student profile characteristics, affective factors, and environmental factors. Consequently, visionary nurse educators are challenged to structure quality student-centered experiences that are maximally valued, optimally utilized, and mutually desired. Nurse educators are also challenged to solicit support from colleagues and truly integrate student-centered interactive learning experiences throughout the curriculum with the specific aim of promoting positive and productive peer partnerships. The purpose of this chapter is to describe strategies for promoting such partnerships. Benefits, barriers, solutions, and strategies will be presented.

NURSE EDUCATOR AS ACTIVE PROMOTER

Professional partnerships are a crucial part of future professional nursing roles (Vance and Olson, 1998; Young & Diekelmann, 2002). Students must not only be introduced to the concept of professional partnerships but must acquire the necessary skills and learn to value partnerships throughout the educational process and a career as a professional nurse (AACN, 1998). This necessitates innovative strategies and sincere commitment on the part of nurse educators, who must be willing to become coparticipants and develop connections or partnerships with students. These connections can create communities of learners who are partners in the learning process whereby the nurse educator shifts the focus from teaching to learning (Bevis, 1989; Diekelmann, Swenson, & Sims, 2003). In this student-centered philosophy of learning, the role of the teacher is to guide, support, and coach learners throughout their educational journey and become active promoters of positive and productive peer partnerships.

As mentioned earlier, nurse educators exert powerful influence on students. If faculty do not value partnerships for their own professional development, then they are unlikely to encourage student interaction, partnerships, or friendships. Similarly, if nurse educators are actively involved in professional partnerships, yet are not vocal about their participation, students will be deprived of positive professional role modeling in this important area.

Comparable to faculty self-appraisal in the previous chapter, faculty self-assessment as active promoters of positive and productive peer partnerships is a necessary precursor for strategy development. Table 12.1 provides a guide for appraising values, beliefs, and actions and for determining whether one is an active promoter. It is proposed that the "actions taken" are what makes one an active promoter. Table 12.1 can also provide a guide for nursing curriculum self-assessment to determine if nursing programs actively promote positive and productive peer partnerships through their program philosophy, learner outcomes, and planned interventions or if there are obstacles present. Intentional planning in coordinated activities aimed at capturing the power of the peer group within the classroom should be a priority and is instrumental in developing a community of learners (Kuh, 2001).

After self-assessment, nurse educators who have not optimally shared positive views, values, beliefs, and experiences with students should make a concerted effort to do so. However, it is not enough to profess values and beliefs to students; nurse educators must be sincerely committed and take positive actions. They need to recognize actual and potential barriers to students' development of positive and productive peer partnerships, propose solutions or goals, initiate strategies to remove barriers, and offer incentives.

Although numerous barriers may exist, only the major ones will be highlighted here. Barriers may be practical or psychosocial. Practical

TABLE 12.1   Self-Assessment: Active Promoter of Positive and Productive Peer Partnerships

Promoter	Values, Beliefs, and Actions	Promoter
Yes	Views professional partnerships as important in own life *and shares beliefs with students**	No
Yes	Views positive and productive peer partnerships as important in undergraduate students' education, professional development, and retention *and shares view with students*	No
Yes	Views encouragement by friends in class as important in undergraduate students' education, professional development, and retention *and shares view with students*	No
Yes	Views own nurse educator role to include active involvement in promoting positive and productive peer partnerships among undergraduate students *and shares view with students*	No
Yes	Maintains professional partnerships *and shares positive and relevant experiences with students*	No
Yes	Updates own knowledge and skills about professional partnerships routinely *and shares relevant information with students*	No
Yes	Recognizes actual and potential barriers hindering students' development of peer partnerships *and initiates strategies to remove barriers*	No
Yes	*Implements strategies to encourage student development of positive and productive peer partnerships*	No
Yes	*Evaluates implemented strategies designed to encourage student development of positive and productive peer partnerships*	No

* Active promoter/facilitator actions are indicated by italics.

barriers include: (1) insufficient background information and/or skills, (2) insufficient in-class opportunities, (3) insufficient out-of-class opportunities, and (4) curricular inconsistency (see Table 12.2). Psychosocial barriers include perceived irrelevance to immediate educational goals, perceived irrelevance to future professional goals, stress, and fear of isolation (see Table 12.3). Students are often faced with a combination of practical and psychosocial barriers.

PRACTICAL BARRIERS: RECOGNITION, SOLUTIONS, STRATEGIES, AND INCENTIVES

Insufficient Background Information and/or Skills

Students, especially beginning (novice) students, may lack sufficient background knowledge and skills necessary for developing positive and productive peer partnerships in nursing. Even more advanced students may need supplementary information to nurture, foster, and expand the knowledge and skills needed to sustain positive and productive peer partnerships throughout the formal educational process and beyond. Nurse educators must integrate the necessary background information and/or skills at various levels in the nursing curriculum.

Congruency between course objectives, prerequisite assignments, course topics, class activities, and methods of evaluation (with clear evidence of partnership development throughout) will help students integrate the necessary knowledge, skills, and attitudes needed to optimize positive and productive peer partnerships as an educational and professional outcome. For example, prerequisite readings related to group dynamics, communication, and group process, supplemented by an in-class video about professional collaboration and followed by an in-class discussion, can assist students in synthesizing information prior to initiating a small-group interactive teaching–learning strategy. Additionally, if students are to develop positive and productive peer partnerships, they must have sufficient background knowledge about a select topic to contribute equally as partners. Careful selection of prerequisite assignments that correspond with intended interactive activities is a necessary precursor for success.

Insufficient In-Class Opportunities

Perhaps one of the greatest barriers to students' development of positive and productive peer partnerships is insufficient in-class opportunity for quality student interaction. The most effective solution is to carefully integrate learner-centered student interactive teaching–learning strategies

TABLE 12.2   Positive and Productive Peer Partnerships: Practical Barriers,
Solutions, Strategies, and Incentives

Barriers	Solutions	Strategies and Incentives
Insufficient background information and/or skills	Integrate adequate learning of the knowledge and skills necessary for developing positive and productive peer partnerships	Course outline Course objectives Course prerequisite assignments Course topics
Insufficient in-class opportunities	Integrate learner-centered student interactive teaching–learning strategies Maximize opportunities for positive and productive peer partnerships within class	Small group discussion Large group discussion Case study Gaming Group simulation Simulated role play Role play Debate Group presentation (oral, PowerPoint) Interview Storytelling Group film (video) production Group poster Paired writing draft critique Paired problem-based learning Paired computer-based learning Paired technical skills practice Paired technical skills testing Paired or group clinical assignment *For Web-based courses:* 　Paired or group e-mails 　Paired or group course discussion boards 　Paired or group chat rooms
Insufficient out-of-class opportunities	Integrate learner-centered student interactive out-of-class activities Maximize opportunities for positive and productive peer partnerships outside of class	Assignments involving all of the above Library literature review Paired or group computer-assisted instruction Professional event participation Professional memberships Enrichment programs Nursing student resource centers
Curricular inconsistency	Integrate learner-centered student interactive activities, opportunities, and incentives throughout the nursing curriculum	Systematic curriculum evaluation Concept mapping Curricular threads Faculty development workshops

TABLE 12.3   Positive and Productive Peer Partnerships: Psychosocial Barriers, Solutions, Strategies, and Incentives

Barriers	Solutions	Strategies and Incentives
Perceived irrelevance to immediate educational goals	Demonstrate relevance to immediate educational goals	Link with course objectives Link with course assignments Link with test questions Provide background information PEW Commission recommendations Low-stakes writing assignments Reflection
Perceived irrelevance to future professional goals	Demonstrate relevance to future professional goals	Faculty role models Student role models Professional role models Link with legal and ethical issues Link with criteria for a profession Benefits to self and others Educational mobility Career mobility
Stress	Eliminate stress Reduce stress Manage stress	Stressor identification Realistic appraisal of strengths Realistic appraisal of weaknesses Strength enhancement Weakness remedies Student role models Judicious, positive feedback Realistic goals
Fear of isolation	Eliminate fear of isolation Minimize fear of isolation Promote feelings of inclusion	Acknowledge fears Open, caring, trusting environment Value of all learners Initial student self-selection Appraisal of strengths and weaknesses Assigned partners or groups

throughout the course, building upon previous interactive activities. Active learning is crucial for peer interaction. Because students have diverse learning needs, strengths, values, and beliefs, weaving multidimensional active learning activities throughout the course will be most beneficial. Students' cultural values and beliefs (CVB) will influence how various strategies are valued, interpreted, and used; therefore nurse educators should take this into consideration when planning, implementing, and evaluating activities (see chapter 3).

Learner-centered interactive strategies may involve students working in pairs, small groups, and/or large groups. Table 12.2 lists several examples. In general, strategies should involve collaborative or cooperative learning, in which all participating students are partners in the process. Collaborative learning experiences positively impact on learning outcomes, academic achievement, satisfaction, stress reduction, motivation, self-efficacy, and retention, especially among diverse student populations (Bean & Eaton, 2001; Cabrera et al., 2002; Gumbs, 2001). Additionally, problem-based collaborative learning corresponds with PEW Commission competency recommendations (PEW Health Professions Commission, 1995), further impressing upon nurse educators reasons to offer generous in-class opportunities.

Specific strategies have advantages and disadvantages. Pairing students eliminates the potential for an audience and enhances the potential for in-depth quality student interactions that can foster cognitive and affective growth (Christiaens & Baldwin, 2002). Groups, however, provide greater opportunities for diverse thinking. Outcome benefits can be maximized with clear directions, group rules, well-matched group composition, effective leadership, immediate feedback and guidance, reflection, and adequate time allocation (Huff, 1997). Story telling with reflection is another effective strategy, especially among culturally diverse learners (Davidhizar & Lonser, 2003; Koenig & Zorn, 2002). For many students, gaming, debates, and role play are effective mechanisms for active, enjoyable learning that results in positive cognitive, psychomotor, and/or affective outcomes. However, individual competitiveness may be contrary to some students' CVB. Currently, the Internet (Web-based courses) provides opportunities for interactive learning in pairs, small groups, and large groups via individual e-mail, group e-mails, course chat rooms, and course discussion boards. Students must be computer literate, confident, and motivated if computer-based strategies are to be effective. Conclusively, nurse educators have many learner-centered student interactive strategies from which to choose; however the educator must be adequately prepared, knowledgeable about student variables, committed, and caring.

In-class opportunities for positive and productive peer partnerships critically depend upon a caring, safe, open environment that is intentionally shaped to embrace all students as unique, individual, and valuable contributors to the learning process. This is essential for optimizing student success and retention, especially among nontraditional students (Tinto, 1997). First, faculty attitudes and actions that demonstrate caring are powerful role models to students. Next, faculty guidance, feedback, and intervention structure and nurture caring environments within the classroom, clinical, or laboratory setting. Both faculty and peers play a meaningful role in creating a caring, supportive environment (Nora, 2001).

Insufficient Out-of-Class Opportunities

In-class opportunities are major factors in the initiation of positive and productive peer partnerships that can be overseen and guided by nurse educators. However, such partnerships can be enhanced greatly through ongoing out-of-class interactions as well. One benefit of out-of-class student interactions is that students may feel freer to share ideas, thoughts, and opinions without the educator present. Partnerships, social networks, and friendships can develop, increasing academic and psychological benefits for all participants. One major drawback is that the potential for distraction may be greater.

Nurse educators have the opportunity and responsibility to provide incentives to enhance the quality of student interactions outside class. Extra-credit options provide an incentive for some, but not all, resulting in positive and productive peer partnerships developing among a more homogeneous group of self-selected students rather than a more diverse group. A homogeneous group is self-limiting because diversity in learning ability, culture, age, and gender may not be present. Out-of-class required assignments have a greater potential for success.

Assignments involving the learner-centered student interactive strategies mentioned in the preceding section and listed in Table 12.2 provide a menu of strategies available to educators. For example, a literature review or survey of resources in the library may be one out-of-class paired or small-group activity. Paired or small-group use of computer-assisted instructional programs can encourage critical thinking. Incentives for promoting student interaction via participation in professional events and memberships provide another aspect of professional socialization (see chapter 11). Enrichment programs (EPs) and Nursing Student Resource Center (NSRC) services offer additional opportunities for high-quality peer interaction, positive and productive peer partnerships, and encouragement by friends (see chapters 13 and 14). Active encouragement of student participation in EPs and NSRC services should be ongoing, especially during major transitional points in the educational process.

Curricular Inconsistency

Inconsistent and/or insufficient integration of activities, opportunities, and incentives throughout the nursing curriculum restricts professional development, confounds educational outcomes, and is confusing to students. Curricular inconsistency is incongruent with the creation of a true community of nursing learners, which is essential for professional socialization, development, and growth. It is also counterproductive to earlier partnership-promoting efforts. In contrast, consistent vertical and horizontal threads, critically woven throughout the curriculum, can support student success via positive academic and psychological outcomes.

Systematic curriculum evaluation using quantitative and qualitative methods helps identify program strengths, weaknesses, inconsistencies, and gaps. Reflective self-appraisal on an individual and a program level is necessary for enhancing the scholarship of teaching (Drevdahl, Stackman, Purdy, & Louie, 2002; Young & Diekelmann, 2002). Concept mapping that focuses on partnership as a concept helps trace the concept throughout the curriculum. Strategy-mapping that traces various student-centered learning approaches will assess another necessary dimension. Curricular vertical and horizontal threads should be complementary, consistent, and appropriate for each educational level. Finally, faculty development workshops targeting identified need areas assist faculty to integrate learner-centered student interactive activities, opportunities, and incentives throughout the nursing curriculum with the specific aim of promoting positive and productive peer partnerships and encouragement by friends in class.

PSYCHOSOCIAL BARRIERS: RECOGNITION, SOLUTIONS, STRATEGIES, AND INCENTIVES

Perceived Irrelevance to Immediate Education Goals

The perceived irrelevance to immediate educational goals is a major obstacle to student participation in positive and productive peer partnerships. Adult learners typically place importance on tasks directly and immediately related to the achievement of educational and/or career goals (Brookfield, 1986; Knowles, 1984). Consequently, the nurse educator is challenged to change existing values and beliefs that negate or minimize the significance of peer partnerships and interactive student activities in achieving immediate goals. For the undergraduate student, immediate goals usually refer to successful achievement at the individual course level. Nurse educators can begin by sparking students' motivation at the immediate course level.

Communication can change the course of action (decisions and behaviors) and influence outcomes in the educational path toward professional socialization and development. Clearly identifying goals as student expected outcomes in a course outline clarifies any ambiguities and communicates the importance of positive and productive peer partnerships in nursing. The course outline can delineate participation in positive and productive peer partnerships as a course objective that complements other course objectives and the course description. Opportunities to develop positive and productive peer partnerships should take place as part of required class activities. For example, a topical outline may list the students' expected outcomes as follows:

At the completion of this class session, the student will be able to

1. Define positive and productive peer partnerships
2. Discuss examples of positive and productive peer partnerships in nursing
3. Identify desirable educational and professional outcomes (benefits)
4. Discuss the potential impact of desirable educational and professional outcomes on students, the academic institution, the nursing profession, the health care system, and society
5. Identify strategies for promoting positive and productive peer partnerships
6. Demonstrate skills for developing positive and productive peer partnerships in nursing

Multiple choice, short answer, and/or essay questions based on learning outcomes via student-interactive activities further validate the time engaged in quality student interaction and partnerships. A written assignment grade, test item points, or test grade that directly impacts upon the course grade validates interactive participation as significant enough to award a quantitative measure that will affect the immediate course grade and progression in the nursing curriculum. Assigning a portion of the course grade based on participation in student-interactive class activities and projects directly demonstrates relevance to immediate educational goals. Communicating consistency between a program's desired educational outcomes and PEW Commission (1995) recommendations concerning educational strategies, desired outcomes, and professional partnerships provides a broader view to students.

Communication may not be sufficient in changing students' attitudes toward valuing the potential of positive and productive peer partnerships and interactive student experiences. Students need to understand and appreciate the conditions under which specific learning strategies may be more or less effective, rather than assuming that certain ones are best (Pintrich & Garcia, 1994). Because reflection is essential for affective learning (Schon, 1987), and affective learning is most crucial for professional development (Bevis, 1989), engaging the student through in-class or out-of-class learner-centered interactive activities should include an individual reflective component. For example, students can be asked to write a "low stakes" reflection of their in-class group experience. Low-stakes writing minimizes the pressure of grading associated with high-stakes writing (Elbow, 1997) and optimizes affective learning outcomes. Reviewing and highlighting the immediate educational benefits obtained from positive and productive peer partnerships further confirms immediate relevance. Discussing the role of positive and productive peer partnerships and encouragement by friends in class in enriching learning, satisfaction, and stress management provides another important dimension to the achievement of immediate educational goals.

Perceived Irrelevance to Future Professional Goals

Often, students' focus on short-term educational goals impedes their ability to recognize the long-range benefits of developing positive and productive peer partnerships. This limited perspective is another barrier to maximizing peer partnership possibilities. Discussions that appraise the relationship between professional standards, employer expectations, and professional partnerships illustrate relevance to future professional goals. PEW Commission (1995) recommendations, along with international, national, and local nursing guidelines, document partnerships as a professional nursing practice expectation, providing further justification.

Personal testimonies about the numerous benefits associated with positive and productive peer partnerships are a powerful incentive to students. For example, a nurse educator engaged in collaborative research can discuss both the personal and professional benefits of such a collaborative partnership. Sharing a story about patient-care benefits and staff satisfaction resulting from a collaborative partnership between two staff nurses provides a different, yet relevant perspective to students. Asking advanced students to share their positive experiences and how these experiences enhanced and facilitated achievement of their educational goals and future professional goals further substantiates the nurse educators' position. Professional role models such as clinical preceptors or invited guest speakers during class time can provide additional testimonies. Finally, asking students to explore their own individual goals can personalize educational and career mobility options and assist them in their understanding of professional relevance.

Stress

Stress related to student interactive learning experiences threatens the development of positive and productive peer partnerships and adversely affects student academic outcomes, satisfaction, persistence and retention (see chapter 7). There may be several different underlying causes of stress associated with student interactive learning experiences; the major goal is stress reduction or elimination. Identifying the underlying causes of stress is an important precursor for stress reduction strategy development. For example, students may experience stress due to the need for self-disclosure or perceptions that group work is difficult (Drevdahl & Dorcy, 2002), high responsibility for learning and/or negative perspectives concerning active-learning strategies (Martens & Stangvik-Urban, 2002). Sources of stress are also interrelated with affective factors such as cultural values and beliefs (CVB), self-efficacy, and motivation. CVB that do not comprehend and/or embrace student-centered interactive activities may cause stress. Inefficacious students may perceive their knowledge and skills as inadequate for successful student interactive experiences, positive and productive peer partnerships, and in-class friendships. Motivation will adversely be affected by stress (see chapter 3).

Acknowledging that students have diverse learning styles, strengths, needs, values, and sources of stress should be followed by case examples of how other students have effectively reduced or eliminated stress associated with student interactive learning experiences. Hearing from diverse students who successfully managed stress, altered negative views, developed positive attitudes, built upon existing personal strengths, remedied personal weaknesses, enjoyed learning, and ultimately developed positive and productive peer partnerships is an inspiring incentive for students. Shared experiences, student interaction, and role modeling facilitate the development of effective coping strategies and positive self-efficacy (Bean & Eaton, 2001). Offering a variety of teaching–learning strategies best accommodates the learning style preferences and needs within a diverse class.

Judicious, immediate, and caring feedback for positive behaviors from educators and peers increases self-efficacy and motivation and reduces stress (Bandura, 1986; Bean & Eaton, 2001). Mutual assistance or reciprocation of academic and nonacademic (emotional) support by peer partnerships can enhance confidence and independence and result in friendships. Friendships that encourage mutual reciprocation and individual independence rather than dependence can help with professional integration, growth, and development.

Fear of Isolation

Fear of isolation or actual feelings of disconnection, difference, detachment, or separateness from other students obstructs the development of quality student interactions, positive and productive peer partnerships, and friendships. Students who perceive themselves as "different" are less likely to engage in interactive behaviors that would promote a sense of belonging (Astin, 1975; Chaney, Muraskin, Cahalan, & Goodwin, 1998). Perceived differences may be based on academic ability and preparedness, motivational levels, age, gender, culture, economic status, neighborhood, and/or other characteristics. Students who perceive themselves as similar frequently tend to congregate when faced with interactive activities. This phenomenon has been referred to as ingrouping (Cravener, 1996) or banding together syndrome (Hummel & Steele, 1996). Although initially students may feel comfortable with the self-selected group, generally such homogeneous groups are counterproductive to the overall goals of interactive learning experiences, professional socialization, and positive and productive peer partnerships. In contrast, diverse, interactive groups have the greatest potential for maximizing outcomes (Brookfield, 1986).

Minority students with a sincere desire to engage with the larger, diverse college community will be more successful in meeting their personal, educational, and professional goals than minority students in predominantly white institutions who are hesitant or reluctant to do so (Bessent, 1997; Tidwell & Berry, 1997). Nurse educators must be aware of the actual, potential, and perceived barriers stemming from past and present experiences with racism and discrimination that serve as barriers to inclusion. Good peer interaction with other students in an inclusive environment where students from all backgrounds experience equality and opportunity maximizes success through positive psychological outcomes, enhanced educational opportunities, and positive academic outcomes (Bessent, 1997; Tidwell & Berry, 1997).

The literature abounds with techniques designed to maximize interpersonal group dynamics, learning outcomes, and psychological outcomes by offering suggested patterns of matching learners. Student self-selection of group members/partners has obvious advantages and disadvantages; however, premature nurse educator-determined groups/partners selection also has some limitations. Cravener (1996) cautions against predicting student learning behavior on an ethnic, racial, or cultural basis rather than in individual evaluation. Antonio (2001) points out that often "surface segregation" occurs in which outwardly a group may seem ethnically homogeneous, but may actually represent diverse ethnic groups. For example, a non-Asian educator may label a group of "Asian" students as homogeneous; however, the students within the group may perceive great diversity among group members. In another perspective, Pintrich & Garcia (1994) propose that psychological mediators, such as self-efficacy and motivation, are more definitive than student demographic characteristics. Conclusively, nurse educators are challenged to select strategies that aim to replace the fear of isolation with feelings of inclusion and connection.

One strategy may be to allow students to self-select group members or partners during the first in-class student interactive activity. The nurse educator has the opportunity to observe individual student strengths and weaknesses in both the learning process and learning product. Additionally, opportunities to facilitate learning, group process, and satisfaction will help students to develop positive and productive peer partnerships. During future student interactive activities, pairing or grouping students based on individual student strengths and weaknesses will enhance learning outcomes via positive and productive peer partnerships. Ongoing efforts to foster a caring, supportive, trusting, and open learning environment must be actively implemented throughout the nursing curriculum. Acknowledging that fears may occur yet can be effectively overcome accentuates the positive. Actions that sincerely strive to foster feelings of inclusion, equality, trust, and connection demonstrate a commitment to all learners.

FOSTERING OTHER PARTNERSHIPS

Creating networks of students who are socially connected to the academic community and have a commitment to learning, persistence, and success can make a marked difference in student retention (Skahill, 2002). Nurse educators are in a key position to foster peer partnerships and class friendships. Friends in class have the ongoing opportunity to discuss class expectations, course requirements, challenges, successes, difficulties, and career plans. They perceive a connection with each other because they are in the same stage of educational and professional development; struggles and joys of learning are mutually experienced.

One limitation, however, is that friends in class are unable to comprehend the broader perspective, rationale for prerequisites or sequencing of courses, benefits of course assignments within the whole scope of the educational process, preparation for RN licensing exam, next course, employment as a RN, or continued education. Interconnectedness between courses and future professional role is frequently limited, skewed, or unknown. Partnership connections with peer mentor-tutors who are further advanced in the educational process can minimize this limitation. Nurse educators can "make a difference" in nursing student retention and success by fostering peer-mentor-tutor partnerships. Chapter 13 will describe peer mentor-tutor partnerships as part of an enrichment program.

KEY POINTS SUMMARY

- The NURS model proposes that encouragement by friends in class will actively promote positive psychological outcomes, self-efficacy, professional socialization, persistence, and retention.
- Nurse educators can make a difference by designing a series of carefully patterned and interwoven student-centered interactive experiences throughout the nursing curriculum structured to promote positive and productive peer partnerships.
- Positive and productive peer partnerships are those purposeful affiliations, alliances, and connections among peers that result in constructive, generative, creative, and desirable outcomes.
- Positive and productive peer partnerships are valuable precursors to class friendships and to fostering encouragement by friends in class.
- Nurse educators must be willing to become coparticipants and develop connections or partnerships with students.
- Faculty self-assessment as active promoter of positive and productive peer partnerships is a necessary first step.
- Nurse educators must recognize actual and potential barriers to students' development of positive and productive peer partnerships, propose solutions or goals, initiate strategies to remove barriers, and offer incentives.
- Practical barriers include insufficient background information and/or skills, insufficient in-class opportunities, insufficient out-of-class opportunities, and curricular inconsistency.
- Psychosocial barriers include perceived irrelevance to immediate educational goals, perceived irrelevance to future professional goals, stress, and fear of isolation.
- In-class opportunities for positive and productive peer partnerships critically depend upon a caring, safe, open environment that

is intentionally shaped to embrace all students as unique, individual, and valuable contributors to the learning process.
- Creating caring communities of learners is essential for optimizing student success and retention.

EDUCATOR-IN-ACTION

Professor Webb has designed a series of carefully patterned and interwoven student-centered interactive experiences throughout the advanced medical-surgical nursing course. They are structured to encourage positive and productive peer partnerships, enhance critical thinking, maximize learning, promote satisfaction, minimize stress, and therefore promote retention. On the first class day, Professor Webb reviews the course outline, elaborates on the multidimensional teaching–learning strategies integrated throughout the course, and emphasizes their purposes and desired outcomes. First he describes some lively, personal experiences in which professional partnerships enhanced his professional development, program of nursing research, teaching, and clinical practice. He briefly reminds students about the communication skills and interpersonal group dynamics essential to facilitating productive collaboration (learned last semester). A one-page handout summarizes major points. An overhead cartoon illustrates student behaviors that interfere with achieving positive learning outcomes and satisfaction. This serves as an icebreaker and students laugh and comment on several of the cartoon scenarios. Next, Professor Webb informs students that the next class will incorporate a small-group activity based on the assigned textbook reading "Nursing Care of the Client with AIDS" and the handout "Opportunistic Infections, Clinical Manifestations, Diagnostic Tests, and Drug Treatment."

On the second class day, Professor Webb allows students to self-select groups. Each five-member group is assigned a specific AIDS-related opportunistic infection and a specific drug used for treating the infection. Group tasks include determining: (1) nursing interventions indicated for each clinical manifestation associated with the infection, (2) nursing implications indicated for each drug, and (3) relevant nursing diagnoses. Professor Webb circulates throughout the room and guides students as needed, noting individual and group strengths and weaknesses. This information can guide future group activities and assignments. After twenty minutes, each group briefly presents on their assigned topic while the remaining students take notes, ask questions, and provide additional suggestions. Professor Webb elaborates and comments as necessary, inviting further student comments and questions. During the two-hour class, all of the groups complete their presentations. However, five other unassigned opportunistic infections and 10 drugs have not yet been discussed. Professor Webb proposes that a manageable option can be that groups meet outside of class and work together before next week. Students unanimously agree and volunteer to take specific topics.

At the beginning of the next class, students present their topics more quickly, accurately, and comprehensively than before. Next, Professor Webb asks students to individually reflect and write about their group activity experience. Select comments include:

Svetlana: "At first I didn't want to do a group activity because I didn't know anyone in my group. Because I had done the reading, I could contribute to the group and then everything was OK. As we discussed each clinical manifestation, everyone realized that it was nursing interventions and implications that were most important to know. I didn't focus my reading this way. Now I will read differently. Our group worked together after clinical to prepare for the next week. We finished up quicker than the first time so we decided to meet every week to prepare for class."

Mina: "The group activity made the topics more fun and realistic. The book seems so abstract. Talking about nursing diagnoses and nursing interventions with my classmates will help me remember the information in clinical and on a test. Not everyone in our group met before class to work on the second assignment, but those of us who did meet got a lot accomplished. We even had time to review last week's class notes."

Ken: "Working in the group in class made me feel like I wasn't alone in my questions, stress, or struggles. Dividing up the infections and drugs and sharing information about the nursing process made the content more manageable."

Willa: "Two people in my group were really smart. I thought I understood the material but after the group activity, I realized that I was trying to memorize instead of thinking critically like a nurse. Later I asked one of those students how she studies. She was really nice and offered to help me if I need it."

Throughout the semester, Professor Webb implements and evaluates subsequent student-centered interactive activities that complement and build upon each other.

REFERENCES AND BIBLIOGRAPHY

Albaili, M. A. (1997). Differences among low-, average- and high-achieving college students on learning and study strategies. *Educational Psychology, 17*(1 and 2), 171–177.

American Association of Colleges of Nursing. (1998). *The essentials of baccalaureate education for professional nursing practice.* Washington, DC: Author.

Antonio, A. L. (2001). Diversity and the influence of friendship groups in college. *Review of Higher Education, 25*(1), 63–89.

Astin, A. W. (1975). *Preventing students from dropping out.* San Francisco: Jossey-Bass.

Bandura, A. (1986). *Social foundations of thought and action: A social cognitive theory.* Englewood Cliffs, NJ: Prentice-Hall.

Baumberger-Henry, M. (2003). Practicing the art of nursing through student-designed continuing case study and cooperative learning. *Nursing Educator, 28*(4), 191–195.

Bean, J. P., & Eaton, S. B. (2001). The psychology underlying successful retention practices. *Journal of College Student Retention: Research, Theory, & Practice, 3*(1), 73–90.

Beck, C. T. (2001). Caring within nursing education: A metasynthesis. *Journal of Nursing Education, 40*(3), 101–109.

Bessent, H. (Ed.). (1997). *Strategies for recruitment, retention, and graduation of minority nurses in colleges of nursing.* Washington, DC: American Nurses Publishing.

Bevis, E. O. (1989). *Curriculum building in nursing: A process* (2nd ed.). New York: National League for Nursing.

Bevis, E. O., & Watson, J. (1989). *Toward a caring curriculum: A new pedagogy for nursing.* New York: National League for Nursing.

Bolan, C. M. (2003). Incorporating the experiential learning theory into the instructional design of online courses. *Nurse Educator, 28*(1), 10–14.

Brady, M., Leuner, J. D., Bellack, J. P., Loquist, R. S., Cipriano, P. F., & O'Neil, E. H. (2001). A proposed framework for differentiating the 21 PEW competencies by level of nursing education. *Nursing and Health Care Perspectives, 22*(1), 30–35.

Braxton, J. M., & McClendon, S. A. (2001). The fostering of social integration and retention through institutional practice. *Journal of College Student Retention: Research, Theory, & Practice, 3*(1), 57–72.

Braxton, J. M., & Mundy, M. E. (2001). Powerful institutional levers to reduce college student departure. *Journal of College Student Retention: Research, Theory, & Practice, 3*(1), 91–118.

Brookfield, S. D. (1986). Understanding and facilitating adult learning. San Francisco: Jossey-Bass.

Cabrera, A. F., Crissman, J. L., Bernal, E. M., Nora, A., Terenzini, P. T., & Pascarella, E. T. (2002). Collaborative learning: Its impact on college students' development and diversity. *Journal of College Student Development, 43*(1), 20–34.

Candela, L., Michael, S. R., & Mitchell, S. (2003). Ethical debates: Enhancing critical thinking in nursing students. *Nurse Educator, 28*(1), 37–39.

Chaney, B., Muraskin, L. D., Cahalan, M. W., & Goodwin, D. (1998). Helping the progress of disadvantaged students in higher education: The federal student support services program. *Educational Evaluation and Policy Analysis, 20*(3), 197–215.

Christiaens, G., & Baldwin, J. H. (2002). Use of dyadic role-playing to increase student participation. *Nurse Educator, 27*(6), 251–254.

Christianson, L., Tiene, D., & Luft, P. (2002). Web-based teaching in undergraduate nursing programs. *Journal of Nursing Education, 27*(6), 276–282.

Churchill, J., Reno, B., & Batchelor, N. (1998). The learning communities concept: Increasing student involvement. *Nurse Educator, 23*(6), 7–8.

Coffman, D. L., & Gilligan, T. D. (2002). Social support, stress, and self-efficacy: Effects on students' satisfaction. *Journal of College Student Retention: Research, Theory, & Practice, 4*(1), 53–66.

Cowen, K. J., & Tesh, A. S. (2002). Effects of gaming on nursing students' knowledge of pediatric cardiovascular dysfunction. *Journal of Nursing Education, 41*(11), 507–509.

Cravener, P. (1996). Multicultural education: A second look. *Nurse Educator, 21*(4), 6–7.

Crow, K. (1993). Multiculturalism and pluralistic thought in nursing education: Native American world view and the nursing academic world view. *Journal of Nursing Education, 32*(5), 198–204.

Davidhizar, R., & Lonser, G. (2003). Storytelling as a teaching technique. *Nurse Educator, 28*(5), 217–221.

Delgado, C., & Mack, B. (2002). A peer-reviewed program for senior proficiencies. *Nurse Educator, 27*(5), 212–213.

DeYoung, S., & Adams, E. F. (1995). Study groups among nursing students. *Journal of Nursing Education, 34*(4), 190–191.

Diekelmann, N., Swenson, M. M., & Sims, S. L. (2003). Reforming the lecture: Avoiding what students already know. *Journal of Nursing Education, 42*(3), 103–105.

Doane, G. A. H. (2002). Beyond behavioral skills to human-involved processes: Relational nursing practice and interpretive pedagogy. *Journal of Nursing Education, 41*(9), 400–403.

Drevdahl, D. (2001). Teaching about race, racism, and health. *Journal of Nursing Education, 40*(6), 285–288.

Drevdahl, D. J., & Dorcy, K. S. (2002). Using journals for community health students engaged in group work. *Nurse Educator, 27*(6), 255–259.

Drevdahl, D. J., Stackman, R. W., Purdy, J. M., & Louie, B. Y. (2002). Merging reflective inquiry and self-study as a framework for enhancing the scholarship of teaching. *Journal of Nursing Education, 41*(9), 413–418.

Duchscher, J. E. B. (2001). Peer learning: A clinical teaching strategy to promote active learning. *Journal of Nursing Education, 26*(2), 59–60.

Elbow, P. (1997). High stakes and low stakes in assigning and responding to writing. *New Directions for Teaching and Learning, 69,* 5–13.

Gaffney, K. F. (2000). Encouraging collaborative learning among culturally diverse students. *Nurse Educator, 25*(5), 219–221.

Grams, K., Kosowski, M., & Wilson, C. (1997). Creating a caring community in nursing education. *Nurse Educator, 22*(3), 10–16.

Greene, B. A., & Miller, R. B. (1996). Influences on achievement: Goals, perceived ability, and cognitive engagement. *Contemporary Educational Psychology, 21,* 181–192.

Gumbs, J. (2001). The effects of cooperative learning on students enrolled in a level 1 medical-surgical nursing course. *Journal of Cultural Diversity, 8*(2), 45–48.

Harden, J. K. (2003). Faculty and student experiences with web-based discussion groups in a large lecture setting. *Nurse Educator, 28*(1), 26–30.

Hayden-Miles, M. (2002). Humor in clinical nursing education. *Journal of Nursing Education, 41*(9), 420–424.

Hoffman, M., Richmond, J., Morrow, J., & Salomone, K. (2002). Investigating "sense of belonging" in first-year college students. *Journal of College Student Retention: Research, Theory, & Practice, 4*(3), 227–256.

Huff, C. (1997). Cooperative learning: A model for teaching. *Journal of Nursing Education, 36*(9), 434–436.

Hummel, M., & Steele, C. (1996). The learning community: A program to address issues of academic achievement and retention. *Journal of Intergroup Relations, 23*(2), 28–33.

Ironside, P. M. (2003). New pedagogies for teaching thinking: The lived experience of students and teachers enacting narrative pedagogy. *Journal of Nursing Education, 42*(11), 509–516.

Jeffreys, M. R. (1991). Time out! Let's play charades. *Nurse Educator, 16*(5), 12, 34.

Kelly, E. (1997). Development of strategies to identify the learning needs of baccalaureate nursing students. *Journal of Nursing Education, 36,* 156–162.

Kennerly, S. (2001). Fostering interaction through multimedia. *Nurse Educator, 26*(2), 90–94.

Knowles, M. (1984). *The adult learner: A neglected species.* Houston, TX: Gulf.

Koeckeritz, J., Malkiewicz, J., & Henderson, A. (2002). The seven principles of good practice: Applications for online education in nursing. *Nurse Educator, 27*(6), 283–287.

Koenig, J. M., & Zorn, C. R. (2002). Using storytelling as an approach to teaching and learning with diverse students. *Journal of Nursing Education, 41*(9), 393–399.

Kramer, N. (1995). Using games for learning. *Journal of Continuing Education in Nursing, 26,* 40–42.

Kuh, G. D. (2001). Organizational culture and student persistence: Prospects and puzzles. *Journal of College Student Retention: Research, Theory, & Practice, 3*(1), 23–40.

Labun, E. (2002). The Red River College Model: Enhancing success for native Canadian and other nursing students from disenfranchised groups. *Journal of Transcultural Nursing, 13*(4), 311–317.

Leininger, M. M., & McFarland, M. R. (2002). *Transcultural nursing: Concepts, theories, research, and practice* (3rd ed.). New York: McGraw-Hill.

Lepp, M., & Zorn, C. R. (2002). Life circle: Creating safe space for educational empowerment. *Journal of Nursing Education, 41*(9), 383–385.

MacIntosh, J., MacKay, E., Mallet-Boucher, M., & Wiggins, N. (2002). Discovering co-learning with students in distance education sites. *Nurse Educator, 27*(4), 182–186.

Martens, K. H., & Stangvik-Urban, L. (2002). Views on teaching-learning: Lessons learned from nursing education in Sweden. *Nurse Educator, 27*(3), 141–146.

Martens, R., & Dochy, F. (1997). Assessment and feedback as student support devices. *Studies in Educational Evaluation, 23*(3), 257–272.

Napoli, A. R., & Wortman, P. M. (1998). Psychosocial factors related to retention and early departure of two-year community college students. *Research in Higher Education, 39*(4), 419–455.

Nora, A. (2001). The depiction of significant others in Tinto's "Rites of Passage": A reconceptualization of the influence of family and community in the persistence process. *Journal of College Student Retention: Research, Theory, & Practice, 3*(1), 41–56.

O'Neil, E. H., & The Pew Health Professions Commission. (1998). *Recruiting health professional practice for a new century.* San Francisco: Pew Health Professions Commission.

PEW Health Professions Commission. (1995). *Health professions education and managed care: Challenges and necessary responses.* San Francisco: Center for the Health Professions.

Pimple, C., Schmidt, L., & Tidwell, S. (2003). Achieving excellence in end-of-life care. *Nurse Educator, 28*(1), 40–43.

Pintrich, P. R., & Garcia, T. (1994). Self-regulated learning in college students: Knowledge, strategies, and motivation. In P. R. Pintrich, D. R. Brown, & C. E. Weinstein (Eds.), *Student motivation, cognition, and learning: Essays in honor of Wilbert J. McKeachie* (pp. 113–133). Hillsdale, NJ: Erlbaum.

Schön, D. (1987). *Educating the reflective practitioner.* San Francisco: Jossey-Bass.

Schunk, D. (1987, August/September). *Self-efficacy and cognitive achievement.* Paper presented at the Annual Meeting of the American Psychological Association, New York, NY. ERIC Document Reproduction Service No. ED287880).

Schunk, D. (1995). Self-efficacy and education and instruction. In J. E. Maddux (Ed.), *Self-efficacy, adaptation, and adjustment: Theory, research, and application* (pp. 281–304). New York: Plenum Press.

Seifer, S. D. (2002). From placement site to partnership: The promise of service-learning. *Journal of Nursing Education, 41*(10), 431–432.

Skahill, M. P. (2002). The role of social support network in college persistence among freshman students. *Journal of College Student Retention: Research, Theory, & Practice, 4*(1), 39–52.

Snyder, M. D., & Weyer, M. E. (2002). Facilitating a collaborative partnership with a homeless shelter. *Journal of Nursing Education, 41*(12), 547–549.

Soldner, L., Lee, Y., & Duby, P. (1999). Welcome to the block: Developing freshman learning communities that work. *Journal of College Student Retention: Research, Theory, & Practice, 1*(2), 115–130.

Sternberger, C. S. (2002). Embedding a pedagogical model in the design of an online course. *Nurse Educator, 27*(4), 170–173.

Tidwell, R., & Berry, G. (1997). Higher education and the African American experience: Barriers to success and remedies for failure. In H. Bessent (Ed.), *Strategies for recruitment, retention, and graduation of minority nurses in colleges of nursing* (pp. 55–62). Washington, DC: American Nurses Foundation.

Tinto, V. (1997). Classrooms as communities. *Journal of Higher Education, 68*(6), 599–623.

Tinto, V. (1998). College as communities: Taking research on student persistence seriously. *Review of Higher Education, 21,* 167–177.

Tinto, V. (2000). Linking learning and leaving: Exploring the role of the college classroom in student departure. In J. M. Braxton (Ed.), *Reworking the student departure puzzle* (pp. 81–94). Nashville, TN: Vanderbilt University Press.

Tucker-Allen, S., & Long, E. (1999). *Recruitment and retention of minority students: Stories of success.* Lisle, IL: Tucker.

Vance, C., & Olson, R. K. (1998). *The mentor connection in nursing.* New York: Springer.

Williams, R. P., & Calvillo, E. R. (2002). Maximizing learning among students from culturally diverse backgrounds. *Nurse Educator, 27*(5), 222–226.

Winters, C., & Owens, R. (1993). Alternative teaching strategies: Using a health fair to meet tribal college and nursing program needs. *Journal of Nursing Education, 32*(5), 237–238.

Yoder, M. K. (2001). The bridging approach: Effective strategies for teaching ethnically diverse nursing students. *Journal of Transcultural Nursing, 12,* 319–325.

Yoder, M. K., & Saylor, C. (2002). Student and teacher roles: Mismatched expectations. *Nurse Educator, 27*(5), 201–203.

Young, P., & Diekelmann, N. (2002). Learning to lecture: Exploring the skills, strategies, and practices of new teachers in nursing education. *Journal of Nursing Education, 41*(9), 405–412.

Chapter 13

Enrichment Program Design, Implementation, and Evaluation*

A n enrichment program (EP) is a formally designed multiservice program that aims to enrich the total nursing student experience by maximizing strengths, remedying weaknesses, promoting positive psychological outcomes, facilitating positive academic outcomes, and nurturing professional growth and development. Services may include several of the following: orientation, mentoring, tutoring, newsletters, career advisement and guidance, workshops, study groups, networking, transitional support, financial stipends, and referral. Services are best facilitated through a collaborative partnership in learning and professional development among nursing faculty, other professional nurses, and students. The ongoing opportunities for professional integration and socialization offer tremendous possibilities for optimizing academic and psychological outcomes. Nurse educators can make a difference in nursing student retention and success through a carefully designed EP.

The main purpose of this chapter is to describe the process of designing, implementing, and evaluating an enrichment program. An illustrative case exemplar, using the Prenursing Enrichment Program (PEP), will complement each step of the process. The PEP consisted of free services for students: orientation, mentoring, tutoring, career advisement and guidance, workshops, networking, and transitional support services

---

* This chapter was excerpted and adapted from Jeffreys, M. R. (2003). Strategies for promoting nontraditional nursing student retention success. In M. Oermann & K. Heinrich (Eds.), *Annual Review of Nursing Education: Volume I*. New York: Springer.

facilitated through a collaborative partnership in learning and professional development. Evaluation of EP components, including academic outcomes, psychological outcomes, and variables influencing retention, will conclude the chapter.

ENRICHMENT PROGRAM DESIGN, IMPLEMENTATION, AND EVALUATION

Enrichment program design, implementation, and evaluation should be a well-planned process. This involves time, energy, money, commitment, collaborative partnerships, and a systematic plan. Figure 13.1 presents an eleven-step process that can guide EP development. Each step will be described, followed by a case exemplar. The Prenursing Enrichment Program (PEP) case exemplar illustrates how this process can be adapted by other nurse educators interested in developing diagnostic-prescriptive enrichment programs for undergraduate nursing students. Although the PEP was designed for nontraditional undergraduate nursing students, the case exemplar has applicability for traditional students as well.

The first phase of the process might appear to be "design," but there is really a predesign phase. This involves five steps: assessing the current situation, reviewing the literature, searching for grants, drafting a plan, and soliciting support. Each step will be described individually and within the context of the PEP case exemplar.

Step 1—Assess Current Situation

A retention strategy or enrichment program should be designed for a specific situation and have empirical support (National League for Nursing Accrediting Commission, 1999). The first step is to systematically assess the current situation, including student profile variables, retention rates, success rates, departmental support, administrative support, and the existing college resources.

A systematic assessment of the targeted student population can be initiated using the NURS model. The realization that there are multidimensional variables influencing retention and success is often overwhelming; yet it is essential to evaluate them before designing the EP. The assessment of student profile variables can give a general description of the student population or can help the nurse educator target a specific student group. For example, a nursing program with many English-as-second-language (ESL) students may need to incorporate language enhancement strategies into an EP.

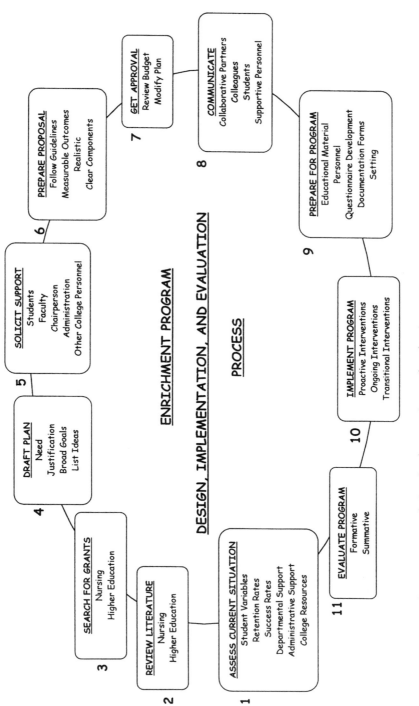

FIGURE 13.1 Enrichment program design, implementation, and evaluation process.

In the PEP case example, student perceptions had been assessed in a previously funded study. Descriptive results from the study of first semester nontraditional associate degree nursing students found that environmental variables were perceived as more influential for academic achievement and retention than academic variables (Jeffreys, 1993, 1995, 1998). Students felt that family, faculty, and friends greatly influenced retention; however family responsibilities were thought to be severely restrictive. Overly confident students who rated their academic factors as greatly supportive had significantly lower nursing course grades. Students with a more conservative self-appraisal of academic and environmental factors had higher nursing course grades. This suggested that some students did not have realistic self-appraisals of strengths and weaknesses, or accurate comprehension of the skills needed for professional nursing education. Because inaccurate perceptions could be detrimental to student retention and success, it was believed that an EP consisting of proactive, ongoing, and transitional interventions would be most effective.

Assessment of current retention rates should differentiate between course retention, ideal program retention, continuous program retention, and interim program retention. (See Table 1.1). Course retention is the easiest to assess. Comparison of course retention rates across various semesters and between courses can help identify trends within the overall program. However, tracking nontraditional students throughout the program is difficult for a variety of reasons. First, nontraditional students often attend college part-time, and therefore a cohort group for analysis is difficult to identify. Second, nontraditional students often must "stop out" for nonacademic reasons such as pregnancy, child care, care of a sick family member, financial strain, employment constraints, and numerous other examples. Traditional students may also stop out for nonacademic reasons. Third, the institution's computer capability for tracking such nontraditional students who frequently attend college part-time and stop out one or more times may be limited. Fourth, the individual tracking of students who stop out and attend part-time is labor-intensive, costly, at increased risk for human error, and results in a small number of students in many different cohorts. A small sample cohort becomes problematic when trying to use inferential statistical analyses.

One recommendation would be to calculate four different program retention rates: ideal program retention, continuous program retention, interim program retention and total program retention. After several semesters, a trend and student profile would emerge. This assessment could guide EP design to specific groups. For the purposes of the PEP, course retention rates across various semesters and for each of the clinical nursing courses was the primary focus.

Assessment of current success rates should differentiate between total and ideal program success (see Table 1.1). Additionally, the various components of "success" should be operationalized, measured, and compared for several semesters to look for common trends and/or gross disparities in trends. This means measuring graduation rates, RN licensing exam pass rates, employment rates, and enrollment rates in more advanced nursing program. A problem in one area could have an impact on other areas. For example, failing the RN licensing exam will affect employment and enrollment in a more advanced nursing program because a RN license is usually required for both options. Inclusion of program success was beyond the scope of the PEP; however, with future expansion of student support strategies and ongoing measurement strategies, it could be possible to evaluate the entire process of retention and success.

Determining departmental support should address both conceptual and instrumental support. Conceptual support refers to the support of the idea of an EP and can range from passive (listening without offering opinions and suggestions) to active (advocacy, suggestions, and verbal commitment). It is valuable to have conceptual support from the chairperson, deputy chairperson, faculty, and staff. Instrumental support refers to allocation of resources such as expertise, money, released time, secretarial services, supplies, space, and teaching load distribution.

After appraising departmental support, administrative support should be assessed. Determining administrative support first requires a comprehensive understanding of the institution's administrative structure, organizational culture, politics, policy, and procedures. Formal meetings with key administrators can provide a valuable guide for EP development. Careful review of current and proposed college resources available to all college students and the adequacy or inadequacy of such services for nontraditional undergraduate nursing students is important to avoid duplication of existing services, substantiate the need for absent or insufficient services, and explore partnership possibilities and pooling of resources.

After assessing each of these areas individually, the overall strengths and weaknesses in the already existing college resources can be evaluated. This overall assessment should reveal areas that need development and provide some basis to determine costs and feasibility. Without the conceptual support of the department and administration, there are too many obstacles that would impair feasibility and implementation. Conceptual support without some commitment to instrumental support also would pose obstacles, although with generous grant funding this difficulty could be overcome.

Before designing the PEP, collaboration with the department chairperson resulted in both conceptual and instrumental support. The chairperson readily gave active support by offering encouragement for the idea and advocating the pursuit of the project. Instrumental support ranged from the chairperson's sharing her expertise to acknowledging future access to secretarial services and supplies. Administrative support was assessed during formal meetings with the divisional dean and vice president of the college. College resource assessment revealed the absence of college tutoring services for nursing courses and the presence of several support services for student referral, such as personal counseling. College resources for the project director such as services by the institution's office of grants and research, were identified. Collaborative partnerships with measurement experts and the director of institutional research were discussed in anticipation of the evaluation phase of the PEP. Conclusively, the overall assessment revealed that the institutional climate was favorable toward PEP development.

Step 2—Review Literature

Next, a review of the nursing and higher education literature should be conducted. Materials should be reviewed for gathering background information about student retention, nontraditional students, retention strategies, evaluation methods, and funding sources. Choice of a relevant conceptual framework can be instrumental to the organization. When reviewing literature concerning other student support strategies, educators should determine strategy strengths, limitations, and appropriateness of fit to the targeted population. One must be aware, however, that there is no panacea; enrichment programs will not solve all problems, nor will they help every student succeed. Realistically weighing the possible benefits against the risk of doing nothing can help in the decision-making process.

In the PEP, a previous compilation of literature on retention necessitated an updated review of the nursing and higher education literature. Published journal articles and books were reviewed and organized into specific categories, expanding the current literature files and making future retrieval and updates easy.

Step 3—Search for Grants

The search for grant resources can be conducted via computer by the nurse educator or by requesting assistance from the institution's office of grants and research. For the PEP, one specific funding source was selected. The funding was specifically allocated for public institutions, associate degree programs, and vocational education. Additionally, specific populations of students were targeted. Prior assessment of student variables in Step 1 supported the observation that many students fell into the targeted categories, therefore it was appropriate to pursue this grant opportunity.

Step 4—Draft Plan

Next, a written draft is developed. Familiarity with the grant's terminology, goals, format, funding capabilities, and guidelines is important prior to drafting a plan. Grant specifications must guide the draft development. Relevant issues reported in the literature and assessment findings (Step 1) also should be incorporated throughout the plan. Clear identification of the need and justification based on the literature and assessment findings is a necessary precursor to establishing goals. At this point, goals should be broad and relate directly to the identified need. The draft should include an "idea" list, leaving details for later consideration.

In the case example, data from the preliminary study of nontraditional associate degree nursing students strongly supported the need for the PEP. The use of a conceptual model as a proposed organizing framework for designing a retention strategy was an added strength. This suggested that the strategy would not haphazardly use a trial and error approach but, based on available conceptual and empirical literature, would use a systematic and detailed approach. The broad goal was to improve student retention. Brainstorming resulted in a list of possible retention strategy components. Reviewing the list for feasibility eliminated some strategies. Finally, prioritizing the remaining components provided an outline of ideas that could be a starting point for soliciting support.

Step 5—Solicit Support

Although soliciting support can be time consuming, the benefits of conceptual and instrumental support commitments are invaluable and help build alliances and partnerships. Although both are important here, soliciting a significant number of instrumental support commitments is an essential precursor to preparing a proposal.

Although this step may seem similar to the assessment of support in Step 1, it has many important differences. First, it builds on the collaborative relationship, initiated in Step 1, that should then evolve or be nurtured into a collaborative partnership. A collaborative partnership can have varying degrees of direct or indirect supportive involvement but all could be potentially critical to the funding of an EP and ultimately its success.

At this point of more formalized commitment to specific tasks, the anticipated time line for the tasks should be mentioned. This gives the program more structure and organization. If the time line is not realistic, it can be adjusted now before writing it into the proposal and setting the plan up for failure. Before preparing a proposal, it is important to tease out which strategies are feasible and realistic and which would be problematic. In this way, the presence or absence of support will result in a modified list of possible strategy components. Instrumental support cannot occur without conceptual support; however, conceptual support without instrumental support greatly limits the possibilities of EP success. Evaluating student support for various components is crucial before entering the design phase (proposal preparation and approval).

The following examples were applicable to the PEP:

- Students agree to use PEP services actively and/or encourage their use.
- Faculty members agree to make announcements in class to encourage students to use PEP services.
- Chairperson agrees to reserve an empty adjunct office to be used for possible peer mentor-tutoring.
- Administrators commit to support released time for project director.
- Director of institutional research agrees to actively assist with transcript data retrieval and data analysis.
- Colleagues agree to review questionnaire drafts and serve as expert reviewers for content validity.

Step 6—Prepare Proposal

In the PEP, the broad goals listed in the draft plan (Step 4) needed to be rewritten to fit the terminology used in the grant proposal guidelines. The initial draft was decreased to pilot several of the strategy components first, followed by an evaluation. This was done for three main reasons. First, there would not be enough time for the project director to carry out all interventions, along with teaching and other faculty responsibilities, even with released time. Second, students would be overwhelmed with so many choices that it would be confusing and would encourage fragmented use of many services rather than promote a concentrated effort and consistency in one or two services. Third, financial constraints limited what could be done.

PEP strategy components were organized to include proactive, ongoing, and transitional interventions. Theoretical and empirical support for this approach and its components were documented in the proposal.

Using grant-specific guidelines and terminology, the evaluation plan included formative and summative evaluation measures. Although the grant's guidelines focused primarily on quantitative results documenting improved academic outcomes, the measurement of students' psychological outcomes (satisfaction) and perceived variables influencing retention were written into the evaluation plan. The justification for their inclusion was based on prior research and the underlying conceptual model. Instrument development and evaluation (reliability and validity studies) were accordingly incorporated into the proposal. Several revisions resulted in a final proposal that was submitted on time according to the procedure at the educational institution.

Step 7—Get Approval

When a project or grant proposal is approved, it is important to review the budgetary allocations for specific categories and check if there are any restrictions or added guidelines. Budgetary constraints may require some modifications from the original proposal plan. These modifications should be finalized before entering the next phase of pre-implementation. The pre-implementation phase acknowledges that there are two essential steps before program implementation: communication and preparation. For the PEP, no major changes from the original proposal were noted.

Step 8—Communicate

Once grant funding is awarded and the budgetary plan modifications are finalized, the project director should communicate that funding has been received. The important questions to consider are with whom to communicate, what needs to be communicated, and how to communicate. Essentially, what must be communicated is the fact that a grant was received and how this will involve the other collaborative partner(s).

Collaborative partners or those individuals who committed time, expertise, service, or some other instrumental support toward the proposed project should be contacted personally. A telephone contact followed by a written memo or copy of the grant award and proposal may be indicated, depending on the type of partnership required and level of involvement. Memos that communicate the necessary details reinforce the verbal communication.

A copy of the grant award may be forwarded to the administration as part of the grant notification process. If not, a copy should be forwarded to all administrators. Announcements made at faculty, curriculum, and other pertinent meetings can be made both verbally and in the form of a written memo or information sheet. Students can be notified about the upcoming services via classroom announcements, memos, and student club meetings.

In the PEP, announcement of the grant award was automatically forwarded to administrators by the institution's office of grants and research. A scheduled meeting with the department chairperson tried to build on the communication, commitments, and partnerships established in Steps 1 and 5. Because the grant was awarded after classes had ended, chairperson support for communicating with students by letter was greatly welcomed. A letter outlining the main features of the PEP was mailed to all students listed as prenursing or associate degree nursing students, along with an application for an orientation session and study group sessions. A letter explaining the funded project was also mailed to all full-time nursing faculty members.

Students already enrolled in the associate degree or RN to BS program received an invitation to apply for a peer mentor-tutor position. Job qualifications and responsibilities were included, along with a blank application form. Peer mentor-tutor qualifications included (1) current enrollment in an upper-level associate degree nursing course or in the baccalaureate program after completion of the college's associate degree program, (2) above-average grades in prenursing and nursing courses and in clinical evaluations, and (3) excellent communication skills. Responsibilities included assistance with orientation sessions, tutoring for prenursing and/or nursing courses, individual and small group mentoring sessions, and collaborating with the project director. Hours were advertised as flexible and negotiable, with wages set at a rate competitive with other college assistants, work-study, and unlicensed hospital personnel wages. Copies of all letters were posted on bulletin boards.

Step 9—Prepare for Program

Allocating a sufficient amount of time for program preparation is important. Making a list of what needs to be done, by whom, and the needed date of completion can help prioritize program preparation components. Preparation may include creating or obtaining educational materials and documentation forms, selection and orientation of personnel, questionnaire development and evaluation, and arranging the physical setting.

In the PEP, a time line was originally submitted with the project proposal and served as a valuable guide. Two tasks that had the highest priority because they involved a series of steps, were time-consuming, and involved several people, were questionnaire development and the selection and orientation of personnel (project assistants and peer mentor-tutors).

Questionnaire Development

Several instruments were developed, as proposed in the grant proposal. A cover letter explaining some background information and the purpose of the instruments, the requested due date, a self-addressed stamped envelope, and an instruction sheet for rating content validity accompanied the instruments. The ratings and comments of the content reviewers provided the basis for minor revisions. Review by a psychometric expert confirmed that the instruments were in a format that could easily be scanned, interpreted, and analyzed, using the SPSS statistical program. The instrument drafts were then given to a project assistant who had computer expertise in creating optical scanning instruments, scanning, and conversion into SPSS. All instruments needed a trial run for scanning to assure ease with future data processing.

Selection and Orientation of Peer Mentor-Tutors

The selection of peer mentor-tutors (PMT) first involved a review of completed applications by the requested due date. The next step involved review of student transcripts and clinical evaluations for each course completed so far. The review of clinical evaluations was quite time consuming but provided insightful information, such as a record of the student's verbal communication and interaction with others, attendance, tardiness, and other important qualities and skills.

The highest-ranking applicants were then invited for an interview. Scheduling, arranging, and conducting the interviews were also time consuming, yet essential to the selection process. During interviews it was emphasized that a collaborative partnership among PMTs, students, and the project director was an important goal.

The next priority was to organize and prepare the educational and documentation materials needed for the PMT orientation. A 90-minute orientation session was held with the PMTs. The overall purposes and goals of the enrichment program, particularly detailing the significance of mentoring in nursing and the role of PMT and student as partners in learning, was described (Figure 13.2). The expected benefits of specific PMT roles and interventions were discussed. This discussion clarified the scope of the PMT role and emphasized the importance of conveying this information during the first contact meeting with students.

Documentation forms for recording the study group's activities and anticipated plans for the next meeting were reviewed with PMTs. The documentation forms would serve as a weekly communication between the PMT and project director. Strategies for enhancing student survival skills addressed such issues as academic support strategies, time management,

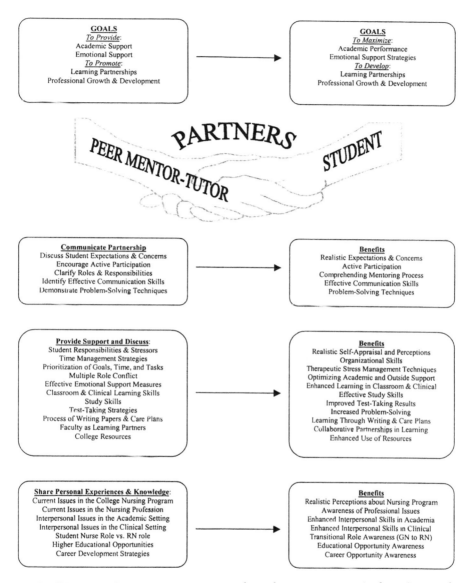

FIGURE 13.2   Peer-mentor-tutor and student as partner in learning and professional development.

Select information obtained from Alvarez, A., & Abriam-Yago, K. (1993). Mentoring undergraduate ethnic-minority students; A strategy for retention. *Journal of Nursing Education, 32*(5), 230–232.

stress reduction techniques, assisting students throughout the educational process, promoting professional growth, and balancing multiple role responsibilities. Handouts and lists of referral resources within the college complemented this discussion.

Next, the simulated situations and group discussion provided an opportunity for PMTs to use problem-solving strategies for academic and nonacademic problems that could potentially arise. Decision-making dilemmas and varying opinions identified areas that required further clarification and guidance. It was emphasized that the PMT would have an ongoing collaborative relationship with the project director throughout the semester.

Finally, PMT study group schedules were confirmed. Because several study groups would occur at the same time, finding sufficient space necessitated organizing room arrangements and reservations via the college's protocol. A written evaluation of the PMT orientation concluded the meeting.

Step 10—Implement the Program

A well-developed and detailed proposal, accompanied by an itemized time line, can be the guide for program implementation. To facilitate implementation, the program should be divided into various intervention categories: proactive, ongoing, and transitional. Each category should complement the others and easily flow among them. There may be some eventual overlap in categories as students participate in an enrichment program throughout several semesters.

Proactive interventions are implemented before the beginning of the semester and aim both to prepare students academically, psychologically, and practically, and to enhance performance, satisfaction, and success. Preparation may allow for opportunities to review previously learned skills, ask questions, review pertinent information, assist with time management strategies specific to the new nursing course, interact with students who previously completed the course, and informally meet the new course instructors.

Ongoing interventions aim to maximize student success by the early identification of strengths and weaknesses before academic difficulties, role conflicts, or stress arises. Early identification of the at-risk student can prevent failure or withdrawal. Often students do not seek help until difficulty arises, and then it is too late to improve an academically precarious situation.

Another benefit of ongoing interventions is that collaborative and productive partnerships can flourish. For example, the PMT-student partnership can only develop with consistent and frequent contacts. Students also can feel more at ease with study group peers, offering both emotional and academic support strategies. This peer interaction helps develop professional socialization, integration, and acculturation into the nursing student role and future RN role. (Alvarez & Abriam-Yago, 1993; Baldwin & Wold, 1993; Bessent, 1997; Perry, 1997; Ramsey, Blowers, Merriman, Glenn, & Terry, 2000; Tucker-Allen & Long, 1999; Vance & Olson, 1998). The opportunity to share experiences and watch role models and peers struggle with similar academic and nonacademic challenges can help increase self-efficacy and motivation to persist (Bandura, 1986; Zimmerman, 1995).

As students move from one phase of the educational process to the next, *transitional interventions* should be implemented (Schön, 1987). Transition from preprofessional to professional education (first nursing course) and one nursing course to the next level nursing course challenges students to embark on a new, unknown path in their journey toward becoming a registered nurse. Guidance at these transitional stages is crucial to encourage retention, enhance achievement, promote satisfaction, and minimize stress.

The PEP encompassed the various stages of the educational process and included proactive, ongoing, and transitional interventions. Activities will be described in the sections that follow.

Orientation

The piloted program included a 2½ hour orientation program before the start of the semester. Although the orientation targeted prenursing students not yet enrolled in a clinical nursing course, several students already in the first nursing course attended. All students were invited to bring a family member, friend, or support person. Each student was personally greeted by a PMT. Everyone received an orientation folder, calendar, and study skills handouts. Several of the participants had just enrolled at the college for the first time; other prenursing students had completed all prenursing required courses.

The agenda included: (1) purposes and goals of the PEP, (2) nursing program requirements, (3) student information, (4) family, friend, and faculty support network, (5) time management strategies, (6) enhancing textbook reading comprehension, (7) enhancing learning skills in the classroom including taking notes effectively, and (8) collaborating with the PMT. Prenursing students then met with their PMT. Following a brief introduction, a follow-up meeting date or phone call was set up based on the individual needs of the student.

Next, students completed a satisfaction questionnaire. All students found the orientation session to be "very helpful and informative." Written and verbal comments by students provided additional information. For example, one student commented that the mentor encouraged her to keep trying. Many students commented that it was helpful to have someone to talk to who had already been through the nursing courses. A few students realized the need to resolve personal and/or family issues before trying to take a full-time course schedule. Most students commented that the handouts and orientation session provided them with new study skills and time management strategies. One student commented that she would share the handouts on family-student-faculty partnerships with her family so that her requests for assistance with household responsibilities would be respected and honored.

Newsletter

A newsletter was created to enrich the prenursing and nursing program experience by broadening information access to students. The biannual newsletter addressed relevant issues such as requirements of the nursing program, student responsibilities, strategies for enhancing academic success, career advisement and guidance, management of work and family responsibilities, and services available to assist students. Announcements concerning workshops, tutoring, and nursing application dates, and notices about the enrichment program were included.

Feature article sections were presented. Questions frequently asked or submitted by students were selected for answers in the featured section "What Enquiring Students Want to Know." The "Stories from the Field" feature provided some clinical case scenarios and attempted to showcase how nursing students can make a positive difference in the clinical setting. Tear-off application forms for PMT study groups comprised the last two pages of the newsletter.

Study Groups

The study groups, led by PMTs, were in great demand. Application forms submitted by the deadline exceeded available openings. Registration was done on a first-come, first-served basis on the assigned registration date and time before the beginning of the semester. Students who submitted applications by the deadline had first choice in selecting study group sessions and were required to commit to regularly scheduled group meetings (usually weekly) starting at the beginning of the semester. The study group registration session also allowed for informal meeting among peers, PMTs, and the project director.

Students in the study groups developed a working partnership with the PMT and other group members. Study groups usually consisted of five students per one PMT. Additional in-person meetings, telephone meetings, and/or referrals were individualized as needed. Frequently, the project director met with referred students about academic and nonacademic problems. The project director was informed about group activities weekly, either through personal visits and/or study group documentation forms. These forms focused the group on the day's tasks or topics, identified specific areas for the following week's session, and documented attendance. Additionally, a PMT comment section informed the project director about individual and group concerns, strengths, weaknesses, and other pertinent academic and nonacademic issues. The documentation forms also helped maintain consistency and structure between and within groups on a regular basis, while keeping the project director informed.

Transitional Workshop

All nursing students were invited to attend a brief transitional workshop prior to the beginning of the next semester. Although there was some overlap between proactive and transitional interventions, the main difference was that transitional interventions targeted students who had already participated in the PEP. The agenda included the purposes and goals of the PEP, the nursing student transitional process, strategies for successful transition, collaborating with a PMT, and study group selection. The workshop addressed the transitional process and issues that nursing students often face when moving from one phase of their professional nursing education to another. Each phase offered different challenges and required students to modify previous successful study strategies to accommodate these new challenges.

For example, study time allocation for a six-credit, fifteen-week course would have to be adjusted to meet the demands of a nine-credit course or a five-credit, half-semester course. Sometimes students needed assistance in changing the focus from an adult client with medical or surgical problems to pregnant clients, children, or mentally ill clients. Although many of the essential underlying professional skills had been learned previously, guidance through the transition from one phase (course) to another could be eased by acknowledging that a transitional process existed and by learning effective strategies to meet transitional challenges. Nursing students stated that working with a PMT has assisted them through this transitional process.

Other transitional support measures included the PEP Nursing Skills Lab Practice Sessions prior to the beginning of the new semester. Nursing students were encouraged to practice any previously learned and evaluated technical skills during the supervised PEP practice session in preparation for clinical. New students accepted into the first clinical course were invited to participate in a Nursing Skills Lab and Educational Resources Tour led by a PMT guide. The tour familiarized students with their new environment and showed them what resources were available to assist them throughout their educational experience.

Step 11—Evaluation

A carefully orchestrated evaluation should be tied explicitly to the proposal's measurement plan and should include both formative and summative components. Formative evaluations assess the process of a program rather than its outcomes. They can be monitored as the program is implemented and can document specific activities, identify difficulties, and allow for diagnostic-prescriptive modifications based on participants' feedback, using both quantitative and qualitative data.

Summative evaluations should be monitored every semester and compared globally at the completion of the program to assess the achievement of desired program outcomes. Because student retention is a dynamic and multidimensional phenomenon, the success of any teaching, support, or enrichment strategy requires a multidimensional evaluation strategy.

The NURS model may be used to identify program outcomes as academic, psychological, and affective. Academic outcomes may include course retention, course success, course withdrawal, continuous program retention, interim program retention, ideal program retention, total program retention, total program success, and ideal program success. Psychological outcomes may include measures of satisfaction or stress; affective outcomes may include self-efficacy (confidence) perceptions.

Following the preestablished plan for data collection and analysis consistently and rigorously will make the evaluation results more valid and reliable. This includes working diligently with previously established partners in the evaluation process, such as the data collectors, director of institutional research, project assistant, and psychometric expert. Once the results are obtained and reviewed for statistical and practical significance, inferences from the data can guide future enrichment program activities, outcome measures, and desired outcomes.

The process of evaluation naturally leads into the beginning of the enrichment program design process (Step 1) again in which the nurse educator would assess the current situation and compare it with the EP evaluation just completed. Assessment would include the appropriateness of generalizing findings to the new situation. The ultimate goal of the EP design, implementation, and evaluation process is that empirical and conceptually based enrichment programs will address the holistic needs of students.

A study was undertaken to evaluate select aspects of the PEP among students who participated in PMT-led study groups throughout the semester. The evaluation addressed academic outcomes, psychological outcomes (satisfaction), and perceived variables influencing retention. Academic outcomes targeted course retention by measuring course success rates, course failure rates, and course withdrawal rates for the intervention group and a control group. Comparisons were done between the clinical nursing courses, within courses, and throughout several semesters.

Overall, the intervention (PEP) group had lower failure rates, lower withdrawal rates, higher course success rates, and positive psychological outcomes (satisfaction). Students also perceived that environmental variables were more influential than academic variables in influencing retention. Social integration variables such as faculty advisement and helpfulness, tutoring, and the EP were perceived as highly supportive. Details concerning the PEP evaluation, including instrumentation, are described in two recently published articles (Jeffreys, 2001, 2002).

High student satisfaction with the PEP and perceptions that the PEP supported retention emphasize the continued need for strategies that enrich the nursing student experience. Formative evaluations of EP interventions and comments on the Satisfaction Questionnaire (Appendix C) also provided valuable information to guide future enrichment strategies. For example, students' written requests for extended study group hours, especially in the beginning nursing courses, substantiated the need for greater allocation of resources to beginning students. Additionally, requests for longer study group sessions increased the sessions from an average of 45 to 90 minutes.

KEY POINTS SUMMARY

- An enrichment program (EP) is a formally designed multiservice program that aims to enrich the total nursing student experience by maximizing strengths, remedying weaknesses, promoting positive psychological outcomes, facilitating positive academic outcomes, and nurturing professional growth and development.
- Enrichment program design, implementation, and evaluation should be a systematic and well-planned process.

- The eleven-step process includes: assess current situation, review literature, search for grants, draft plan, solicit support, prepare proposal, get approval, communicate, prepare for program, implement program, and evaluate program.
- The Prenursing Enrichment Program (PEP) case exemplar illustrates each step individually, describes PEP activity components, and highlights the main benefits of peer mentor-tutor partnerships and other essential partnerships.
- The PEP consisted of free services for students: orientation, mentoring, tutoring, career advisement and guidance, workshops, networking, and transitional support services facilitated through a collaborative partnership in learning and professional development.
- Evaluation included the assessment of academic outcomes, psychological outcomes, and variables influencing retention.

EDUCATOR-IN-ACTION

Professor Bridges is the project director of an enrichment program that includes weekly study groups led by peer mentor-tutors (PMTs). Although the PMT orientation addressed roles and responsibilities of study group participants as well as PMT roles and responsibilities, PMTs expressed concern that study group participant expectations were often different and sometimes inappropriate. To address this issue, Professor Bridges prepared a handout on "Study Group Etiquette; Dos and Don'ts to Maximize Success" (see Table 13.1). After reviewing the handout with PMTs, she distributed it to first-semester nursing students, briefly reviewed it, and invited students to sign up for study groups. PMTs reviewed the handout again with students on the first study group meeting day and clarified any ambiguities. PMTs reported positive results from this approach:

Maura: "Because I did this on the first day, students knew more what to expect from the study group. When one student asked me about what might be included on an exam, another student was quick to say that this was inappropriate. Besides, I could just refer to the handout if it came up again. I felt more comfortable with setting limits."

Lynn: "Overall, students seemed to come to the study group on time and more prepared than last semester. They didn't expect me to summarize their readings, but came prepared to ask me specific questions about the readings."

TABLE 13.1 Study Group Etiquette: Dos and Don'ts to Maximize Success

Do

1. Join a study group at the beginning of the semester.
2. Attend group meetings regularly.
3. Complete prerequisite class readings.
4. Expect to contribute to the group discussion.
5. Plan to study individually in addition to the group study.
6. Respect each individual group member.
7. Ask questions related to the group focus topic.
8. Bring notes and other necessary materials to group sessions.
9. Tell the group facilitator if the study session is meeting your needs.
10. Set a target plan for the next meeting.

Don't

1. Wait until after the first exam to join a study group. Your success can be enhanced by group study.
2. Attend groups intermittently. This disrupts group effectiveness and cohesiveness.
3. Expect that others will read the chapters for you. Actively reading chapters *before* enhances classroom learning and group interaction.
4. Expect everyone else to do all the discussion. Actively discussing material identifies your strengths and weaknesses. Everyone has strengths and weaknesses. Remedying weaknesses *before* an exam maximizes your chances for success. *The group facilitator is a RESOURCE person available to ASSIST you. The group facilitator is not a lecturer.*
5. Substitute group study sessions for individual reading, writing, and studying. Study groups should *supplement, complement, and enhance* your individual study time. Study groups are not a substitute for meeting with your course instructor when you have difficulty or class-specific questions.
6. Make biased assumptions about individual group members or treat some members with less respect. Mutual respect enhances group interpersonal dynamics and interaction effectiveness.
7. Ask questions just to show off, change the topic, challenge the group facilitator, or obstruct the group process. Questions asked for the right reasons should always be asked; questions asked for the wrong reasons should be avoided.
8. Leave notes, study guides, care plan information, and so on at home. It is an unnecessary disadvantage to you and other group members when essential materials are not available.
9. Expect the group facilitator to read your mind. Your input is not only valuable, it is essential.

(continued)

TABLE 13.1 Study Group Etiquette: Dos and Don'ts to Maximize Success *(continued)*

Don't (continued)

10. Leave the group session without having an idea about what will occur at the next meeting. This will save time at the beginning of the next meeting. Additionally, everyone should be focused on what needs to be done before the next meeting (reading) and what essential materials should be brought.

Don't Ask the Group Facilitator—(Peer Mentor-Tutor)

1. "What's going to be on the exam?" This is unethical. Besides, it is unknown. Remember, you are studying to become a qualified, safe, registered professional nurse who will care for human lives. Therefore, you are not simply studying for an exam but for a lifelong career.
2. "Can I see the paper/care plans you did when you were in Nursing _____ Class?" Again, this is unethical. The most valuable learning occurs from the *process* of learning to write a paper, rather than simply the finished product.
3. "Can I copy your notes from when you took the Nursing _____ Class?" You will learn more by active note taking and immediate review of notes after class.

Tony: "Last semester a student kept asking me for my old care plans. Although I knew I was doing the right thing by refusing, I still felt uncomfortable. With these written guidelines, I'm more comfortable about this issue. This semester students showed me parts of their care plan as they were working on it and asked me for guidance when they got stuck. They didn't expect the answer but rather were satisfied when I asked them a series of questions to help them come up with the answer."

Student study group participants also reported positive responses:

Tamika: "I always studied on my own before so I didn't really know what to expect about a study group. The handout and explanation set everything straight at the beginning."

Tomas: "Last semester I was in the enrichment program study group. Some of the people just listened and never contributed anything. After a while three of us just dropped out and formed our own study group without the PMT but we missed her guidance and mentoring. This semester everyone is contributing in some way. Everyone has learned a lot and we enjoy studying together."

Dominique: "I'm a person who needs structure so the guidelines of dos and don'ts really helped me."

Professor Bridges continually evaluates the multidimensional aspects of the enrichment program, using student feedback and academic outcome measures to guide future interventions.

REFERENCES AND BIBLIOGRAPHY

Alvarez, A., & Abriam-Yago, K. (1993). Mentoring undergraduate ethnic-minority students: A strategy for retention. *Journal of Nursing Education, 32,* 230–232.

Baldwin, D., & Wold, J. (1993). Students from disadvantaged backgrounds: Satisfaction with a mentor-protégé relationship. *Journal of Nursing Education, 32,* 225–226.

Bandura, A. (1986). *Social foundations of thought and action: A social cognitive theory.* Englewood Cliffs, NJ: Prentice-Hall.

Bessent, H. (Ed.). (1997). *Strategies for recruitment, retention, and graduation of minority nurses in colleges of nursing.* Washington, DC: American Nurses Publishing.

Braxton, J. M. (Ed.). (2000). *Reworking the student departure puzzle.* Nashville, TN: Vanderbilt University Press.

Christman, L. (1997). Socialization to professional nursing roles. In B. Kozier, G. Erb, & K. Blais (Eds.), *Professional nursing practice: Concepts and perspectives* (p. 127). New York: Addison-Wesley.

Jeffreys, M. R. (1993). *The relationship of self-efficacy and select academic and environmental variables on academic achievement and retention.* Unpublished doctoral dissertation, New York, Teachers College, Columbia University.

Jeffreys, M. R. (1995). Joining together family, faculty, and friends: New ideas for enhancing nontraditional student success. *Nurse Educator, 20*(3), 11.

Jeffreys, M. R. (1998). Predicting nontraditional student retention and academic achievement. *Nurse Educator, 23*(1), 42–48.

Jeffreys, M. R. (2001). Evaluating enrichment program study groups: Academic outcomes, psychological outcomes, and variables influencing retention. *Nurse Educator, 26*(3), 142–149.

Jeffreys, M. R. (2002). Students' perceptions of variables influencing retention: A pretest and post-test approach. *Nurse Educator, 27*(1), 16–19 [Erratum, 2002, 27(2), 64].

Jeffreys, M. R. (2003). Strategies for promoting nontraditional student retention and success. In M. Oermann & K. Heinrich (Eds.), *Annual review of nursing education: Volume I* (pp. 61–90). New York: Springer.

Jeffreys, M. R., & Smodlaka, I. (1996). Steps of the instrument-design process: An illustrative approach for nurse educators. *Nurse Educator, 21*(6), 47–52; (Erratum, 1997, 22(1), 49).

National League for Nursing Accrediting Commission. (1999). *Criteria and guidelines for the evaluation of associate degree programs in nursing 1999.* New York: National League for Nursing.

Patterson, C., Crooks, D., & Lunyk-Child, O. (2002). A new perspective on competencies for self-directed learning. *Journal of Nursing Education, 41*(1), 25–31.

Perry, L. (1997). The bridge program: An overview. *Association of Black Nursing Faculty Journal, 8*(1), 4–7.

Ramsey, P., Blowers, S., Merriman, C., Glenn, L. L., & Terry, L. (2002). The NURSE Center: A peer mentor-tutor project for disadvantaged students in Appalachia. *Nurse Educator, 25*(6), 277–281.

Schön, D. (1987). *Educating the reflective practitioner.* San Francisco: Jossey-Bass.

Schwitzer, A., & Thomas, C. (1998). Implementation, utilization, and outcomes of a minority freshman peer mentor program at a predominantly white university. *Journal of the Freshman Year Experience, 10,* 31–50.

Tinto, V. (1993). *Leaving college: Rethinking the causes and cures of student attrition.* Chicago: University of Chicago Press.

Tinto, V. (1997). Classrooms as communities. *Journal of Higher Education, 68*(6), 599–623.

Tinto, V. (1998). College as communities: Taking research on student persistence seriously. *Review of Higher Education, 21,* 167–177.

Tucker-Allen, S., & Long, E. (1999). *Recruitment and retention of minority nursing students: Stories of success.* Lisle, IL: Tucker.

Vance, C., & Olson, R. (1998). *The mentor connection in nursing.* New York: Springer.

Zimmerman, B. J. (1995). Self-efficacy and educational development. In A. Bandura (Ed.), *Self-efficacy in changing societies* (pp. 202–231). New York: Cambridge University Press.

Chapter **14**

The Nursing Student Resource Center: A Place for Linking Strategies Together

A ll students, regardless of background, age, academic preparedness, or other influencing factors, will benefit from coordinated,
interactive, and multimedia student support services and resources.
Support services and resources may encompass a variety of strategies
based on students' diverse needs. According to Tinto (1993), effective
strategies must demonstrate commitment to the welfare and education of
all students above other institutional goals and aim to integrate all students
as full members into a cohesive learning community. In professional
programs, students benefit from discipline-specific strategies for easing
the transition from preprofessional educational into professional education and then into the profession (Schon, 1987).

Unfortunately, nursing student services that are fragmented rather
than complementary and centrally located may discourage student use.
For example, services that are scattered throughout the campus isolate
users by physically distancing students and preventing the development
of nursing discipline-specific group solidarity. Absent or inconsistent
faculty commitment to the promotion of resources and services available
confuses students and discourages ongoing enrichment strategies throughout the curriculum. Unused or underused student services are tragic;

their untapped potential in enhancing student academic and psychological outcomes could have a significant positive impact on nursing student retention and professional development.

There is no single solution or strategy for improving student retention; therefore, an approach that links multiple strategies is most effective. The well-designed nursing student resource center (NSRC) offers a place for effectively linking multiple strategies together. Nurse educators are in the key position to develop and coordinate complementary nursing student support strategies through the design of a NSRC. The main purpose of this chapter is to describe the process of designing, operating, and evaluating a nursing student resource center. Key definitions, concepts, decisions, and considerations will be discussed.

NURSING STUDENT RESOURCE CENTER DEFINED

A center is a "place of concentrated activity, influence, or importance" (*Roget's Thesaurus*, p. 147). The word "place" indicates that the center is a space designated for a specific purpose. A NSRC is the heart or focus for specifically designed and coordinated resources and activities that are important in influencing student outcomes. The NSRC is a central place where learning, resources, support, peer interaction, professional socialization, and other activities enrich other learning experiences and settings separate from the classroom, clinical, and nursing skills laboratory. It is a place where students can seek help, support, and guidance through a coordinated effort among several activities and multimedia resources to enhance success, enrich learning, and promote positive academic and psychological outcomes. The positive benefits of organized student support interventions within a central location or NSRC has been discussed in the literature (Ankele, Lohner, & Masiulaniec, 2001; Ramsey, Blowers, Merriman, Glenn, & Terry, 2000).

The philosophy behind designing a "center" is that creating a place for nursing students will promote professional socialization, satisfaction, positive academic outcomes, persistence, and stress reduction. The word "room" is avoided as more passive, suggesting a storage facility of resources rather than a philosophy that promotes active learning and ongoing interaction. A center promotes active engagement of learners at various levels of the educational and professional development process and actively and purposefully coordinates multidimensional and multimedia efforts and strategies to maximize learning and satisfaction and minimize stress. The center is where all points come together, that is, all phases and components of nursing education become integrated appropriately and in a complementary fashion that seeks to elevate learning to a higher level (synthesis) among all components. This is enhanced by the positive influences of peers and students in more advanced levels of the educational and professional process.

ANTICIPATING STUDENT NEEDS: INTEGRATING COMPUTER TECHNOLOGY

In a seamless retention system, student needs and profile characteristics are anticipated well in advance (Burr, Burr, & Novak, 1999). Preparing graduates of nursing programs who are computer-literate and who exercise critical thinking, clinical decision making, and reflection is an absolute necessity (Mueller, Pullen, & McGee, 2002). Empirical evidence shows that computer-assisted instruction (CAI) can enhance self-efficacy in clinical decision making, and create a link between theoretical and clinical learning without the fear of jeopardizing client safety (Madorin & Iwasiw, 1999; Weis & Guyton-Simmons, 1998). Students may have guided practice without the instructor present (Boyce & Winne, 2000). Especially for adult learners who are self-directed and desire immediate feedback for performance, CAI offers a forum for independent learning, immediate feedback, clinical decision making, and critical thinking in a nonthreatening environment. Additionally, computer-based learning tools can influence lifelong learning (Zinatelli, Dube, & Jovanovic, 2002).

Previous computer experience and faculty promotion of software programs have a direct impact on student use (Thede, Taft, & Coeling, 1994). Previous computer experience may include degree of comfort and familiarity with computer use, satisfaction with software programs, correlation of CAI material with course content and immediate goals, self-efficacy about computer skills, easy access to CAI, satisfaction, and support services associated with CAI use. For example, the quality of the software program can influence student learning, interest, and motivation. A high quality program is one that is interactive, stimulating, uses multimedia format, permits user control, and provides immediate and descriptive feedback in questioning (Khoiny, 1995). If software programs are to be perceived as user friendly, programs must be promoted consistently by faculty throughout the curriculum, beginning students must be introduced to CAI early in the curriculum, and software programs must complement and enhance learning via other educational media (film, video, reading, lecture, etc). Using a standardized, reliable, and valid evaluation tool for appraising instructional software can enhance the probability that programs will meet overall curricular objectives (Boyce & Winne, 2000).

Unfortunately, the growing numbers of minority students and new immigrants in higher education have limited resources. Furthermore, limited access to computer technology is characteristic of many minority and lower income students (Burr, Burr, & Novak, 1999). Consequently, integrating computer technology throughout the nursing curriculum must be accompanied by strategies to enhance nursing students' computer technology access, skills, use, and values.

The nontraditional student is older, with multiple role responsibilities competing with academic demands. For such students, the opportunity for social integration, professional socialization, professional development, and exploration of new educational technology resources is usually limited. These students mainly attend classes, with little interaction outside the classroom. Furthermore, their organized study time and opportunities to use educational resources are often limited. Frequently, students are inefficacious in using computers and other educational resources; interaction with student peers and more advanced students who use nursing resources and equipment effectively can assist them to achieve academic success and positive psychological outcomes (satisfaction).

Additionally, minority students in predominantly white institutions may experience social isolation and therefore require extra measures to encourage interaction with nonminority students and among culturally different minority peers, explore new technologically enriched learning strategies, and feel integrated within the college and nursing profession. Socialization and interaction across racial and ethnic groups can have a strong positive impact on retention by increasing satisfaction and self-confidence (Astin, 1993).

Traditional students may feel isolated from older students or other nontraditional students. Although traditional students may not have multiple role responsibilities or other barriers typically faced by minority students, they often require assistance with college adjustment, time management, developmental issues related to adolescence and young adulthood, and transition into professional responsibilities and expectations. Such issues may detract from the traditional students' integrated use of CAI and/or their perceived value of CAI. Interaction and coordinated support strategies can have a positive impact on CAI use and overall traditional student retention.

LINKING STRATEGIES TOGETHER: A HOLISTIC APPROACH

The literature supports interaction as the key to effective learning (Kennerly, 2001). Students, especially adult learners, demand student-centered learning and environments that are multidimensional, flexible, nurturing, and holistic. Holistic factors address academic and nonacademic needs. Student-centered learning encourages interaction. Interaction implies that the student is in contact with information, resources, and/or people so that opportunities for information exchange and new experiences are accessible (Kennerly, 2001). Nurse educators have the responsibility to structure student-centered experiences that enhance the potential for interaction.

The NSRC can enhance student interactions with peers, resources, and information. Developing a social environment that engages students and enhances student interaction is crucial, especially for commuter students (Braxton & Mundy, 2001). The NSRC offers such an environment of opportunities. Additionally, the presence of a NSRC demonstrates to students that the institution cares and is committed to nursing students success by providing them with a special place of their own. Institutional commitment to student success and student needs and concerns helps foster positive attitudes toward the institution. The organizational environment impacts greatly on student persistence and retention through student perceptions (Berger, 2001).

Linking strategies together in a flexible yet complementary fashion will not only enhance learning opportunities but can influence student choice, use, persistence, satisfaction, and outcomes. Choices that respond to the multidimensional nature of learning, learning styles, time constraints, multiple role responsibilities, and other factors influencing persistence and retention will enhance student use (Bork, 2000). For example, offering workshops on days and times that complement students' class schedules without requiring an additional trip to campus may increase opportunities for many nontraditional commuter students.

Meeting the needs of learners in various stages of the educational process necessitates a NSRC that holistically accommodates students' changing academic and nonacademic needs. The mentoring needs and types of partnerships change over time, necessitating flexibility, anticipatory planning (Vance & Olson, 1998), and attention to the quality of student interaction (Ishitani & DesJardins, 2002). The quality of interaction influences (professional) socialization, academic integration, psychological growth, self-efficacy, and motivation. Such factors influence student persistence, academic outcomes, satisfaction, and levels of stress (Bean & Eaton, 2001).

Creative means of bringing together students in ongoing contact with one another and with various educational resources, working with students in cohorts, and creatively linking beginning and advanced students not only captures the power of peer group interaction and develops a supportive environment outside of the classroom but provides the foundation for initial and ongoing (lifelong) professional socialization, mentoring, and commitment. The literature repeatedly states that peer interaction and a supportive environment outside the classroom are vital (Kuh, 2001; Nora, 2001). Kuh (2001), for example, speaks about "academic neighborhoods" and Tinto (1997, 2000) talks about "learning communities." Successful learning communities strategically link faculty, students, staff, and other resources into a cohesive network; students take responsibility for peers (Soldner, Lee, & Duby, 1999). The concept of creating an environment conducive to learning and socialization outside the classroom underlies these and other similar terms. It is proposed that the NSRC is a place that creates a caring, local nursing neighborhood of learners that holistically fosters professional growth, development, and socialization by the careful integration of various strategies, thereby enhancing student persistence and retention through the attainment of positive academic and psychological outcomes (satisfaction and decreased stress). Creating such an environment requires strategic planning, careful decision making, flexibility, and ongoing commitment.

DESIGN DECISIONS AND PLAN

Similar to the design of an enrichment program (see chapter 13), the predesign phase involves five steps: assessing the current situation, reviewing the literature, searching for grants, drafting a plan, and soliciting support. Readers are encouraged to review chapter 13 for details and rationale about these steps as overlapping areas will not be repeated here. Briefly, the first step is to assess the current situation, including student profile variables, retention rates, success rates, departmental support, administrative support, grant opportunities, and the existing college resources. The NURS model can provide a systematic guide for assessing factors affecting student retention and success in a particular institution.

Together, literature support and student survey responses can justify the need for designing a NSRC. For example, among several student sample populations, survey responses indicated great interest in and need for student support services, including study assistance, workshops, career advisement, computer and educational resources, and peer support (Jeffreys, 1998, 2001, 2002a). Easy access to current nursing resources and assistance with educational equipment (books, computers, etc.) were also identified needs. Furthermore, grant opportunities existed for the development of nursing student retention strategies. This vital information strengthens justification for a NSRC when soliciting support and preparing a proposal.

Conceptual and instrumental support by the nursing faculty and administrators is essential. Although conceptual support is fundamental to promoting success of a NSRC, accurately appraising the amount of instrumental (monetary and service) support is crucial. Inaccurate estimates of needed services or funds will obstruct or prevent the eventual development and operation of a NSRC. Consequently, systematic decision making sets the framework for a realistic and feasible plan. Suggestions for systematic decision making will follow.

First, a checklist approach offers a quick appraisal of desired resources, activities, and services that can later be revised and/or refined when the overall checklist results are reviewed. After deciding upon desired educational resources, educators need to consider the necessary equipment and furniture (see Figure 14.1). For example, computer-assisted instructional programs with videos require earphones. A listening center composed of earphones, jack box with individual volume controls, rack, and plastic cover will allow groups of students up to four to view CAI videos together or individually and to keep equipment clean and well organized. An adequate sized work station for the computer, large monitor, listening center, and enough seats will therefore be needed.

Consideration of desired student support activities precedes the decisions on needed personnel, required furniture and equipment, and miscellaneous materials for enhancing these activities (see Figure 14.2). For example, a telephone link to a peer mentor or tutor may provide opportunities for easy and quick access to social and academic support that does not necessitate lengthy intervention. Often, the knowledge that a caring peer mentor or tutor is available by telephone to answer a quick question, verify a study group meeting, offer positive encouragement for continued study behaviors, offer a suggestion on prioritizing assignments, and suggest ways of balancing multiple role responsibilities is valuable in minimizing stress, enhancing satisfaction, and promoting positive academic outcomes. Especially for commuter students and nontraditional students with multiple role responsibilities, quick access to support without commuting is comforting. Obviously a peer mentor, telephone, telephone jack box, and telephone service are necessary.

If a nursing skills practice laboratory does not already exist within a school of nursing, nurse educators may wish to allocate a separate section of the NSRC for technical skills practice. A separate, sufficiently large area is recommended to accommodate equipment and minimize the noise associated with technical skills practice. Many schools of nursing have a separate classroom and laboratory for teaching and practicing technical skills; therefore the NSRC design in this chapter will exclude the details necessary in planning a nursing skills practice laboratory. The

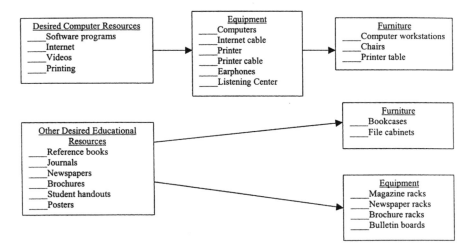

FIGURE 14.1 Planning the nursing student resource center: Checklist of desired educational resources, equipment, and furniture.

philosophy behind a NSRC is to complement, enrich, and coordinate learning in various course components (classroom, clinical, nursing skills laboratory); thus the assumption is that a nursing skills practice laboratory already exists. Interested readers are referred to sources in the literature discussing the teaching and learning involved in technical nursing skills and laboratory design.

It is especially important to evaluate the actual, potential, and hidden costs and services sometimes overlooked in design planning that underlie the desired resources and activities. For example, the need to rewire a room that is going to be converted into a NSRC to accommodate computer stations will require electricians and possibly contractors and painters, if walls and ceilings need to be opened and expanded. An architect and a campus planning expert will need to evaluate fire and building safety issues and prepare a floor plan. Installation of computer software programs requires institutional and technical support. Special security measures may be necessary. Construction of a new building or an addition to an already existing building will require more time, consultation, services, and money.

Once the checklists are completed, revisions and refinement will be required. Deleting unrealistic resources or activities based on insufficient conceptual and instrumental support or available space may be necessary. Detailing the amount, type, and cost of desired resources, equipment, furniture, activities, and personnel may necessitate arriving at more

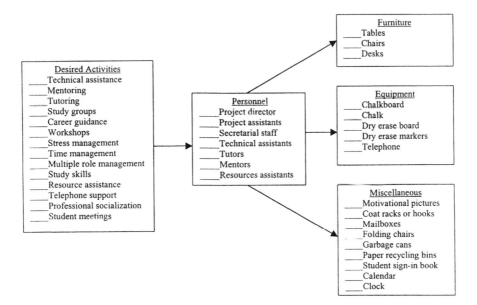

FIGURE 14.2   Planning the nursing student resource center: Checklist of desired student support activities, needed personnel, equipment, furniture, and miscellaneous items.

feasible and realistic cost estimates. Soliciting support via formal commitment to specific tasks, time allocation for specific tasks, and ongoing availability to assist/consult with specific tasks should be finalized in written follow-up letters or memos.

Willingness to further refine details and make additional revisions is important. However, a sparse selection of resources, services, and activities without the potential opportunity for future expansion will probably not make a significant impact on nursing student retention. With a large one-time grant or benefactor, a NSRC may need to be clearly delineated with a final plan. However, allocation of funds for its ongoing operation needs to be realistically appraised. With the distribution of funds over several years, it may be important to delineate several phases in the overall development of the NSRC. For example, purchase of five computers each year over a four-year-period will lead to twenty computers. Advanced planning concerning sufficient space, electrical requirements, and technical support is therefore important. Modifications based on grant proposal guidelines and/or institutional guidelines should be strictly followed to optimize funding opportunities and approval.

Once the NSRC project or grant is approved, it is important to review the budgetary allocations for specific categories and check if there are any restrictions or added guidelines. Budgetary constraints may require some modifications from the original proposal. Once modifications are finalized, the project director should communicate to faculty, administrators, students, support personnel, and collaborative partners that funding has been received. Collaborative partners (those individuals who committed time, expertise, service, or some other instrumental support toward the proposed project) should be contacted personally. A telephone contact followed by a written memo or copy of the grant award and proposal may be indicated, depending on the type of partnership or services required and the level of involvement. Memos that communicate the necessary details reinforce the verbal communication. Publicizing available job openings for positions associated with the NSRC should be done early to permit a large pool of applicants for best selection. Written and verbal announcements should describe roles and responsibilities, qualifications, hours, wages, and any other important information.

PREPARATION

Coordination of all tasks, services, and activities associated with developing, operating, and evaluating the NSRC is a complex responsibility of the project director. Allocating a sufficient amount of time for program preparation is essential. Adequate released time for the project director is integral to the overall success of the NSRC. Making a list of what needs to be done, by whom, and the needed date of completion can help prioritize program preparation components. If a time line was originally submitted with the NSRC proposal, it can be a valuable guide for organization. Preparation may include ordering furniture and equipment, creating or obtaining educational materials and documentation forms, selection and orientation of personnel, questionnaire development and evaluation, and arranging the physical setting. Dividing tasks among NSRC development, operation, and evaluation can help prioritize them.

Tasks associated with the NSRC setting and development take first priority. Minor remodeling, reconstruction, electrical work, painting, floor waxing, security measures, and cleaning need to be completed before furniture and equipment can be set up. Therefore, early initial contact and ongoing contact and collaboration with associated services will be necessary. Anticipating that work schedules may fall behind due to unexpected complications will ease frustration and stress. For example, a leak discovered during remodeling may delay further action until plumbers are contacted and subsequently complete their work.

After contacting appropriate personnel for remodeling/reconstruction or construction, the project director should order equipment, furniture, and educational resources. Sometimes delays in processing purchase order requests may occur; early submission enhances the probability that ordered items will arrive well before the anticipated NSRC opening date. Previewing and reviewing educational resources before proposal preparation decreases preparation time now; however, if previews and reviews were not done previously, the project director will need sufficient preview and review time for self and/or other faculty members. Prearranging for a safe and secure storage area for equipment and furniture is advisable in the event that the NSRC remodeling is delayed.

While waiting for the NSRC setting to be completed, the project director can move to the high priority tasks involved with operation and evaluation. Two tasks that usually have the highest priority because they involve a series of steps, are time-consuming, and concern several people are the selection and orientation of personnel who will work in the NSRC (operation) and questionnaire development (evaluation).

Selection and Orientation of NSRC Personnel

The desired activities checklist (Figure 14.2) provides a guide for the selection of NSRC personnel. Criteria for selection may include: (1) current enrollment in an upper-level nursing course, (2) above-average grades in prenursing and nursing courses, (3) above-average clinical evaluations, (4) excellent communication skills, (5) knowledge of basic computer skills, and/or (6) recommendation from a previous course instructor. For the purposes of this chapter, a student personnel worker employed in the NSRC will be referred to as a Nursing Student Resource Assistant (NSRA). The application form, the applicant's written statement of reason for interest, college transcripts, clinical evaluations, written recommendations, prior work history, and experience provide baseline information about the applicant prior to an invited interview. The interview process should allow for dialogue concerning expected responsibilities and necessary skills.

If assistance with CAI is an expected responsibility, noting applicants' technical finesse with computers and their attitude concerning the value of CAI is important. Willingness, motivation, and eagerness to build upon existing computer skills to accommodate new software programs are helpful assets. An applicant's sensitivity to students inefficacious in their learning abilities and/or computers is an important quality to note. Scheduling, arranging, and conducting interviews are time consuming, yet essential to the selection process. During the interview it should be emphasized that a collaborative partnership among NSRC personnel and the project director is an important goal.

The next priority is to organize and prepare the educational and documentation materials needed for the NSRA orientation and the operation of the NSRC. A NSRC brochure detailing hours of operation, services, equipment, NSRA role, and CAI programs should succinctly convey the main features of the NSRC and can easily be distributed to students. A separate CAI brochure or NSRC brochure insert listing alphabetized topics, names of the corresponding computer software programs, icons, method for accessing, and suggestions for use is another valuable tool for guiding students through the use of various software programs throughout the educational process. Noting the recommended user level assists users in avoiding programs that are too advanced while minimizing the risk that available and appropriate programs are inadvertently overlooked. Maximizing CAI use appropriate to the target learner audience will minimize stress and dissatisfaction. Other necessary educational support materials may include handouts on time management, stress reduction, balancing multiple roles, test-taking strategies, study skills, college adjustment, and other college resources. Documentation forms for recording attendance, CAI use, study group topics, and other proposed NSRC activities and resources should be well designed to enhance the efficiency of record keeping, data management, and data analysis.

Orientation offers structure and direction for NSRAs; it assists in organizing and coordinating NSRC activities, services, and resources via the NSRA role. An orientation session should review the overall purposes and goals of the NSRC, particularly detailing the significance of mentoring in nursing and the role of NSRA and student as partners in learning. The expected benefits of specific NSRA roles and interventions should be highlighted, clarifying the scope of the NSRA role, and emphasizing the importance of conveying this information to students. Documentation forms for recording the study group's activities and for recording anticipated plans for the next meeting and other activities must be clearly reviewed with NSRAs. Some documentation forms can serve as a weekly communication between the NSRA and the project director. Strategies for enhancing student survival skills may address such issues as academic support strategies, time management, stress reduction techniques, assisting students throughout the educational process, promoting professional growth, and balancing multiple role responsibilities. Handouts and lists of referral resources within the college should complement this discussion, along with detailed procedures for contacting technological support personnel (for computers, software, e-mail, telephones) and security personnel. Hands-on practice with various CAI software programs and other educational media helps develop NSRA confidence and familiarity with new equipment.

Simulated situations and NSRA group discussion provide opportunities for NSRAs to use problem-solving strategies for academic, nonacademic, and computer technology-related problems that could potentially arise. Simulated situations related to computer technology include dealing with students who: (1) misuse the Internet for nonacademic purposes, (2) misuse the Internet to obtain papers via on-line papermills, (3) misuse the Internet for other unethical and/or illegal purposes, (4) are afraid to use the computer, (5) are reluctant to do RN licensing practice questions for fear of being wrong, and (6) see little value in CAI. Decision-making dilemmas and varying opinions identify areas that require further clarification and guidance. Continued emphasis that the NSRA will have an ongoing collaborative relationship with the project director throughout the semester offers reassurance. A written evaluation of the orientation by the NSRA provides information to guide future orientations.

Questionnaire Development

Evaluation measures should include academic and nonacademic components. Measures of satisfaction, stress, student perceptions concerning strategy components on retention, or self-efficacy may all be appropriate; however, the evaluation measures should be carefully selected based on predetermined desired outcomes. The review of existing instruments for use and/or adaptation as part of the initial review of the literature in the predesign, decision, and planning phase can save time when deciding upon evaluation measures. If existing instruments are selected, collaboration with content and psychometric experts will further determine if instrument selection is appropriate. Obtaining permission for instrument use from its author should be initiated early, combined with a request to possibly collaborate regarding intended use. Sometimes, existing questionnaires may require minor or major adaptations, necessitating permission from the author. Determining collaboration or negotiation with the author concerning intended changes, method of administration, scoring, data collection, data analysis, and/or final adapted questionnaire revision should be done early to avoid delays in evaluation. Development and evaluation of a new questionnaire is time consuming and requires a systematic plan. Review by a psychometric expert should affirm that the format will be easily scanned, interpreted, and analyzed, using statistical software programs. A project assistant with computer expertise in creating optical scanning instruments, scanning, and conversion into SPSS can format the instrument. However, all instruments need a trial run for scanning to assure ease with future data processing. Reliability and validity tests must be routinely conducted with each sample whether old, new, or adapted questionnaires are used; therefore additional time for data collection and analysis should be allocated.

OPERATION

Operation of the NSRC consists of proactive, ongoing, and transitional interventions. A smoothly operating NSRC begins with excellent publicity and reliable, conscientious, and caring NSRAs. Proactive announcements of NSRC services, resources, and hours available offer assurance that nursing student support services are available and should be used throughout the semester before academic difficulties arise. Before the beginning of the semester, information can be distributed via the nursing Webpage, listserv, group e-mail, postal mail, presemester orientation meetings, registration, and bulletin boards. At the beginning of the semester, distribution of NSRC brochures accompanied by an in-class personal greeting and invitation from the project director and/or NSRA will serve as a reminder to use services proactively and throughout the semester. Highlighting the main features and benefits of select services, resources, and activities pertinent to each course will help optimize effective use of coordinated resources and activities within the NSRC and throughout the curriculum. An orientation or introduction to the NSRC can be scheduled for new students.

Early formation of weekly study groups, weekly practice test question groups, CAI user groups, care plan groups, student peer support groups, and other student groups will maximize student success by the early identification of strengths and weaknesses before academic difficulties, stress, or role conflicts arise. Early identification of the at-risk student can prevent failure or withdrawal. Often students do not seek help until difficulty arises, and then it is often too late to improve an academically precarious situation. (See chapter 13 for details concerning enrichment programs and study group strategies.) Early planned scheduling for weekly individual tutoring, self-CAI study, and other self-directed study strategies can also maximize success and facilitate contact with NSRAs and other students at various stages of the educational and professional development process.

NSRA-student partnerships cannot develop without consistent and frequent contacts. Ongoing contact can evolve into interactions that flourish into collaborative and productive partnerships. Students also can feel more at ease with group peers, offering emotional, academic, and technological support strategies. This peer interaction helps develop professional socialization, integration, and acculturation into the nursing student and future RN roles. The opportunity to share experiences and watch role models and peers struggle with similar academic, technological, and nonacademic challenges can help increase self-efficacy and motivation to persist (Bandura, 1986; Zimmerman, 1995).

By linking various strategies, the NSRC offers the unique opportunity for students at various stages of the educational and professional development process to share experiences and watch role models and peers use multimedia approaches to learning with varying levels of ease and satisfaction. More advanced students can be role models to guide students through transitional stages and encourage persistence through personal, academic, and professional challenges typically associated with various transitional points. Guidance at these transitional points is crucial to encourage retention, enhance achievement, promote satisfaction, and minimize stress. As students move from one level of the educational process to the next, publicizing activities, resources, and services particularly important for this new level (course) helps spark ongoing energy to persist and build upon previously used NSRC services. A brief orientation session can complement an announcement. Activities, services, and resources should be intricately woven together in a pattern that has easily identifiable vertical and horizontal curricular threads that create a strong and durable fabric necessary for the positive academic and psychological outcomes of nursing student persistence and success.

Ongoing collaboration between NSRAs and the project director is crucial to the smooth operation of the NSRC. Collaboration may occur during regularly scheduled intervals and/or as needed via in-person meetings, telephone calls, e-mail, documentation forms, or other written communication. It may not be feasible for the project director to be on site during all NSRC hours; however, open channels of communication are necessary to facilitate success and create an atmosphere of the "nursing learning neighborhood." Anticipating problems, facing existing problems immediately, suggesting solutions, and verbally praising NSRAs for positive actions will enhance the function of the NSRC and maximize efficient use of the project director's time.

EVALUATION

A carefully orchestrated evaluation should be tied explicitly to the NSRC's plan and should include both formative and summative components.

Formative evaluations assess the functioning or operation of the NSRC (rather than outcomes); can be monitored as the program is implemented; and can document specific activities, identify difficulties, and allow for diagnostic-prescriptive modifications based on participants' feedback, using both quantitative and qualitative data. Formative evaluations can provide immediate feedback for initiating needed changes at any point in the semester.

Summative evaluations should be monitored and compared globally at the completion of each semester to assess the achievement of desired outcomes over a period of time. The NURS model may be used to identify academic, psychological, and affective program outcomes. Academic outcomes may include course retention, course success, course withdrawal, continuous program retention, interim program retention, ideal program retention, total program retention, total program success, and ideal program success. Psychological outcomes may include measures of satisfaction or stress; affective outcomes may include self-efficacy (confidence) perceptions.

Because student retention is a dynamic and multidimensional phenomenon, the NSRC evaluation should include academic and nonacademic (psychological and/or affective) outcomes. In one evaluation study, academic outcomes (nursing course grade and withdrawal) were measured by the student transcript record and compared with the previous year's retention rates (Jeffreys, 2002b). During the second year of NSRC operation, student NSRC use, course pass rates, and course retention rates increased; failure rates and course withdrawal rates decreased. Results demonstrated a 6% increase in course retention from one spring semester group to the next spring semester group. For the fall semester groups, an 8% increase in course retention was noted. Course retention greatly impacted upon program retention as greater numbers of students successfully completed courses and could therefore progress in the program.

In the same study, student psychological outcome (satisfaction) was measured by a satisfaction questionnaire (see Appendix D). To maintain consistency in data collection, the project director administered the satisfaction questionnaire at the end of the semester during lecture class sessions. Overall, students were satisfied with nursing and/or prenursing courses, nursing discipline as a career choice, college, and NSRC services. Qualitative comments on student questionnaires further attested to their general satisfaction with the NSRC. Requests for continued and expanded NSRC services and hours were noted (Jeffreys, 2002b).

Following the preestablished plan for data collection and analysis consistently and rigorously will help make the evaluation results more valid and reliable. This includes working diligently with previously established partners in the evaluation process, such as the data collectors, director of institutional research, project assistant, and psychometric expert. Once the results are obtained and reviewed for statistical and practical significance, inferences from the data can guide future NSRC activities, resources, services, outcome measures, and desired outcomes. The ultimate goal of the NSRC is for empirical and conceptually based retention strategies to continue to address the holistic needs of changing student populations.

KEY POINTS SUMMARY

- The NSRC is a central place where learning, resources, support, peer interaction, professional socialization, and other activities enrich other learning experiences and settings separate from the classroom, clinical, and nursing skills laboratory.
- The philosophy behind designing a "center" is that creating a place for nursing students will promote professional socialization, satisfaction, positive academic outcomes, persistence, and stress reduction.
- The well-designed nursing student resource center (NSRC) offers a place for effectively linking multiple strategies.
- The predesign phase involves five steps: assessing the current situation, reviewing the literature, searching for grants, drafting a plan, and soliciting support.
- An appraisal of desired resources, activities, and services serves as a planning guide and must be reviewed for feasibility and expansion opportunities.
- Preparation may include ordering furniture and equipment, creating or obtaining educational materials and documentation forms, selecting and orientating personnel, developing and evaluating a questionnaire, and arranging the physical setting.
- Operation of the NSRC consists of proactive, ongoing, and transitional interventions.
- As students move from one level of the educational process to the next, publicizing activities, resources, and services particularly important for this new level (course) helps spark ongoing energy to persist and build upon previously used NSRC services.
- Because student retention is a dynamic and multidimensional phenomenon, the NSRC evaluation should include academic and nonacademic (psychological and/or affective) outcomes.

EDUCATOR-IN-ACTION

Professor Booke is the project director of a newly funded nursing student resource center (NSRC). Furniture and equipment include eight small study tables, sixteen computers with nursing interactive and multimedia programs, two printers, two bookcases with resource books, two small sofas, a file cabinet, a large chalkboard, motivational pictures, a bulletin board, a telephone, and a small desk. Student services include enrichment program study group sessions, individual peer-tutoring, peer-mentoring, career guidance, computer-assisted instruction and practice test questions, and workshops. The new project is publicized to students via in-person announcements in class and by flyers.

As part of the evaluation plan, Professor Booke prepares to evaluate the functioning of the NSRC after six weeks of operation. Her formative evaluation targets both the student users and the student workers and includes both qualitative and quantitative assessments. For example, all students using the NSRC during week six are asked to complete an anonymous ten-item satisfaction questionnaire and write additional comments in the comment section. Student workers are asked to complete a similar survey concerning the NSRC equipment, facilities, and overall functioning. A quick scan of survey responses and written comments indicates overall satisfaction; however several emerging themes are apparent. To gain further insight, Professor Booke invites ten students in the NSRC to a brief, 30-minute open roundtable discussion about the NSRC services and facilities. Several student comments and subsequent educator actions follow below:

Nori: "The NSRC is a great place. I can come and practice NCLEX questions and discuss them with my classmates and mentor. We can look up information in the resource book if we get stuck. Everything is right here."

Jean-Paul: "The NSRC is a place to stop in before class or after class, study, talk about our stress, or practice questions. You always see someone you know. It helps us nursing students feel like one big family. That doesn't happen in the library—it's too big. There's always someone here in the NSRC to answer a nursing question."

Susanna: "Sometimes it gets really crowded and noisy so I can't really concentrate to do reading or answer practice test questions. Sometimes I have to wait to use a computer. There are no other computers on campus with the nursing computer programs."

Martine: "I wish the NSRC were open on weekends, especially before test days. The peer mentor-tutor and the study groups really help me a lot.

Ebony: "Samantha, one of the peer mentor-tutors, is the best. She offered to help me outside of the study group during the NSRC morning hours. It's quiet at the NSRC in the mornings. My grades have really improved with the extra tutoring. I even enjoy learning!"

Nancy: "I live far away so I can't come in extra to use the NSRC. A few times I got stuck at home and called the NSRC. Samantha was able to guide me through by asking me a series of questions until I figured out the answer myself. That's what's good about the peer mentor-tutors—they help you through the process; they don't give you the answer. I was able to continue studying at home without any problems."

Discussions with the student peer mentor-tutors (PMTs) indicated that the NSRC was noisy and crowded on certain days and times. During these times, PMTs felt that students could not use resources and services optimally and individual attention to students was impossible. Based on the formative evaluation findings, Professor Booke implements the following actions:

- gathers detailed data on student use of different types of services, time, and day
- schedules open NSRC hours on alternating weekend days
- schedules additional open hours closely before midterms and final exams
- schedules two PMTs during busy hours
- explores the possibilities for expanding the facility, equipment, and services

Summative evaluation (academic outcomes, retention rates, and student satisfaction) will provide valuable outcome data that can substantiate ongoing and/or expanded student services via the NSRC.

REFERENCES AND BIBLIOGRAPHY

Alvarez, A., & Abriam-Yago, K. (1993). Mentoring undergraduate ethnic-minority students: A strategy for retention. *Journal of Nursing Education, 32*(5), 230–232.

Ankele, R., Lohner, L., & Masiulaniec, B. A. S. (2001). Innovative teaching within the nursing resource center: A blueprint for student success. *Journal of Multicultural Nursing & Health, 7*(3), 6–9.

Astin, A. (1993). Diversity and multiculturalism on campus: How are students affected? *Change, 25*(2), 44–49.

Baldwin, D., & Wold, J. (1993). Students from disadvantaged backgrounds: Satisfaction with a mentor-protégé relationship. *Journal of Nursing Education, 32,* 225–226.

Bandura, A. (1986). *Social foundations of thought and action: A social cognitive theory.* Englewood Cliffs, NJ: Prentice-Hall.

Bean, J. P., & Eaton, S. B. (2001). The psychology underlying successful retention practices. *Journal of College Student Retention: Research, Theory, & Practice, 3*(1), 73–90.

Berger, J. B. (2001). Understanding the organizational nature of student persistence: Empirically based recommendations for practice. *Journal of College Student Retention: Research, Theory, & Practice, 3*(1), 3–22.

Bessent, H. (Ed.). (1997). *Strategies for recruitment, retention, and graduation of minority nurses in colleges of nursing.* Washington, DC: American Nurses Publishing.

Bork, A. (2000). Futurespective. *Technological Horizons in Education, 27*(6), 49.

Boyce, B. A. B., & Winne, M. D. (2000). Developing an evaluation tool for instructional software programs. *Nurse Educator, 25*(3), 145–148.

Braxton, J. M., & McClendon, S. A. (2001). The fostering of social integration and retention through institutional practice. *Journal of College Student Retention: Research, Theory, & Practice, 3*(1), 57–72.

Braxton, J. M., & Mundy, M. E. (2001). Powerful institutional levers to reduce college student departure. *Journal of College Student Retention: Research, Theory, & Practice, 3*(1), 91–118.

Burr, P. L., Burr, R. M., & Novak, L. F. (1999). Student retention is more complicated than merely keeping the students you have today: Toward a "seamless retention theory." *Journal of College Student Retention: Research, Theory & Practice, 1*(3), 239–253.

Ishitani, T. T., & DesJardins, S. L. (2002). A longitudinal investigation of dropout from college in the United States. *Journal of College Student Retention: Research, Theory, & Practice, 4*(2), 173–202.

Jeffreys, M. R. (1998). Predicting nontraditional student retention and academic achievement. *Nurse Educator, 23*(1), 42–48.

Jeffreys, M. R. (2001). Evaluating enrichment program study groups: Academic outcomes, psychological outcomes, and variables influencing retention. *Nurse Educator, 26*(3), 142–149.

Jeffreys, M. R. (2002a). Students' perceptions of variables influencing retention: A pretest and post-test approach. *Nurse Educator, 27*(1), 16–19 [Erratum, 2002, 27*(2), 64].

Jeffreys, M. R. (2002b). *Evaluation of the nursing student resource center.* Unpublished report.

Jeffreys, M. R. (2003). Strategies for promoting nontraditional student retention and success. In M., Oermann & K. Heinrich (Eds.), *Annual review of nursing education: Volume I* (pp. 61–90). New York: Springer.

Jeffreys, M. R., & Smodlaka, I. (1996). Steps of the instrument-design process: An illustrative approach for nurse educators. *Nurse Educator, 21*(6), 47–52 [Erratum, 1997, 22(1), 49].

Kennerly, S. (2001). Fostering interaction through multimedia. *Nurse Educator, 26*(2), 90–94.

Khoiny, F. E. (1995). Factors that contribute to computer-assisted instruction effectiveness. *Computers in Nursing, 13*(4), 165–168.

Kuh, G. D. (2001). Organizational culture and student persistence: Prospects and puzzles. *Journal of College Student Retention: Research, Theory, & Practice, 3*(1), 23–40.

Madorin, S., & Iwasiw, C. (1999). The effects of computer-assisted instruction on the self-efficacy of baccalaureate nursing students. *Journal of Nursing Education, 38*(6), 282–285.

McCannon, M., & O'Neal, P. V. (2003). Results of a national survey indicating information technology skills needed by nurses at time of entry into the work force. *Journal of Nursing Education, 42*(8), 337–340.

McNeil, B. J., Elfrink, V. L., Bickford, C. J., Pierce, S. T., Beyea, S. C., Averill, C., & Klappenbach, C. (2003). Nursing information technology knowledge, skills, and preparation of student nurses, nursing faculty, and clinicians: A U. S. survey. *Journal of Nursing Education, 42*(8), 341–349.

Mueller, S. S., Pullen, R. L., & McGee, K. S. (2002). A model nursing computer resource center. *Nurse Educator, 27*(3), 115–117.

Nora, A. (2001). The depiction of significant others in Tinto's "Rites of Passage": A reconceptualization of the influence of family and community in the persistence process. *Journal of College Student Retention: Research, Theory, & Practice, 3*(1), 41–56.

Perry, L. (1997). The Bridge Program: An overview. *Association of Black Nursing Faculty Journal, 8*(1), 4–7.

Ramsey, P., Blowers, S., Merriman, C., Glenn, L. L., & Terry, L. (2000). The NURSE Center: A peer mentor-tutor project for disadvantaged nursing students in Appalachia. *Nurse Educator, 25*(6), 277–281.

Roget's II: The New Thesaurus (3rd ed.). (1995). Boston: Houghton Mifflin.

Schön, D. (1987). *Educating the reflective practitioner.* San Francisco: Jossey-Bass.

Schwitzer, A., & Thomas, C. (1998). Implementation, utilization, and outcomes of a minority freshman peer mentor program at a predominantly white university. *Journal of the Freshman Year Experience, 10*(1), 31–50.

Soldner, L., Lee, Y., & Duby, P. (1999). Welcome to the block: Developing freshman learning communities that work. *Journal of College Student Retention: Research, Theory, & Practice, 1*(2), 115–130.

Thede, L. Q., Taft, S., & Coeling, H. (1994). Computer-assisted instruction: A learner's viewpoint. *Journal of Nursing Education, 33*(7), 299–305.

Tinto, V. (1993). *Leaving college: Rethinking the causes and cures of student attrition.* Chicago: University of Chicago Press.

Tinto, V. (1997). Classrooms as communities. *Journal of Higher Education, 68*(6), 599–623.

Tinto, V. (1998). College as communities: Taking research on student persistence seriously. *Review of Higher Education, 21,* 167–177.

Tinto, V. (2000). Linking learning and leaving: Exploring the role of the college classroom in student departure. In J. M. Braxton (Ed.), *Reworking the student departure puzzle* (pp. 81–94). Nashville, TN: Vanderbilt University Press.

Tucker-Allen, S., & Long, E. (1999). *Recruitment and retention of minority students: Stories of success.* Lisle, IL: Tucker.

Vance, C., & Olson, R. K. (1998). *The mentor connection in nursing.* New York: Springer.

Weis, P. A., & Guyton-Simmons. (1998). A computer simulation for teaching critical thinking. *Nurse Educator, 23*(2), 30–33.

Zimmerman, B. J. (1995). Self-efficacy and educational development. In A. Bandura (Ed.), *Self-efficacy in changing societies* (pp. 202–231). New York: Cambridge University Press.

Zinatelli, M., Dube, M. A., & Jovanovic, R. (2002). Computer-based study skills training: The role of technology in improving performance and retention. *Journal of College Student Retention: Research, Theory, & Practice, 4*(1), 67–78.

Chapter 15

Future Directions: A Vision for Tomorrow

T he most persistent trend in nursing student persistence research is that nursing student attrition persists. Current and future enrollment trends predict a more academically and culturally diverse nursing student population, suggesting that nursing student persistence, retention, and success will be even more complicated in the future. Furthermore, the escalating nursing shortage and rising health care needs urgently demand immediate and future attention toward promoting nursing student retention and success. Every nurse educator has the potential to make a positive impact on nursing student retention. Nurse educators will always be in the most strategic position to influence retention positively. Unfortunately, the predicted nursing faculty shortage; the declining number of nurses who will be adequately prepared for the educator role; the growing need to defend, define, and redefine the "scholarship of teaching"; compounded by the substantial gaps in nursing student retention research present grave obstacles for the future. The purpose of this chapter is to propose future directions and create a positive vision for tomorrow. Recommendations for nurse educators will be introduced.

FUTURE DIRECTIONS

Stimulate Interest and Commitment

Without deep commitment and sincere interest in nursing student retention, the future of nursing education, nursing, and health care will be bleak. Nurse educators of today are challenged to look beyond their immediate daily educator responsibilities, beyond tomorrow, and toward the vast future ahead for nursing education and nursing. This necessitates a broader world view in which all nurse educators must see their role as important and significant for promoting nursing student retention. Visionary nurse educators are further challenged to spark interest in others by sharing insights, disseminating information, questioning, and mentoring. Nurturing beginning levels of commitment, invigorating ongoing interest, and clarifying conflicting values will present continual challenges in the future.

Value Retention Research

Nursing student retention research must be valued especially by nurse educators, nurse researchers, nurses in clinical agencies, undergraduate nursing students, graduate nursing students, college administrators, members of tenure and promotion committees, funding agencies, and legislators. The value of educational research, including retention research, must become equitable with other areas of research. Unfortunately, not everyone believes that student retention or other educational research is a serious research priority or legitimate area for scholarly research (Diekelmann & Ironside, 2002; Drevdahl, Stackman, Purdy, & Louie, 2002; McLaughlin, Brozovsky, & McLaughlin, 1998; Tinto, 1998).

One controversy concerns the association of research value with the amount of funding received. The expenses of retention research may be significantly less than those of clinical research; therefore, comparison based on financial cost is invalid. The amount of funding available for educational research is also significantly less. The value of the research must not be equated with the amount of grant funding received. If college administrators or members of tenure and promotion committees view retention research as less important than clinical research, despite evidence of a well-designed, rigorous research study, then nurse educators/researchers may be discouraged from pursuing research in nursing education and retention. In the future, the active valuing of retention research through the publicized, tangible benefits of career advancement, grant funding, tenure, and promotion must complement the intangible benefits of positive morale, satisfaction, and self-actualization. This visionary future must begin with all members of the nursing profession valuing its rich diversity, including nursing educational research and scholarship.

Expand Specialized Knowledge Base

Expanded knowledge of the complex process of undergraduate nursing student retention should be systematically organized so that concepts, constructs, and variables are linked in a comprehensive fashion and are specific to undergraduate nursing student retention. Both conceptual and empirical literature must be routinely reviewed and synthesized so that increasing quality of knowledge will sufficiently complement its increasing quantity. Specialized knowledge must build on previous nursing knowledge, as well as interdisciplinary conceptual and empirical knowledge. In this book, the Nursing Undergraduate Retention and Success (NURS) model presented an organizing framework for examining the multidimensional factors that affect undergraduate nursing student retention and success that can be used to guide further knowledge expansion and literature reviews.

Test Conceptual and Theoretical Directions

Theory testing and new theory development will add richness to the current paucity of retention theory and research. The NURS model was proposed as a new organizing framework that will need modification and repatterning when new data become available. The model is flexible enough to allow for the introduction and testing of new variables. Researchers may wish to test select components of the model and validate existing directional propositions or propose alternative patterns of indirect and direct relationships. Future research on indirect relationships will enrich the comprehension of the retention process (Bean & Metzner, 1985).

Testing components of the model, or the model in entirety with different student populations, is also needed. At first, local studies are advocated to control for extraneous variables. Multi-institutional studies should be disaggregated based on program type or other pertinent differing characteristics (Bean & Eaton, 2000). Past retention studies in higher education and nursing frequently lacked the guidance of an underlying conceptual framework, thus confounding comparison between studies. In the future, it will become increasingly crucial for nurse educators to develop a program of nursing student retention research using the same conceptual framework. The benefit of using the same model to guide research is the ability to compare results between various student groups over time, thus adding depth to retention research.

Adopt Consistent Definitions

Adopting consistent conceptual and operational definitions within and between nursing student retention studies will promote valid and reliable data analysis, multistudy and multisite comparison, meta-analysis studies, and advancement of the state of nursing science. The higher education literature advocates the development of student retention databases (McLaughlin, Brozovsky, & McLaughlin, 1998). In the future, databases on nursing student retention will be compiled and will provide valuable direction for future research, teaching innovations, nursing curricula, and institutions. Today, retention and other nursing educational studies are often disconnected from each other due to lack of definitions, ambiguous or inconsistent definitions, and/or different definitions. Optimally, consistent terminology would encourage the opportunity for multidisciplinary collaboration, comparison, and research. The definitions presented in Table 1.1 and other definitions provided throughout this book seek to provide a beginning point for possible adoption or adaptation in the future.

Identify At-Risk Students

Historically, retention (or attrition) research has allocated much attention to the identification of at-risk students using post hoc studies or autopsy studies after students have already left the academic institution (Braxton, Brier, & Hossler, 1988). Retention studies in the future must shift the focus from autopsy studies to prospective studies, in which the early identification of at-risk students allows for early intervention, maximizing opportunities for achievement and success. Although at-risk students have been identified on the basis of select student profile characteristics, early identification measures of the future will need to take into account the interaction among many variables, necessitating a different approach. The NURS model may guide a systematic process for identifying at-risk students. Quantitative approaches using questionnaires (Appendices A and B) or qualitative approaches such as focus groups can provide valuable data in identifying at-risk students at the beginning of a semester or nursing program. More approaches are needed that assist students' self-discovery that they are at risk; such approaches may encourage early self-help and/or help-seeking behaviors.

Develop Diagnostic-Prescriptive Strategies to Facilitate Success

The profusion of evidence-based nursing practice must expand still further to include nursing education. The increasing diversity of students demands a concerted effort in developing diagnostic-prescriptive strategies to facilitate success. Accurate appraisal of student strengths, weaknesses, perceptions, and concerns is a necessary precursor for any diagnostic-prescriptive intervention. Such an appraisal extends beyond merely identifying students who are at risk for failure and/or attrition.

Diagnostic-prescriptive strategies may be initiated at the individual, subgroup, or larger group level. Proponents of a psychological approach to student retention presume that persistence decisions occur on an individual level (Bean & Eaton, 2000). Others advocate analysis at the departmental level (McLaughlin, Brozovsky, & McLaughlin, 1998). Past interventions have frequently targeted subgroups of students based on age, ethnicity, nursing program, scholastic aptitude, or other characteristic (Tucker-Allen & Long, 1999). The NURS model is flexible enough to be used to guide assessment at the individual, subgroup, course, program, institution, or multisite level.

In the future, it will be increasingly essential to develop strategies for success based on individual student assessments. Generally, student assessment has centered on aptitude measures; yet current and future research will demonstrate that other forms of student assessment will need to be developed. Practical feasibility and the numerous benefits of student interaction will necessitate clustering and matching students based on strengths and weaknesses in order to create positive and productive cohort strategy intervention groups. The future of diagnostic-prescriptive interventions is contingent upon the development of reliable and valid assessment tools that consider the multidimensional phenomenon of undergraduate nursing student retention. Nurse educators will need to be adequately schooled in educational measurement and/or be prepared to consult with appropriate experts. Additionally, they will need more expertise to develop innovative strategies that address students holistically, especially as diversity among nursing students and faculty increases.

Connect Retention with Innovations in Teaching and Educational Research

One purpose of the NURS model is to guide innovations in teaching and educational research. What this suggests is that every teaching innovation can potentially impact upon nursing student retention either positively or negatively. Visionary nurse educators of the future will need to seriously consider how various teaching innovations will affect different student groups' academic and psychological outcomes. Such considerations necessitate the consistent pairing of teaching innovations and educational research that not only aims to evaluate learning outcomes but also strives to evaluate the direct and/or indirect effects on student retention. The future of nursing and nursing education urgently needs (and will depend upon) the advanced development of the scholarship of teaching (science of nursing education), including theoretically and empirically supported teaching innovations and more educational research (Diekelmann, 2002; Diekelmann & Ironside, 2002; Drevdahl, Stackman, Purdy, & Louie, 2002; Riley, Beal, Levi, & McCausland, 2002; National League for Nursing, 2002a, 2002b; Storch & Gamroth, 2002; Tanner, 2002; Young & Diekelmann, 2002). However, it will be extremely important to advocate a broad view of the science of nursing education that connects the scholarship of teaching with the other dimensions within the scholarship of nursing education.

Evaluate Retention Strategy Effectiveness

Another intended use of the NURS model is to provide a framework for evaluating retention strategy effectiveness. Anecdotal accounts of retention strategy components and their presumed effectiveness are inadequate today and will undermine future efforts to advance the science of nursing education if continued. Additionally, failure to quantitatively demonstrate positive outcomes resulting from retention strategy components will severely limit funding opportunities for future student retention interventions. Although anecdotal accounts and other qualitative data provide important information for nurse educators, current and projected future funding agency criteria will probably continue to emphasize quantitative data. Nurse educators of the future will need to be astute in selecting and gathering valid and meaningful quantitative and qualitative data for future funding, and educational, theoretical, practical, and empirical purposes. Furthermore, nurse educators will need to carefully plan formative and summative evaluations that specifically include academic and psychological outcomes if evaluations are to be truly comprehensive and holistic.

Today's limited number of nursing instruments and methods for evaluating educational innovations (Diekelmann & Ironside, 2002) will continue to severely limit evaluation capabilities unless the number of nursing faculty specifically prepared for the scholarship of nursing education is substantially increased. Whereas development of new, valid and reliable instruments may be indicated, the proliferation of instruments to measure the same phenomena will limit comparative studies, meta-analysis studies, and psychometric studies. Retention strategy evaluation studies of the future must include appropriate psychometric testing of the instruments used. Psychometric study results must be centrally compiled in databases easily accessible to other educators and researchers for future consideration, use, adaptation, and/or testing.

Revitalize Nursing Education

The current shortage of nurse educators is projected to grow well into the future. Furthermore, the number of nurse educators who have been formally prepared in nursing education will continue to decline. For example, the number of graduates specifically prepared in nursing education via masters programs with education tracks declined to only 116 graduates in 2000 (Rizzolo, 2002). Advanced practice nurses (clinical nurse specialists and nurse practitioners) are now hired as part-time, adjunct, or full-time faculty, yet may not have received formal preparation in nursing education, the role of the nurse educator, or academia. Without formal preparation, these nurse educators are poorly equipped to meet the needs of diverse student populations and optimize nursing student retention and success. Nursing students' chance for success should not be jeopardized because of poorly prepared nurse educators.

Formal preparation must include opportunities for students to learn both the science and the art of teaching; a series of educational courses is insufficient (Tanner, 2002). Retention, curriculum, evaluation, and other important educational areas should include didactic learning experiences if educators are to be well prepared to engage in and advance the scholarship of nursing education. Advanced practice nurses who elect to pursue doctoral education in or outside of nursing may also lack formal preparation in nursing education and educational research at the doctoral level, thereby missing the opportunity to develop the necessary skills and expertise to conduct educational research independently. The opportunity to be mentored by expert researchers in nursing education while conducting doctoral research focused on nursing education may also be absent. Consequently, experienced nurse educators and researchers will need to mentor inexperienced faculty and researchers differently than before, especially when novice faculty lack formal courses in nursing education and student teaching experiences.

Presently and in the near future, experienced nurse educators must plan to allocate considerable time in mentoring inexperienced nurse educators and researchers. Mentoring doctoral students interested in pursuing studies in nursing education will extend beyond the doctoral program's faculty. Existing and future technology will make mentoring and collaboration possible beyond the geographic constraints of the past. Because of the current and future shortage of nurse educators, those experienced in retention and other educational research will be in great demand for consultation, collaboration, leadership, and mentoring. Although initially this demand may require substantial time commitment and energy, nurse educators must invigorate the next generation of nurse educators with excitement about nursing education scholarship.

Visionary nurse educators and leaders must also seize the opportunity to invite undergraduate students, peer mentor-tutors, graduate students, and nurses in clinical agencies to seriously consider nursing education (and education research) as a possible career option. Highlighting incentives within the Nurse Reinvestment Act pertinent to nursing faculty development is one strategy. Sharing positive and exciting experiences about nursing education and research is another. Together, nurse educators, other nurses, college administrators, legislators, and policy makers must take action to revitalize nursing education. Revitalization will improve nursing education overall, and nursing student retention will undoubtedly benefit from this process.

CONCLUSION

Today, nurse educators may agree that nursing student retention and success are important, and yet consensus will not make retention and success instantly happen. However, taking appropriate action will make a difference. Whatever is done (or not done) today will influence what happens tomorrow and beyond. Each nurse educator or future nurse educator is empowered to make a difference in the world of nursing education and in the lives of students. As active partners in the complex process of nursing student retention, nurse educators can continually seek to understand the dynamic and multidimensional process of nursing student retention, develop empirically and conceptually supported retention strategies, and make a positive difference.

KEY POINTS SUMMARY

- The most persistent trend in nursing student persistence research is that nursing student attrition persists.
- Every nurse educator has the potential to make a positive impact on nursing student retention today and in the future.
- The NURS model can guide future directions in retention research, theory, and practice.
- Future directions include:
  1. Stimulate interest and commitment
  2. Value retention research

3. Expand specialized knowledge base
4. Test conceptual and theoretical directions
5. Adopt consistent definitions
6. Identify at-risk students
7. Develop diagnostic-prescriptive strategies to facilitate success
8. Connect retention with innovations in teaching and educational research
9. Evaluate retention strategy effectiveness
10. Revitalize nursing education

REFERENCES AND BIBLIOGRAPHY

Adams, C. E., Murdock, J. E., Valiga, T. M., McGinnis, S., & Wolfertz, J. R. (2002). *Trends in registered nurse education programs: A comparison across three points in time—1994; 1999; 2004.* Retrieved on April 2, 2003 from http://www.nln.org/aboutnln/nursetrends.htm.

Bean, J. P., & Eaton, S. B. (2000). A psychological model of student retention. In J. Braxton (Ed.), *Reworking the student departure puzzle* (pp. 48–61). Nashville, TN: Vanderbilt University Press.

Bean, J. P., & Eaton, S. B. (2001). The psychology underlying successful retention practices. *Journal of College Student Retention: Research, Theory, & Practice, 3*(1), 73–90.

Bean, J. P., & Metzner, B. (1985). A conceptual model of nontraditional undergraduate student attrition. *Review of Educational Research, 55,* 485–540.

Braxton, J. M. (Ed.) (2000). *Reworking the student departure puzzle.* Nashville, TN: Vanderbilt University Press.

Braxton, J. M., Brier, E. M., & Hossler, D. (1988). The influence of student problems on student withdrawal decisions: An autopsy on "autopsy" studies. *Research in Higher Education, 28*(3), 241–253.

Chester, E. A., & Espelin, J. M. (2003). Nurture novice educators. *Nurse Educator, 28*(6), 250–254.

DeYoung, S., Bliss, J., & Tracy, J. P. (2002). The nursing faculty shortage: Is there hope? *Journal of Professional Nursing, 18*(6), 313–319.

Diekelmann, N. (2002). "She asked this simple question": Reflecting and the scholarship of teaching. *Journal of Nursing Education, 41*(9), 381–382.

Diekelmann, N., & Ironside, P. M. (2002). Developing a science of nursing education: Innovation with research. *Journal of Nursing Education, 41*(9), 379–380.

Drevdahl, D. J., Stackman, R. W., Purdy, J. M., & Louie, B. Y. (2002). Merging reflective inquiry and self-study as a framework for enhancing the scholarship of teaching. *Journal of Nursing Education, 41*(9), 413–418.

McLaughlin, G. W., Brozovsky, P. V., & McLaughlin, J. S. (1998). Changing perspectives on student retention: A role for institutional research. *Research in Higher Education, 39*(1), 1–17.

National League for Nursing. (2002a). *Nursing Education Research, Technology, and Information Management Advisory Council (NERTIMAC)*. Retrieved on April 2, 2003, from http://www.nln.org/aboutnln/nertimac.htm.
National League for Nursing. (2002b). *Nursing education research priorities*. Retrieved on April 2, 2003, from http://www.nln.org/aboutnln/research.htm.
Riley, J. M., Beal, J., Levi, P., & McCausland, M. P. (2002). Revisioning nursing scholarship. *Journal of Nursing Scholarship, 34*(4), 383–389.
Rizzolo, M. A. (2002). Where have all the teachers gone? Long time passing. . . . *Shaping the Future, 1*(1), 2–4.
Stevenson, E. L. (2003). Future trends in nursing employment. *American Journal of Nursing Career Guide 2003,* 19–25.
Storch, J., & Gamroth, L. (2002). Scholarship revisited: A collaborative nursing education program's journey. *Journal of Nursing Education, 41*(12), 524–530.
Tanner, C. A. (2002). Learning to teach: An introduction to "Teacher Talk: New Pedagogies for Nursing." *Journal of Nursing Education, 41*(3), 95–96.
Tinto, V. (1998). College as communities: Taking research on student persistence seriously. *Review of Higher Education, 21,* 167–177.
Tucker-Allen, S., & Long, E. (1999). *Recruitment and retention of minority students: Stories of success.* Lisle, IL: Tucker.
Young, P., & Diekelmann, N. (2002). Learning to lecture: Exploring the skills, strategies, and practices of new teachers in nursing education. *Journal of Nursing Education, 41*(9), 405–412.

Student Perception Appraisal-1 (SPA-1)—Pretest

SOCIAL SECURITY NO:

⓪ ⓪ ⓪ ⓪ ⓪ ⓪ ⓪ ⓪ ⓪
① ① ① ① ① ① ① ① ①
② ② ② ② ② ② ② ② ②
③ ③ ③ ③ ③ ③ ③ ③ ③
④ ④ ④ ④ ④ ④ ④ ④ ④
⑤ ⑤ ⑤ ⑤ ⑤ ⑤ ⑤ ⑤ ⑤
⑥ ⑥ ⑥ ⑥ ⑥ ⑥ ⑥ ⑥ ⑥
⑦ ⑦ ⑦ ⑦ ⑦ ⑦ ⑦ ⑦ ⑦
⑧ ⑧ ⑧ ⑧ ⑧ ⑧ ⑧ ⑧ ⑧
⑨ ⑨ ⑨ ⑨ ⑨ ⑨ ⑨ ⑨ ⑨

Going to school is one part of your life. Certain factors may restrict or support YOUR successful goal achievement.

Evaluate each item in terms of how it may affect YOUR ability to remain in nursing courses this semester.

Using the scale below, choose a number from (1) to (6) and mark your response accordingly.

1. = Does Not Apply
2. = Severely Restricts
3. = Moderately Restricts
4. = Does Not Restrict or Support
5. = Moderately Supports
6. = Greatly Supports

1) Personal study skills	①	②	③	④	⑤	⑥
2) Faculty advisement and helpfulness	①	②	③	④	⑤	⑥
3) Transportation arrangements	①	②	③	④	⑤	⑥
4) Financial status	①	②	③	④	⑤	⑥
5) Class schedule	①	②	③	④	⑤	⑥
6) Family financial support for school	①	②	③	④	⑤	⑥
7) Hours of employment	①	②	③	④	⑤	⑥
8) Personal study hours	①	②	③	④	⑤	⑥
9) College library service	①	②	③	④	⑤	⑥
10) Family emotional support	①	②	③	④	⑤	⑥
11) Family crisis	①	②	③	④	⑤	⑥
12) Employment responsibilities	①	②	③	④	⑤	⑥
13) Prenursing enrichment program service	①	②	③	④	⑤	⑥
14) College tutoring service	①	②	③	④	⑤	⑥
15) College counseling service	①	②	③	④	⑤	⑥
16) Family responsibilities	①	②	③	④	⑤	⑥
17) Financial aid and/or scholarship	①	②	③	④	⑤	⑥
18) Academic performance	①	②	③	④	⑤	⑥
19) Encouragement by friends outside of school	①	②	③	④	⑤	⑥
20) Encouragement by friends within classes	①	②	③	④	⑤	⑥
21) Computer laboratory service	①	②	③	④	⑤	⑥
22) Child care arrangements	①	②	③	④	⑤	⑥

Student Perception
Appraisal-2
(SPA-2)—Post–test

```
SOCIAL SECURITY NO:
┌──┬──┬──┬──┬──┬──┬──┬──┐
│  │  │  │  │  │  │  │  │
└──┴──┴──┴──┴──┴──┴──┴──┘
 ⓪ ⓪ ⓪ ⓪ ⓪ ⓪ ⓪ ⓪ ⓪
 ① ① ① ① ① ① ① ① ①
 ② ② ② ② ② ② ② ② ②
 ③ ③ ③ ③ ③ ③ ③ ③ ③
 ④ ④ ④ ④ ④ ④ ④ ④ ④
 ⑤ ⑤ ⑤ ⑤ ⑤ ⑤ ⑤ ⑤ ⑤
 ⑥ ⑥ ⑥ ⑥ ⑥ ⑥ ⑥ ⑥ ⑥
 ⑦ ⑦ ⑦ ⑦ ⑦ ⑦ ⑦ ⑦ ⑦
 ⑧ ⑧ ⑧ ⑧ ⑧ ⑧ ⑧ ⑧ ⑧
 ⑨ ⑨ ⑨ ⑨ ⑨ ⑨ ⑨ ⑨ ⑨
```

Going to school is one part of your life. Certain factors may have restricted or supported YOUR successful goal achievement.

Evaluate each item in terms of how it affected YOUR ability to remain in nursing courses this semester.

Using the scale below, choose a number from (1) to (6) and mark your response accordingly.

1. = Does Not Apply
2. = Severely Restricts
3. = Moderately Restricts
4. = Does Not Restrict or Support
5. = Moderately Supports
6. = Greatly Supports

1) Personal study skills ① ② ③ ④ ⑤ ⑥
2) Faculty advisement and helpfulness ① ② ③ ④ ⑤ ⑥
3) Transportation arrangements ① ② ③ ④ ⑤ ⑥
4) Financial status ① ② ③ ④ ⑤ ⑥
5) Class schedule ① ② ③ ④ ⑤ ⑥
6) Family financial support for school ① ② ③ ④ ⑤ ⑥
7) Hours of employment ① ② ③ ④ ⑤ ⑥
8) Personal study hours ① ② ③ ④ ⑤ ⑥
9) College library service ① ② ③ ④ ⑤ ⑥
10) Family emotional support ① ② ③ ④ ⑤ ⑥
11) Family crisis ① ② ③ ④ ⑤ ⑥
12) Employment responsibilities ① ② ③ ④ ⑤ ⑥
13) Prenursing enrichment program service ① ② ③ ④ ⑤ ⑥
14) College tutoring service ① ② ③ ④ ⑤ ⑥
15) College counseling service ① ② ③ ④ ⑤ ⑥
16) Family responsibilities ① ② ③ ④ ⑤ ⑥
17) Financial aid and/or scholarship ① ② ③ ④ ⑤ ⑥
18) Academic performance ① ② ③ ④ ⑤ ⑥
19) Encouragement by friends outside of school ① ② ③ ④ ⑤ ⑥
20) Encouragement by friends within classes ① ② ③ ④ ⑤ ⑥
21) Computer laboratory service ① ② ③ ④ ⑤ ⑥
22) Child care arrangements ① ② ③ ④ ⑤ ⑥

Enrichment Program
Satisfaction Survey

Student feed back is essential for meeting future students needs. Please answer the following questions and mark your response accordingly.

1.   = Strongly Agree
2.   = Agree
3.   = Disagree
4.   = Strongly Disagree
5.   = Unable to Evaluate

1) I am satisfied with nursing as my career choice.   ①   ②   ③   ④   ⑤

2) The nursing and prenursing courses completed so far
    provided me with valuable learning.   ①   ②   ③   ④   ⑤

3) Overall, I am satisfied with learning opportunities at the
    college.   ①   ②   ③   ④   ⑤

Concerning the Enrichment Program:

4) Overall, I was satisfied.   ①   ②   ③   ④   ⑤

5) The faculty advisor was helpful.   ①   ②   ③   ④   ⑤

6) The Peer mentor/tutor was helpful.   ①   ②   ③   ④   ⑤

7) The workshops were informative.   ①   ②   ③   ④   ⑤

8) The newsletter was informative.   ①   ②   ③   ④   ⑤

Social Security Number (Optional)

⓪	⓪	⓪	⓪	⓪	⓪	⓪	⓪	⓪
①	①	①	①	①	①	①	①	①
②	②	②	②	②	②	②	②	②
③	③	③	③	③	③	③	③	③
④	④	④	④	④	④	④	④	④
⑤	⑤	⑤	⑤	⑤	⑤	⑤	⑤	⑤
⑥	⑥	⑥	⑥	⑥	⑥	⑥	⑥	⑥
⑦	⑦	⑦	⑦	⑦	⑦	⑦	⑦	⑦
⑧	⑧	⑧	⑧	⑧	⑧	⑧	⑧	⑧
⑨	⑨	⑨	⑨	⑨	⑨	⑨	⑨	⑨

Comments:

Appendix **D**

Nursing Student Resource Center Satisfaction Survey

Student feedback is essential for meeting future student needs. Please complete the questionnaire. Thank you.

Rate your level of satisfaction for each item using the following scale:

> ① = very satisfied
> ② = satisfied
> ③ = somewhat satisfied
> ④ = not satisfied

1)	Nursing as a career choice	①	②	③	④
2)	Nursing courses completed	①	②	③	④
3)	Overall learning opportunities at the college	①	②	③	④
4)	Opportunity for nursing students to have a Nursing Student Resource Center	①	②	③	④

Rate your level of satisfaction concerning the Nursing Student Resource Center (NSRC) using the following scale:

> ① = very satisfied
> ② = satisfied
> ③ = somewhat satisfied
> ④ = not satisfied
> ⑤ = did not use

5)	Overall Nursing Student Resource Center	①	②	③	④	⑤
6)	Computerized test review	①	②	③	④	⑤
7)	Computer-assisted instructional programs	①	②	③	④	⑤
8)	Internet and other computer educational uses	①	②	③	④	⑤
9)	Listening center	①	②	③	④	⑤
10)	Study groups	①	②	③	④	⑤
11)	Individual study	①	②	③	④	⑤
12)	Nursing Student Resource Assistants	①	②	③	④	⑤
13)	Bulletin board announcements	①	②	③	④	⑤
14)	Workshops	①	②	③	④	⑤
15)	Hours of operation	①	②	③	④	⑤

Appendix E

Student Withdrawal Questionnaire

Student feedback is essential for meeting future students needs. Please answer the following questions and mark your response accordingly.

Part I

How did each item influence YOUR decision to withdraw a nursing course this semester? Using the scale below, choose a number from (1) to (4) and mark your response accordingly.

1. = Strong influence
2. = Some influence
3. = Little influence
4. = No influence

A. Transportation arrangements   ①   ②   ③   ④

B. Financial status   ①   ②   ③   ④

C. Class schedule   ①   ②   ③   ④

D. Family crises   ①   ②   ③   ④

E. Employment responsibilities.   ①   ②   ③   ④

F. Family responsibilities   ①   ②   ③   ④

G. Academic difficulty or failure   ①   ②   ③   ④

H. Child care arrangements   ①   ②   ③   ④

I.   Change in health status   ①   ②   ③   ④

J. Uncertainty or change in major   ①   ②   ③   ④

Part II

From the above items, please select the ONE major reason for your withdrawal from a nursing course this semester. Make your response accordingly.

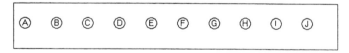

Ⓐ   Ⓑ   Ⓒ   Ⓓ   Ⓔ   Ⓕ   Ⓖ   Ⓗ   Ⓘ   Ⓙ

Comments:

Demographic Data Survey

SOCIAL SECURITY NO:

Student Background Information:

Direction: Please mark one choice for each category.

1.   Sex:

    Ⓐ   Female   Ⓑ   Male

2.   Age:

    Ⓐ   Under 25
    Ⓑ   25 to 29
    Ⓒ   30 to 34
    Ⓓ   35 to 39
    Ⓔ   40 to 44
    Ⓕ   45 to 49
    Ⓖ   Over 49

3.   Number of credits this semester :

    Ⓐ   3 or 4
    Ⓑ   5 to 8
    Ⓒ   9 to 11
    Ⓓ   12 or 13
    Ⓔ   over 13

4.   Which of the following categories
    best describes you?

    Ⓐ   Alaskan Native or American Indian
    Ⓑ   African-American/Black
    Ⓒ   Asian or Pacific Islander
    Ⓓ   Puerto Rican
    Ⓔ   Other Hispanic
    Ⓕ   White
    Ⓖ   Other (specify) _____

5.   Is English your first language?

    Ⓐ   Yes   Ⓑ   No   (please turn over for questions 6 - 11)

6.   Are you the first member of
     your family to attend college?

     Ⓐ   Yes   Ⓑ   No

7.   Previous healthcare experience?

     Ⓐ   None
     Ⓑ   LPN
     Ⓒ   Other

8.   Marital Status :

     Ⓐ   Single
     Ⓑ   Married
     Ⓒ   Divorced/Separated
     Ⓓ   Widowed
     Ⓔ   Single living with partner

9.   Number of dependent children living
     with you :

     Ⓐ   None
     Ⓑ   One
     Ⓒ   Two
     Ⓓ   Three
     Ⓔ   Four
     Ⓕ   Five or more

10. Number of hours weekly you are
     employed to work :

     Ⓐ   None
     Ⓑ   1 to 10
     Ⓒ   11 to 20
     Ⓓ   21 to 30
     Ⓔ   31 to 40
     Ⓕ   Over 40

11. Family's total yearly income
     before taxes :

     Ⓐ $0   to $9,999
     Ⓑ $10,000   to $19,999
     Ⓒ $20,000   to $29,000
     Ⓓ $30,000   to $39,000
     Ⓔ $40,000   to $49,000
     Ⓕ   Over $50,000

Index

Absenteeism
  monitoring of, 67
  relation to academic retention, 67–69
Academic factors, defined, 8
Academic factors in student attrition,
    64–77
  academic services, 70–71
  attendance, 67–71
  class schedule, 69–70
  study hours, 66–67
  study skills, 65–66
Academic outcomes, defined, 8
Academic outcomes of nursing
    educational experience, 125–127
  meanings of, variation in, for
    different students, 127
  methods of evaluation, 126
  numerical calculation, complexity
    beyond, 127
  pass rate calculations, advantages of,
    126
  variations, between courses,
    instructors, 126
Academic preparation, of college
    applicants, 3
Academic services, relation to academic
    retention, 70–71
Accelerated track, stress associated
    with, 133
Accidental disasters, impact of, 144
Action plan, development of, 174–181
Active military duty, student called
    into, 145
Advanced practice nurses, direct
    reimbursement to, 148

Advisement, faculty, 167–187
  culturally incongruent, vs. culturally
    congruent, 176
African-American students, 19, 29
  cultural values/beliefs, 54–56
  family support, 84
  student profile characteristics, 19
Age, 15–17
  as barrier for older students, 15
  myths about, 15
  older students, 15
    additional role responsibilities of, 16
    impact on classroom environments,
      16
  as predictor of academic achievement,
    16
  social integration, 15
Ages of children, of nursing students,
    86–87
Aging patient population, impact of,
    150
Aging practicing nurse population,
    impact of, 150
American Association of Critical Care
    Nurses, membership in, 108
Announcements of nursing student
    resource center services, 264
Anxiety, as source of self-efficacy
    information, 56
Application, professional memberships,
    195
Approval of, nursing student resource
    center project, 259–260
Asian American students, 17, 19, 27,
    45–50

297

CPSIA information can be obtained at www.ICGtesting.com
Printed in the USA
LVOW080619290212

270922LV00006B/33/A